CRUDE FUEL
MONKEY
FOOD DIET

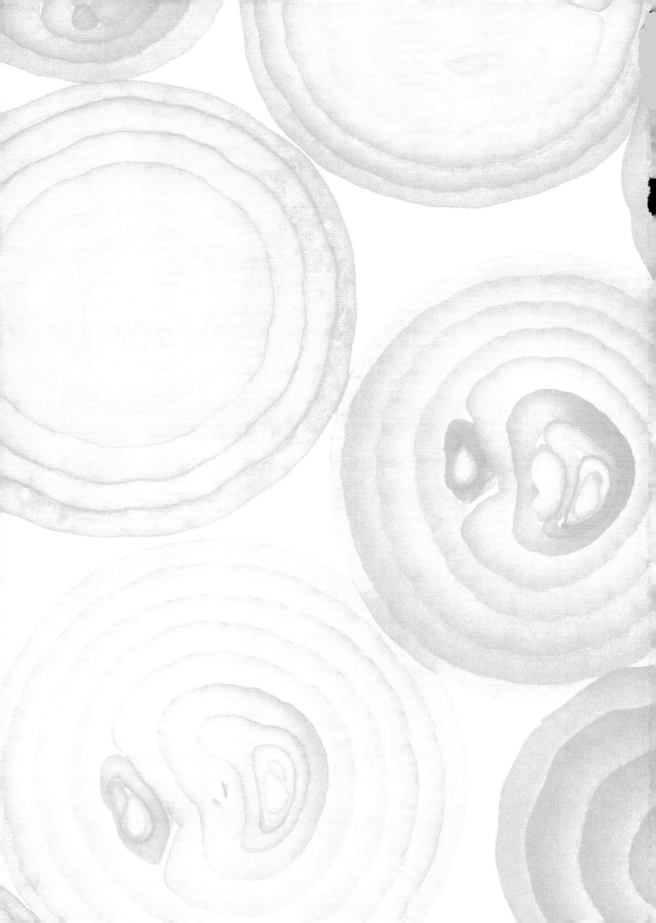

CRUDE FUEL MONKEY FOOD DIET

THE NON-MAINSTREAM HEALTH BOOK TO CHANGE YOUR LIFE FOR THE BETTER

GEORGE ZAHREBELSKI, MS, MD

GEORGE ZAHREBELSKI PUBLISHING, LLC
HOFFMAN ESTATES, ILLINOIS

PUBLISHED BY GEORGE ZAHREBELSKI PUBLISHING, LLC
Hoffman Estates, Illinois

Printed in the United States of America on acid-free paper

ISBN-13: 978-0-578-40306-9 (pbk)
ISBN-13: 978-0-578-40307-6 (ebk)

Library of Congress Control Number: 2018913203

The information provided herein is intended to empower individuals by increasing personal health awareness and understanding to improve lifestyle choices that maximize quality existence and lead to genuine lifelong health and a greater sense of well-being.

This publication is not intended to sell drugs, health supplements, food recipes, specialized health services, or commercial health products; it is, on the contrary, intended for the mass of humanity that falls under the commercial spell of various for-profit industries.

COVER DESIGN BY Laura Duffy

For my children, wife, and family
and all who are motivated and striving
to be healthy naturally

Trust is a tool to play humanity in the lifetime money game.
You are being played.
It's all about the money.
Consider this work as "sunshine" that enlightens,
and that exposes hidden darknesses
in the nutrition, health, and weight management industries.

Contents

Preface

In this book, I share my understanding of the health and nutritional concepts that I learned over 30 years from science professionals, medical colleagues, and clinical experiences as a physician and practicing gastroenterologist and hepatologist helping patients improve their life quality and achieve healthier lives.

I spent my early childhood years under simpler circumstances while growing up in Brazil, where basic, natural, whole foods were available fresh from growers and farmers who sold produce and domestic animal stock at weekly neighborhood street fairs. During those years, cooking meals at home was the norm, with time dedicated daily to preparing and eating meals with family; dining out in restaurants was an exception reserved only for the most special occasions.

My later childhood years in the United States saw harried routines and tightly scheduled days dominate daily living and consume family time. Convenience food items we purchased prepared from supermarkets and fast-food vendors progressively substituted for home-cooked meals as family demands mounted under growing economic and occupational obligations.

My desire to get back to my roots of living healthily and naturally and to learn the workings of the human body and understand the relationships that individuals share with each other and with their immediate environment and the surrounding world consequently drove my academic interests and pursuits. I studied chemistry at the undergraduate and graduate levels, which led to medical study in internal medicine and, eventually, gastroenterology and hepatology.

Throughout my academic career, I worked with scientists notable in their fields to carry out varied research projects, which included analyzing toenail samples for trace mineral elements to assess human health conditions to synthesizing novel organic chemical agents and characterizing chemical reaction by-products, evaluating the pharmacologic effects of hypnotic agents on sleep in mice, and studying the toxic effects of low oxygen states on liver cells. My research activities have contributed to studies published in major scientific journals. I have maintained a strong interest in teaching, beginning with undergraduate and graduate school teaching assistantships through instruction of supervised junior physicians in training and continuing with the education of patients concerning health matters.

During my thirty years practicing medicine, I have witnessed significantly declining American health despite rising health care costs. In 2017, the United States health care expenditures were nearly 3.5 trillion dollars with estimates for health care spending reaching 5.7 trillion dollars for 2026, while annual Medicare spending growth has accelerated to approximate 5% for 2017. The American health care system has ostensibly deteriorated progressively into a sick care system that has clearly become unaffordable to maintain in its current state.

Rather than working to defend and protect national health, American health care strategies have embarked on promoting the efficient dissemination of expensive commercial industry health care interventions and products to all individuals in society. A great majority of health problems suffered by American society unfortunately arise from modifiable health risk factors unsatisfactorily addressed by the current health care system.

The American public is hungry for real truths that support health and promote the general welfare without exerting a human toll or arriving with hidden costs. I believe that everyone deserves better from the leaders and systems entrusted to safeguard their health.

My professional experiences, personal interest in attaining health naturally, and frustration with worsening societal health despite skyrocketing health care costs have culminated in writing *CRUDE FUEL Monkey Food Diet* to deliver a fresh approach to help people achieve healthier lives more simply and inexpensively, without dependence for assistance from the commercial industry system.

As an insider in the health care system, I highlight the health care industry compromises and shortcomings that impede individuals from living healthier lives and teach how to identify and counter the commercially driven forces surreptitiously controlling and redirecting lifestyle decisions impacting health to generate industry revenues at human expense. I detail the essentials of healthy living based on my professional experiences as a digestive system and liver health specialist. I instruct how individuals can make better behavioral and lifestyle choices and direct personal efforts and resources to achieve and maintain health naturally and maximize longevity and life potential for the lowest lifetime costs.

My book is the culmination of my aspirations and efforts to be pertinently informative and provide truly caring health strategies with simple health-conserving and money-saving solutions to improve and maximize health, which can be implemented easily by everyone within their daily routines for no additional costs to themselves or society.

Acknowledgments

I thank my parents for giving me life and providing me with support and the opportunities that helped shape my life; they taught me many of the basics of nutrition by example.

I must also thank my family for enthusiastically endorsing my efforts to complete this work, while patiently listening to my many impromptu nutritional lectures and tolerating me reading every packaged food ingredient label in the kitchen. My wife, in particular, was selflessly encouraging and supported me to produce this project. I hope my work may serve to help make my children's future truly healthier.

Two important groups of people were instrumental in inspiring me to achieve and complete this accomplishment: my professors and scientific colleagues, whose teaching and devoted efforts toward studying the intricate complexities of human biology and behavior inspired me to create this work, and my patients, who challenged me to teach them basic nutritional concepts creatively so they can attain healthier lives.

Special thanks to

Holly Monteith, my editor at holly.t.monteith@holly-editorial.com, for her painstaking editorial work to make this book more readable and comprehensible, and for helping me launch this book for public distribution.

Laura Duffy, my book cover designer at laura@lauraduffydesign.com, for her brilliant creativity in designing the cover to reflect the feeling and meaning that I intended to convey through this book.

Emily Zahrebelski, my lovely daughter, who patiently taught me some basics of using Excel and helped me generate important graphs included in the book to depict available governmental data on U.S. health care expenditures and per capita consumption of calories from various food products.

Eddie Zahrebelski, my rigorously analytical son, whose review of my earliest book drafts oriented me toward attempting to write more simply, concisely, and intelligibly.

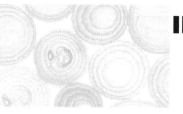

INTRODUCTION

FATNESS **IS EXCESS**

At some point, the overloading burden of living fat prematurely wears out and breaks down the human body system. To prevent a personal demise from living fat requires understanding what fat is and what drives humans to become fat and then living the appropriate lifestyle to avoid a fat demise.

Warning! In life, there are alternative facts and alternative realities that are meticulously designed and strategically employed to control human decisions and interests.

The obvious is what is seen.

The truth is not always obvious.

The obvious is not always true.

Commercial industries create truths to generate business profits. Commercial industry truths are not what is portrayed to be obvious but what is meant to be believed and remembered. Open the mind to see how commercial nutrition, health, and weight management industries profit by making humanity pay.

Do you want to lose excess weight, or are you just paying *lip service* to the "Industry" and are going to die trying to lose weight?

Learn that what you don't really know can kill you slowly and expensively.

Hope exists for personal triumph and transformation to achieve healthier, longer, richer, and more satisfying lives at a fraction of the cost imposed by industry on humanity. Learn to overcome the hidden forces that deviously control human behavior without informed consent.

AWARENESS

Awareness is a human quality that synchronizes personal sensory experiences of the surrounding world with the appropriate interpretation and understanding of those experiences to improve survival choices.

Human survival depends on health and nutrition.

Having nutritional and health awareness can help guide personal life choices to achieve longer, more productive, less expensive, and enjoyable lives free from preventable illnesses and unnecessary, costly dependence on commercial industry products and services.

Powerful industry forces covertly and insidiously manipulate human behaviors to divert focus away from optimal healthy living and toward increasing industry profits. Sophisticated ever-evolving marketing strategies skillfully manipulate the complex interrelationships that exist between nutrition, health maintenance, weight management, industry, money, and human influence to benefit industry systems.

If any life exists in a human body, there is value for commercial industries to use that life force to generate corporate revenues. Impersonal manipulation of humanity to further industry interests is widespread and apparent in daily operations of a commercial world. Commercial interests and the forces of industry continuously labor to control human lives like a commodity to be acquired, traded, and spent. Profiteering commercial enterprises glibly minimize, refute, and dismiss any adverse health consequences and negative socioeconomic impacts of consumer manipulation. Hired industry experts apply fancy statistical and mathematical analyses to promote self-serving commercial agendas that highlight investor profits and societal jobs created from the commercial undertakings that manipulate consumers.

Resistance to the seduction of industry forces requires that these forces be recognized and understood. Awareness levels the playing field between consumers and the industries that use any available means to profit at consumers' expense. Awareness removes the rose-tinted glasses placed on consumers by industry to alter their perspective of the world according to standards designed, persuasively depicted, and promoted by skilled industry operators, who surreptitiously influence humans for money using a multitude of contracted media and communication modalities.

Ultimately, the real basis to resist the powerful forces that negatively influence human behaviors for commercial profit is not only to understand these forces but to have a better understanding of oneself. Understanding how the mind and body both work and how external forces steer humanity can improve personal decisions and lifestyle choices to achieve real health, lower the costs of living, increase personal productivity, and create a happier and more gratifying life.

LIFE IS A HIGHLY COMPLEX BIOLOGICAL SYSTEM

To understand the details and interrelationships among individual components of life's intricate biological systems is a daunting mission that may require generations of scientists to accomplish. The intertwining of incompletely understood scientific complexities of human biology with simple daily living complicates human survival and generates pervasive confusion concerning real basic human needs required for life.

Information and sensory overload, knowledge deficit, limited available time, and desperate human desires to attain personal health and well-being predispose to creating victims of profit industries, which foster confusion that steers consumers to become *lost in the details of nonsense.*

Terms such as sodium, potassium, salt, protein, gluten, carbohydrates, pectin, sugar, starch, high fructose, partially hydrogenated, trans fats, fiber, fat, cholesterol, natural, whole foods, organic, artisan, glycemic index, and FODMAP now occupy daily human vocabulary and govern nutritional behavior. These complicated biological and scientific terms are often poorly understood by most people and even by experts themselves. Even worse, industry frequently intentionally misuses these terms to manipulate and steer human behaviors for commercial profit.

Therefore, it is easy to become lost when attempting to guide healthy behaviors using industry-created terms as directional road signs. The average person should not have to possess a food engineering or nutrition degree to choose nutritious foods to eat.

1 AN OWNER'S MANUAL AND OPERATOR'S GUIDE FOR THE BODY VEHICLE

1.1 THE BODY VEHICLE

The body vehicle is the human body, a complex living, biological, chemical, and physical machine entity having elaborately integrated and interdependent components packaged within one unified structure to perform critical life-sustaining functions for earthly existence.

The human body vehicle comes designed having various characteristic physical sizes, shapes, and abilities possessing limits and qualities strictly defined by signature genetic codes programmed into DNA, which is contained within every individual body vehicle cell and is similarly carried by all body vehicles of humanity.

Complex genetic program codes within DNA are blueprints that run all aspects of body vehicle existence, including growth, development, function, survival, and even death. DNA is ultimately the command center that houses all genetic programming dictating body vehicle existence.

Body vehicle DNA, then, is the common thread that maintains a semblance of constancy to connect and unify all individual body vehicle cells and biological events to work under the recipe toward a shared purpose.

Features and capabilities that apply to the **body** vehicle include:

1. no comparable commercial replacement parts
2. no trade-in value
3. runs on earth air, water, and fuels
4. requires regular maintenance to sustain
5. self-monitoring
6. self-regulating
7. self-repairing
8. self-programming
9. perpetually recharges energy with fueling and rest

The body vehicle has numerous strengths, weaknesses, and limitations.

To maximize personal survival, productivity, and life accomplishments requires keen awareness with all human faculties activated and alert to take advantage of body vehicle strengths, recognize body vehicle limitations, and improve on body vehicle weaknesses.

Often underappreciated facets of the magnificent body vehicle design are its structural symmetry with built-in elements of redundancy and backup for many of the operational aspects carrying out routine as well as specialized and protective body vehicle functions, which provide optionality to accomplish body vehicle survival.

Examples of redundancy and backup for vital body vehicle functions include having two lungs, two kidneys, two lobes of the liver with a dual blood supply, two reproductive gonads, two breasts, two eyes, two ears, two arms, two legs, two sides of the brain, numerous teeth, a complex, overlapping immune system of resistance protecting against incursion by toxic substances and foreign organisms, and numerously layered cellular enzyme systems ensuring completion of critical metabolic, biological operations that keep the body vehicle alive.

General body vehicle resilience to innumerable survival stresses on earth is a testament to the greatness of the body vehicle design.

1.2 BODY VEHICLE COMPONENTS FALL INTO TWO MAIN CATEGORIES

HARDWARE: Encompasses all physical structures that carry out mechanical work and physical, biological actions.

SOFTWARE: Consists of all programs that command and run the hardware performing the physical, biological operations that allow human functioning.

Software includes behavioral programs that run "*subconsciously*" to control and execute hardware actions automatically without conscious awareness or voluntary effort and all "*consciously intentional*" or planned directives that orchestrate volitional hardware actions and activities.

Software governing behaviors may come *built-in* at birth for survival or become *acquired* through life experiences.

Biological existence on earth requires that the body vehicle correctly read, interpret, and appropriately respond to all internally and externally transmitted body vehicle signals and information in all surrounding life situations and circumstances.

Body vehicle hardware and software combine to provide the body vehicle with the capability to safely navigate planet earth on a journey much dependent on sensory feedback and the ability to make timely body vehicle physical, metabolic, and behavioral adjustments necessary to survive an expected lifetime.

1.3 THE BRAIN

Body vehicle software exists within a central data processing and command center known as the **brain.**

The adult brain weighs only approximately 1,200–1,300 g (2.75 lbs.), makes up just 1%–2% of total human body vehicle weight and is housed entirely in the protective skullcap cavity called the calvarium. This proportionately tiny body vehicle component has a massive computing network and the capability to interpret all acquired body vehicle information, and then direct and coordinate all body vehicle functions and activities.

From the brain emerge electrochemical hardware circuits and cables called the **cranial** nerves and **spinal** cord, which function as two-way communication portals that help guide body vehicle existence by feeding data to the brain and sending out messages to other body vehicle parts. Twelve pairs of cranial nerves emerge symmetrically from both sides of the brain to send intricately branching nerve networks into the face, eyes, ears, nose, tongue, throat, and voice box. The spinal cord cable runs down the middle of the back and gives rise to 31 pairs of spinal nerves, which exit the spine symmetrically on either side in branches that progressively sprout delicate nerve circuits into the neck, torso, extremities, and chest, abdominal, and pelvic organs.

The cranial nerves and spinal cord transmit data to the brain acquired from the surrounding external environment through the senses of sight, sound, smell, taste, and touch or received from ongoing internal body vehicle chemical and physical experiences. Alternatively, the brain uses the cranial nerves and spinal cord to dispatch commands to body vehicle hardware to execute specific life actions.

Body vehicle system data acquisition and command dispatch also proceed through chemical communication pathways incorporating the release and blood delivery of signaling molecules produced by the brain as well as by various other body vehicle parts interacting with the brain.

The simplest level of direct human interaction with the surrounding world occurs through the stimulation of body vehicle sight, sound, taste, touch, and smell sensory portal receptors that interface with the outside environment. Sensory portal receptors are body vehicle feelers gauging various forms of transmitted energy, with sound coming from vibrational air compression energy, sight from light energy, smell and taste from chemical energy, and touch from temperature variation and pressure energies. Sensory portal receptors are therefore first-line external and internal body vehicle environment receivers of physical and chemical information that can also adaptively amplify or dampen their signal responses to accommodate stimulation intensity. Data collected by sensory receptors feed through communication portals to the brain for interpretation and further processing.

Many navigate the long life journey existing almost exclusively *in the moment* of the *here and now,* continuously reacting physically and emotionally to the sensory portal–delivered information, while committing limited time and energy to contemplate the meaning of their life journeys and personal reactions.

Typical activities plugging human existence into the moment and engaging the body vehicle wholly within immediate responses driven by ongoing here-and-now sensory stimulation include driving a car; eating a meal; cleaning up a mess; engaging in intimate sexual relations; actively listening to music or conversations; operating media devices; playing a sports game; and working in a production line, keeping up with productivity demands, all of which require that attention be focused entirely on responding immediately to activities in progress.

When comprehensively combined, human data acquisition portals form an elaborately complex receptive network that continuously transfers enormous bits of information to the massive computational network of the brain to maintain body vehicle survival.

Processing centers of the brain integrate and make "sense" of information delivered through communication portals from internal body vehicle and external environments. Body vehicle survival on earth depends on brain software to decode and interpret physical, chemical, and social data rapidly to command proper and timely hardware responses. The vast amounts of information continuously fed to the brain are data-mined for pertinence and carefully processed to help navigate the body vehicle on earth. Data-mining software of the brain filters out relevant data from sensory clutter to extract useful information to be acted upon immediately, to dispatch survival directives or to be stored strategically for later retrieval and usage. Actionable sensory information triggers executive brain areas to command appropriate physical and biochemical hardware responses that manifest as complex body vehicle behaviors and metabolic actions.

The brain requires accurate, detailed, and comprehensive information delivery to ensure that brain executive areas order the best survival responses. Consequently, sensors, regulators, and effectors that gauge, integrate, and govern all body vehicle actions, especially those that involve acquiring, processing, and utilizing fuel and vital nutrients to sustain body vehicle life, intricately equip the entire body vehicle physical structure.

Computing brain centers demand constant energy and upkeep to process innumerable data and run body vehicle hardware without interruption. Because the brain has such high energy demands, interrupting the fuel supply to the brain for any significant period measured only in minutes can disastrously lead to permanent brain injury and even death. The body vehicle hardware executing brain commands must also be nutritionally energized appropriately to ensure successful performance of vital body vehicle life actions directed by the brain.

Therefore, body vehicle existence is inseparable from body vehicle nutrition and fueling, which are of prime importance for executive brain functions.

Consequently, the body vehicle elaborately manages the utilization, impact, and fallout of energy infusions delivered into the body vehicle, since physical and chemical repercussions exist with energy deficiencies and excesses. The body vehicle also stringently regulates levels of fuel and vital nutrients to maintain proper function, storing surpluses as necessary to ensure survival through periods of scarcity and deprivation and eliminating excesses when required to avoid body vehicle toxicity. Additionally, body vehicle hardware can manufacture certain essential biologic life substances as needed from nutrient raw ingredients taken into the body vehicle system as food. Body vehicle hardware even includes a purification system that neutralizes, clears, eliminates, and excretes both ingested toxins and wastes generated through life-sustaining body vehicle metabolic processes to prevent poisoning while the body vehicle carries out life operations.

The brain consists of two main structural and functional components that ensure body vehicle survival.

1.3.1 Primitive Brain and Brain Stem

Known as the *reptilian brain,* this controls primal, instinctual urges and impulses and survival drives. The primitive brain manages basic body vehicle survival, which involves sensing the world; discharging primitive emotions, such as pleasure, pain, anger, and fear; and providing immediate reflex behavioral responses.

Human sense organs delivering sight, sound, smell, taste, and oral sensations hardwire directly into the primitive brain and brain stem through the cranial nerves. Ten of the 12 main cranial nerves sensing the external world emerge from the brain stem.

1.3.2 Higher-Order Brain or Frontal Lobe

The frontal lobe governs behavioral choices and controls inhibitions of primal brain impulses and actions by appropriately filtering and making sense of raw sensory data received by the brain.

The higher-order brain processes sensory information by appealing to intellect and reasoning to attribute meaning to internal and external body vehicle sensory experiences and then discharges proper executive orders for the body vehicle to follow. The frontal lobe gauges and guides behavioral responses, tempering and adjusting primal urges and reflexes according to personal motives, societal rules, and social norms, and drives activities such as judgment and planning of actions.

Higher-order brain functions are ultimately responsible for life planning and working out the logistics for executing life goals; they provide color, texture, and shades of meaning to personal decisions and primal emotions, as opposed to primitive brain functioning, which is directly concerned with the here and now and with immediate gratification. Contemplating the meaning of existence occurs in the higher-order brain.

The decision-making networks of the deliberate, conscious-thought, higher-order brain and the automatic subconsciously reactive primitive brain often act as rivals in behavioral choices. Therefore, a brain sensing a piece of chocolate cake may discharge reflex behaviors to devour the cake immediately if no behavioral controls existed. The frontal lobe would act to intercept and restrain reflexive actions from the brain stem to eat the cake if one were on a diet or if the cake were meant to be served later for dessert.[1]

Most behavioral decisions derive from a concerted effort involving both the primitive and higher-order brains. Primitive emotions provide a value system, helping with the reasoning and decision-making of logical thinking.

Initially, humans experience physical **gut** reactions when making decisions. The physiologic states of the body vehicle provide a framework for decision-making, especially during times of stress and anger, when gut feelings guide difficult decisions. Stimulation of body vehicle oral taste and sexual organ physical pleasure zones gains control of emotions, which then guide behaviors.

Existing within the higher-order brain is the **mind,** which encompasses all *acquired behavioral software* running the body vehicle system. Human existence is a cohesive mind–body vehicle experience, with the mind driving the body vehicle.

Learning and life experiences shape the mind and promote the development of intellect and mind awareness, allowing appropriate choice of body vehicle behaviors and actions that best fit personal and societal expectations and life circumstances and goals. Daily experiences become neurochemically encoded and etched into brain hardware for retrieval as necessary.

While human thinking occurs in real time, generated thoughts are timeless and may become permanently programmed into brain memory banks through the physical establishment of new neurochemical communication pathways connecting working brain cells. *Established neurochemical communication pathways* coursing through individual body vehicle brains are known as **connectomes,** which are as unique as fingerprints to individuals. Connectomes are then available patterns of electrochemical flow encoded into brain circuitry that link together how internal and external data stream through the brain for active processing.

Much of the brain programming helping the body vehicle navigate everyday existence as well as survival challenges runs subconsciously on autopilot, filtering through **decision tree algorithms**, which have behavioral default settings generated both from genetically inherited factors and individual life experiences. Algorithms comprise a series of steps or a branching set of potential behavioral options, commands, or unequivocal tasks that lead to a finite endpoint and activate for execution under appropriate external circumstances.

---

1. Various pictorial renditions of the brain's frontal lobe and brain stem components are readily available to view online by searching under "brain frontal lobe and brain stem images."

Behavioral algorithms are embodied physically within the branching patterns of established brain connectomes, which are then continuously modified and cropped as necessary to accommodate newly acquired life experiences. Ultimately, the brain learns and executes behaviors based on best estimates to dispatch and accomplish goals, utilizing established connectomes and algorithms to produce more efficient thought, recognition, and behavioral responses. Learned behaviors with programmed responses become relegated to instinctual or automatic modes for safety and efficiency. Given the brain's intelligence, with its tremendous learning and memory capabilities, learning something new and then forgetting is vastly more valuable than never learning that something in the first place.

The hijacking of body vehicle sensory portals to deliver data designed by commercial industries can direct body vehicle behaviors and choices manipulatively to serve industry interests. "Viral" programming codes can be covertly implanted into higher-order brain software to corrupt and *change the mind* to run mindless programs that control body vehicle behaviors and choices according to provocative and seductive commercial industry triggers and influences.

Commercial industries can prime the mind to decide quickly without thinking, predisposing to impulsive body vehicle actions adversely affecting body vehicle health while profiting industry. Human behavioral clichés identifiable as patterns of repetitive behaviors, generally recognizable as personal habits, personality traits, mannerisms, and individual styles of social interaction, offer some glimpses of programmed thought processes executed by the mind to run the body vehicle system.

Many body vehicle health disorders result from surreptitiously disturbing the mind driving the body vehicle system.

1.4 BIOLOGICAL CLOCK PROGRAMS WITH TIMERS

Biological clock programs with timers govern many of the programmed, routine operations of body vehicle behaviors and biological functions. **Pacemaker cells** exist in the brain and in various body vehicle organs, such as the heart and the digestive tract, to keep the appropriate timing and rhythm of functioning organs. Biological timers regulate behaviors that occur daily within twenty-four-hour day and night cycles or that are programmed to happen within longer time frames or during specific periods of body vehicle lifetime.

Circadian time rhythms coordinate and control cyclically repetitive human behaviors, such as feeding, sleeping, wakefulness, waste elimination, and sexual reproduction activities, according to individual body vehicle and human species needs.

Body vehicle biological clock programs can be trained, manipulated, controlled, exploited, and corrupted by appealing to and enslaving primal survival instincts, which then are commandeered by entrenching surrogate programming that subconsciously operates mindless body vehicle repetitive routines that generate commercial industry revenues with predictable regularity.

Therefore, regular habits, such as patronizing some favorite coffee shop daily to get a cup of specialty coffee and a donut, going out after work regularly for a few drinks, or having pizza and beer at a local restaurant every weekend, may well be displays of commercially reprogrammed body vehicle biological clocks. Some commercial industry business names and marketing campaigns incorporate a specific day of the week ostensibly in an apparent attempt to assimilate commercial behaviors into consumer biological clock programs.

1.5 HUMAN EXISTENCE

While human life is extremely complex, living is simple.

Human biological existence requires that the body vehicle meet basic survival needs consisting of

1. breathing air
2. drinking water
3. eating food
4. moving
5. resting
6. eliminating waste
7. staying warm
8. staying out of danger
9. reproducing to pass the privilege on to a new human being

Human existence is hardwired and governed by

NEEDS ↔ WANTS

↖↘ ↙↗

CRAVES

Needs, wants, and craves are interdependent and profoundly influence each other.

Needs are vital, basic life necessities essential for human survival and without which body vehicle life ceases to exist, for example, food, water, and shelter.

Wants are fanciful desires for life amenities and luxuries not particularly required for body vehicle survival but that can affect an individual's social status and make life more interesting, fun, convenient, and comfortable, for example, luxury automobiles, a high-fashion purse, gourmet chocolate, an automatic dishwasher, air conditioning, and indoor bathrooms.

Craves are irresistible desires, urges, and impulses to acquire or experience something that provides pleasurable sensory stimulation or relieves pain or suffering and temporarily gratifies those drives to acquire, for example, chocolate, sweets, a juicy steak, sex, tobacco, alcohol, and narcotics.

Needs, wants, and craves are driving forces that motivate and move the body vehicle into action. *Unfortunately, humans frequently cave into craves and wants, which govern human behaviors and actions.* Commercial industries exist and opportunely thrive on subverting, perverting, converting, and ultimately hijacking and controlling human needs, wants, and craves.

1.6 SURVIVAL

The body vehicle is a living biological entity animated and driven by an innate life force and requires fuel to exist and function physically. For a human to have the best opportunity to accomplish the ultimate purpose of life existence, the body vehicle must survive.

The body vehicle has a will that continuously makes survival choices to satisfy body vehicle biological needs on the life journey to accomplish the body vehicle life purpose. Chemical, physical, and biological factors working internally and externally to the body vehicle determine vital body vehicle needs for existence.

Ultimately, individual human survival is a combined undertaking critically depending on the choices and efforts of many existing interdependently within various communities under diverse life circumstances. Therefore, ensuring both individual and human species survival is a fundamental objective of the body vehicle.

1.6.1 Feeding and Breeding

Humans energize and reproduce to survive.

The body vehicle serves as the **action center** that accomplishes survival goals, with **feeding, breeding,** and **sensing** forming the basic foundations that sustain and perpetuate human life. If all human males and females were segregated according to biological gender and strictly prevented from interacting and physically engaging, then humanity would become extinct in precisely one human lifetime. Hence, humans need to breed and procreate to ensure that humanity survives. Breeding is the closest human element toward achieving immortality.

A more immediate instinctual survival drive than averting the potential extinction of humanity is to feed and prevent more imminent personal death from occurring in much shorter time frames without food. Most of the physical space and electrochemical circuitry in the human brain is devoted to managing body vehicle physical parts and actions centering on feeding, breeding, and sensing.

Successful body vehicle navigation through the world to accomplish and ensure personal survival and species procreation depends on the brain to process and interpret massive amounts of sensory information continuously acquired through the eyes, ears, nose, mouth, hands, and genitals. Foraging for food, feeding the mouth with nutrients and fuel, and tasting the palatability of nourishment sustaining human survival all critically depend on the abilities to smell, taste, and touch using the nose, mouth, and hands. Humans plug into each other and intimately play during procreative activities, physically coupling through the mouth to kiss and the genitals to copulate and breed while using the hands to hold on and position correctly to ensure optimal physical connection for reproduction.

Consequently, since feeding, breeding, and sensing are fundamental for human survival, the brain invests proportionately more nerve fibers to connect with the lips, tongue, nose, ears, hands, and sexual organs than to areas such as the torso, back, and other extremity parts that are less immediately pertinent for survival. The disproportionate commitment of brain nerve circuitry toward body vehicle components involving feeding, breeding, and sensing is illustrated by the **human homunculus,**[2] a human caricature exaggerating the basic proportions of body vehicle parts relative to the devotion of brain fibers, so that the lips, mouth, tongue, nose, ears, hands, and genitals, which have a higher inflow of brain fibers compared to other body vehicle parts, are displayed proportionately larger.

Overall, most brain circuitry serves informational data processing, interpretation, and storage activities, as well as executive functions, dispatching appropriate physical, emotional, and intellectual body vehicle responses to incoming internal and external body vehicle sensory experiences.

Ultimately, human needs for feeding and breeding make human behaviors predictable and consequently amenable to manipulation by profiteering commercial industries. Through evolutionary design, basic body vehicle behavioral programming to seek pleasure and avoid pain and suffering was more likely to promote successful individual and species survival than avoiding pleasure and seeking pain and suffering, which were more prone to affect survival adversely.

Consequently, body vehicle programming promoting behaviors that ensure personal and species survival, such as feeding and breeding, are hardwired to provide pleasure and emotional gratification and reduce pain and suffering, which, in turn, further reinforces and perpetuates those survival behaviors. Some examples of the many human survival behaviors that produce pleasure or reduce pain and suffering are satisfying hunger, eliminating waste, finding warmth and shelter, engaging in courtship and reproductive sexual activities, providing and having companionship, and nurturing and rearing a child, all of which become self-reinforcing activities that perpetuate human survival.

Regulatory features govern the programming and execution of body vehicle pleasure–pain survival responses and include adaptive acclimation of the

---

2. A search of the internet will reveal many representations.

senses with the numbing and loss of sensitivity that follow repeated exposures to a potent pleasurable stimulus and increased sensitivity with amplification of the pain and suffering that happen after repeated body vehicle exposures to an unpleasant or noxious stimulus. Subsequent noxious stimuli cause pain and suffering sooner and at lower levels of stimulation to alert the body vehicle more quickly to circumstances and activities that are threatening its health and survival.

On the other hand, repeated pleasurable stimulation leads to progressive loss of pleasure-reward intensity to gradually extinguish the desire to continue engaging in a particular activity and essentially release the body vehicle to move on to perform other operations.

Since body vehicle actions often predictably follow some behavioral algorithms based on probabilities to experience pleasure, reduce pain and suffering, and satisfy feed-and-breed survival needs, then usurping and manipulating human drives to seek pleasure and avoid or relieve pain and suffering and to feed and breed provide industry with immensely profitable commercial opportunities.

1.6.2 Competition and Greed

Humans are opportunists and competitive predators.

Basic body vehicle survival programming encoded into DNA working blueprints issues an unsophisticated rudimentary *head start* for the body vehicle to exist successfully on earth, while socioeconomic status, learning, and life experiences provide *competitive edges* that increase the odds for individuals to survive and thrive under complex social circumstances.

Having socioeconomic advantages with monetary backing, available job opportunities, supportive families, safe living environments, better education, and access to coaching, tutors, and inside contacts brings individuals up-to-speed more quickly, to provide a leg up to surpass the pack for scarcer higher-level socioeconomic opportunities.

Given that strength exists in numbers, humans instinctually or intentionally band together to capture more available life opportunities to ensure personal survival and procreation. Social and organizational involvement, strong family bonds, and close friendships and community ties also promote more successful life existences. Competitive and predatory instincts lead humans to develop negative biases and fear toward any entities perceived as threatening to any aspect of personal or belonged group survival. Prejudices develop when human ignorance combines with primal feed-and-breed survival instincts to create unreasonable preconceptions concerning possible body vehicle survival threats imposed by others. Anger and aggression are primal instincts inherent in defending and grabbing opportunities to feed and breed.

Greed, the predacious desire for amassing personal surplus and excess, distinguishes between how humans and other animals fulfill basic feed-and-breed survival needs. Individuals and human-created commercial entities grab opportunities to **feed** and **breed** *with* **greed** to stack survival odds disproportionately in their favor.

Profit industries routinely entice humans to cave into their basic desires to feed and breed with greed to conveniently expand and potentiate commercial industry options to influence and manipulate human behaviors and interests. Basic impulses to feed and breed with greed and fundamental drives to seek pleasure and avoid pain and suffering prime unsuspecting humans for reprogramming of their body vehicle software to fit commercial industry purposes.

Greed regularly blurs decision boundaries between basic needs, wants, and craves, confounding the question of how much is enough. Human greed looks to get something for nothing and dodge responsibility, frequently leading to taking shortcuts and seeking easy fixes to address life obligations, challenges, work, and survival demands. Greed also influences human intentions to maximize individual and system gains at the expense of others and sows distrust into human interactions.

The existence of legal contracts between humans or human-created commercial entities and the profitability of the professional legal system are consequences of existing human greed and distrust. Contracts are created to secure an element of acceptable equity and fairness and to enforce promises and financial obligations involving agreements made between circumspect self-serving humans driven by greed. Attorneys representing bargaining parties help negotiate "fair" settlements and iron out legally binding and societally enforced agreements, acceptably balancing individual human greed tendencies.

1.7 INTELLIGENCE

The lowest level of existence inherent to all living biological organisms encompasses the abilities to feed and to breed or reproduce.

High-level intelligence is a factor that sets humans apart from lower animals. Evolution has built onto feeding and breeding basics to establish ever more complex and sophisticated behaviors, eventually leading to the development of intelligence, which transcends simple physical behaviors to handle progressively more formidable competition as resources become scarce and require sharing for individual and species survival.

Intelligence is the ability to connect and explain related or seemingly disparate ideas and circumstances and then use explanations to simplify existence and gain survival advantages. Intelligence allows for creative and decisive thinking to produce accomplishments more efficiently, permitting better survival decisions and more significant achievements using less time and energy.

Amassing power derives from intelligent leveraging of available opportunities and resources to marshal control and wield greater influence over many on a grander scale. Accumulating wealth and achieving economic domination result from astutely identifying existing human needs or creating new human demands, and then cornering exclusive ownership of the supplies and supply lines fulfilling those needs and demands, as evidenced by the activities of monopolies particularly within the processed food, pharmaceutical, health care, fossil fuel, media, and information technology industries.

1.8 HEALTH

A fundamental goal of human existence is to experience well-being or live feeling well for as long as one lives. **Health** is the experience of biologically transparent body vehicle functioning with smoothly flowing body vehicle life activities.

A transparently functioning body vehicle can actively perform tasks of daily living and accomplish personal life goals without distraction, interruption, or limitation from intrusive, uncomfortable, and distressing signals or experiences from body vehicle sensors, alarms, or physical parts.

Healthy body vehicle rhythms and activities of daily living, such as walking, sleeping, eating, bathing, and dressing, flow uninterrupted without involving much conscious effort or focused attention.

A healthy body vehicle has the optimal structure, function, and ability to adapt continuously to changing life adversities to meet the challenges of daily living. Throughout a human lifetime, health is a dynamic state of being continually influenced to work for or against existence, and humans must learn how to defend and protect health, which is most easily and inexpensively accomplished by choosing the appropriate behaviors and lifestyles.

An optimally maintained and cared for body vehicle exists at the maximal genetically attainable level of health. Maintaining health is about body vehicle upkeep and not body vehicle repair required to correct adverse consequences of body vehicle neglect or disrepair resulting from insufficient, inappropriate, or absent body vehicle attention and maintenance.

Fortunately, the body vehicle is naturally equipped with all the necessary hardware and software to ensure and maintain health. At birth, health is naturally delivered free of charge with most body vehicles.

Keeping health is many orders of magnitude less costly than paying to regain or restore health commercially when lost. Failure to satisfy necessary body vehicle maintenance leads to the progressive deterioration and decline of body vehicle health to proportionately increase survival costs benefiting only commercial industries.

Given the inherent ability of the body vehicle to remain healthy with appropriate care, attending to basic body vehicle maintenance needs minimizes the cost of living by limiting the need to repair the body vehicle to extraneous circumstances when health is unfortunately lost.

Maintaining body vehicle health consumes energy and consequently requires an adequate provision of fuel. Fuel inherently equals life, as without fuel, there can be no body vehicle life.

Fueling is fundamental to living healthy. The quality and quantity of fuel delivered into the body vehicle profoundly affect personal health, well-being, and survival. Selecting better-quality and appropriate quantities of fuel leads to a healthier and longer life with a greater sense of well-being. A healthier life translates to less suffering and lower living expenses.

Therefore, fueling appropriately to power the body vehicle is an investment returning many health and survival benefits.

1.9 REPAIR

Body vehicle hardware components function optimally within their physical, chemical, and biological limitations, and substantially exceeding hardware component tolerances risks inflicting component injury that subsequently requires repair.

The ranges and maximum limits of software capabilities are less defined since the extent of circumstances testing software capabilities is yet to be fully characterized.

Maintaining health lowers the personal need for body vehicle repairs. Continuous and progressive body vehicle cellular and tissue wear and tear dictate body vehicle earthly existence.

Numerous mechanisms cause body vehicle deterioration, including cellular regeneration and operational programming errors; combating the forces of gravity and friction; shuttling around and utilizing reactive fuel energies throughout the body vehicle; and defending body vehicle survival against toxicities and invading biological organisms.

The body vehicle software and hardware work in concert to maintain body vehicle structure and function according to predetermined, genetically defined requisites. **Repair** is the dynamic ability of the body vehicle system to reverse and compensate for body vehicle biological deterioration and physical, chemical, mechanical, thermal, and biological injury. The drive for body vehicle cellular repair is programmed into DNA and other cellular blueprints charged with optimizing cellular functions for survival.

Body vehicle repair programs correct health disrepair, dysfunction, and damage occurring under normal and extreme physical and biological stresses and survival challenges placed on the body vehicle system. Repair programs direct multiple and diverse biochemical and physiologic body vehicle cellular responses that attempt to return the body vehicle to a healthy baseline state, working according to original, "factory-installed" specifications. Repairs can physically restructure hardware components, alter hardware function, and reprogram software to protect the body vehicle against harm and adversity.

One particularly vital cellular repair process, termed **autophagy,** involves cellular housekeeping, whereby cells internally engulf and eat up cellular debris from broken down or extraneous components to clean up, remove, and recycle cluttering elements.

Body vehicle repairs progress through a spectrum of possibilities according to the severity, extent, and reversibility of body vehicle injury and can range from minimal repair, leading to complete restoration of damaged tissues, up to advanced degrees of repair for irreversible damage, which results in the replacement of injured tissues with disfiguring scar formations to cause loss of original tissue elements and function.

Immediately following tissue and cellular injury from any cause, the body vehicle quickly implements repair programs to attempt to correct any detected disturbances detrimental to body vehicle health or survival to rebalance the body vehicle system and restore lost system integrity. Dead and dying body vehicle cells send out biological distress signals that alert other cells of ensuing danger and recruit immune system cells to initiate reparative processes and clear out devitalized cells.

Cellular biological distress signals also activate death programs in neighboring cells in a domino effect that act as a scorched-earth, self-destruct mechanism, especially with an ongoing cellular injury, which can significantly perpetuate and extend the original injury.

Following repeated, persistent, or severe injuries to body vehicle cells and tissues, compensatory repair responses that patch up damages often ineffectively correct injuries and produce excessive scarring, causing outright loss of damaged tissues and cells. Excessively scarred vital organs eventually lose their biological capacity to function.

Some notable examples of body vehicle degradation following injuries and repairs that permanently compromise the original qualities of body vehicle components include disfiguring skin scarring following healing of significant wounds; bone and joint deformity consequent to the mending of advanced injuries and fractures; loss of brain matter following stroke and head trauma; cirrhosis of the liver complicating viral infections, heavy alcohol intake, and excessive ingestion of food calories; heart failure developing from heart attacks, uncontrolled high blood pressure, and dysfunctional heart valves; and deteriorated lung capacity resulting from years of tobacco use and toxic fume damage. Irreparable injury and scarring of body vehicle tissues and organs leads to lasting damage and dysfunction and impairs health to reduce the life-span or accelerate death, as exemplified above by the advanced health disorders.

When managing body vehicle repair responses, the best strategy to pursue to optimize health and survival is to prevent injury or damage in the first place by avoiding toxic behaviors and lifestyles that harm and deteriorate the body vehicle system.

Intervention with primary prevention is the obvious first choice of all health-directed strategies.

The next best course of action to prevent irreversible body vehicle damage with permanent loss of function is to intervene sooner and limit or discontinue activities and behaviors causing injury and harm, thereby limiting repair activation to the lowest levels required to correct damages that are minimally above normal body vehicle wear and tear.

1.10 PLASTICITY

The body vehicle system runs automatic, behavioral, and metabolic functional programs directing and carrying out routine survival activities.

Body vehicle software that controls learned behavioral patterns, such as walking, talking, biking, swimming, and eating, becomes more efficient with training and repetition.

The body vehicle continuously adapts to meet survival challenges better. Both healthy, constructive and harmful, destructive body vehicle stresses influence and reprogram body vehicle survival software and provoke physical changes in hardware to compensate for and meet stress demands.

Plasticity refers to the dynamic capability of original body vehicle software and hardware to physically, chemically, and biologically reformat or remold like plastic to alter the inherent body vehicle structure, function, and activity as necessary to maintain survival in response to the demands of living.

Plasticity changes occur as an adaptive response to internal and external body vehicle pressures driving the expression of inherited genetic body vehicle DNA programs governing body vehicle biology. Some common factors powerfully driving body vehicle plasticity include ingested nutrients, the living environment, and social interactions.

Body vehicle functional program loops have inherent *learning capabilities* and modify as necessary through training and imposed challenges to respond more efficiently and quickly to the demands of daily living.

Most individuals are quite familiar with the concept of plasticity known as "practice makes perfect." Psychological, pharmacologic, and social factors can pressure brain activity to adapt and revise routine behavioral patterns. Under repetitive circumstances, body vehicle software directing behaviors compresses and streamlines programming to accomplish tasks faster using reduced brain activity. Body vehicle plasticity providing fluidity of structure and function recalibrates the body vehicle system to work at alternate levels adapted toward meeting environmental and life stresses more effectively. The capability to reprogram software and reconfigure hardware as necessary helps ensure body vehicle health and survival under diverse circumstances. Without plasticity and the flexibility to adapt to stresses, the body vehicle could potentially die when encountering adversity.

The facility of body vehicle plasticity is dependent on biological age and is more marked during human developmental periods like early childhood and puberty, when body vehicle systems enter states of rapid biochemical and physiological transition, increasing body vehicle susceptibility toward aberrant and mutational transformation from toxic pressures.

Plasticity mechanisms can be intentionally influenced to promote body vehicle health or can be covertly commandeered by outside forces for nefarious purposes. Consequently, commercial industries opportunely tap into body vehicle plasticity, attempting to usurp and reshape natural body vehicle survival programs to control and manipulate human behaviors for commercial profit. Commercial industries often use strategic words, actions, and biological influences to steer human behaviors surreptitiously and, ultimately, engineer behavioral program loops that lock in physical and functional dependence on commercial industry products with every available opportunity.

Conscious human awareness substantially exists within two main domains of experience, which are either a state of pleasure with the absence of pain and suffering or a state of pain and suffering with the absence of pleasure. Neurochemical or sensory portal stimulation of specific brain centers triggers software programming, eliciting pleasure or pain experiences.

Hedonistic pleasure-reward centers of the brain are potent motivators for human behaviors modulated by the brain chemical dopamine. **Dopamine** is the pleasure-reward system chemical neurotransmitter that controls the body vehicle system pull of the *now.*

Dopamine and pleasure-reward centers form a powerful basis for body vehicle motivational programming and survival learning. The experience of instant gratification has a greater emotional pull on the body vehicle than delayed gratification, meaning that the pull of what is happening now is stronger than the pull of what might be in the future.

Exercising willpower and self-control takes more energy than giving in to satisfy immediate desires; and when willpower and energy levels run low, the pull of the *now* to gratify immediate urges usually dictates behavioral choices of action.

Anticipating activities and experiences that lead to pleasure raises brain dopamine to motivate participation in those activities. Feelings of suffering, unhappiness, and pain also increase dopamine to motivate behaviors that readily rectify these unpleasant feelings or avoid the kinds of circumstances and situations creating unpleasant feelings.

Activities that lead to the experience of pleasure and success or escape from pain and suffering also stimulate the release of dopamine to reinforce the anticipation of performing these activities in the future. Therefore, dopamine drives humans into action, and the dopamine pleasure-reward system combines to drive the body vehicle toward pleasure and away from pain and suffering.

Excessive release of dopamine leading to repeated stimulation of pleasure-reward areas of the brain reduces and eventually depletes dopamine necessary for maintaining motivation, emotional balance, and a sense of well-being, resulting in feelings of unhappiness. Humans quickly learn how to "fix" or artificially raise low or decreasing dopamine levels through specific behaviors and by using substances known to produce pleasure or reduce pain and suffering.

When dopamine levels become depleted and produce unhappiness, as commonly occurs with unpleasant hangovers following a night of debauchery and raucous good times, pleasure-reward centers must be hyperstimulated to manufacture and release more dopamine to help correct unpleasant feelings.

Once a behavioral or chemical fix becomes an expected element in the body vehicle repertoire of hedonistic or pain-avoidance drives, then the absence of the fix itself leads to pain and suffering that triggers dopamine release, activating the body vehicle software programs that motivate seeking and acquiring the fix. Anticipating and pursuing the fix boost dopamine levels to further reinforce behaviors that "score" fixes, generating corrective dopamine pulses.

Therefore, excessive pursuit of hedonistic pleasure-reward activities that repeatedly raise or work to replenish dopamine levels can make people behave like "dopes," addicted to continually seeking experiences that reproduce feelings of pleasure-reward or lessen the unhappiness produced by low dopamine levels for any reason. "Dopes" then become biologically trapped within self-perpetuating pleasure-reward-producing or pain-and-suffering-reducing behavioral loops.

Sugar and fat work to potently stimulate hedonistic pleasure-reward centers of the brain, similarly to how heroin, cocaine, nicotine, and alcohol neurochemically activate brain pleasure-reward centers. Human food science has drastically changed the spectrum of commercial foods. Commercial food industries apply food engineering principles in contrived schemes that tap into the understanding of dopamine chemistry to orchestrate control of human eating and predictably drive eating behaviors to increase industry profitability. Even the thought of consuming tasty sugary and fatty substances that produce pleasure and provide an escape from unpleasant feelings triggers the release of dopamine to motivate obtaining those foods.

Processed and refined commercial food products are typically densely packed with sugar and fat and rapidly deliver the "goods" into the body vehicle system upon ingestion to powerfully activate pleasure-reward areas of the brain and create further anticipation and pursuit of these same pleasure-reward experiences. Excessive ingestion of highly processed and refined commercial food products that potently stimulate pleasure-reward centers of the brain with sugar and fat leads to body vehicle biological training that reinforces behaviors to reacquire and consume those food products. Pleasure-reward centers of the brain repeatedly stimulated by sugar and fat undergo adaptive, neurochemical structural and functional changes to desensitize and develop tolerance to the same level of sugar and fat stimulation, which then requires even more sugar and fat to reach anticipated levels of pleasure-reward experiences. Consequently, regular consumption of large amounts of sugar and fat leads to neurochemical reprogramming of hedonistic behavioral program loops to crave even more sugar and fat to achieve the same expected levels of pleasure, motivating the body vehicle and facilitating behaviors to consume even more sugar and fat.

Hence, commercial forces "dupe" consumers to eat processed and refined food products having high sugar and fat content to create "dopes," who become trapped continually anticipating and chasing hedonistic pleasure-reward experiences and seeking to reduce personal unhappiness through consumption of artificially formulated commercial food products.

Developmental stages like early childhood and puberty, with their rapidly transitioning behavioral physiology, increase vulnerability to industry behavioral and chemical programming. Industry traps young victims in behavioral program loops that promote dependence on commercial industry food products to satisfy personal pleasure, create happiness, and relieve suffering and unpleasant feelings. Infants and children going through puberty who are exposed to large amounts of sugar and fat may become hooked lifelong to rely on eating high-sugar and high-fat artificial foods to experience happiness and cope with life's difficulties.

Thus, the body vehicle system undergoes biochemical, physiologic, and behavioral changes to accommodate and automate what it is trained to do. Behaviors having either beneficial or detrimental body vehicle consequences that are carried out repetitively eventually entrench to endure indefinitely and become more automatic, progressively quicker, and more efficient through repetition. Consequently, individuals should consistently steer the body vehicle to execute healthy behaviors that satisfy daily existence needs beneficially, and they should avoid harmful practices that only profit commercial industries while providing no true life benefits in return to behaviorally trapped individuals.

2 INDUSTRY

Industry exists for and because of humanity.

Industry comprises the conglomeration of producers and suppliers of commercial products and services supplying the demands, needs, wants, and craves of humanity for profit.

Industry systems are intricately complex and encompass many elaborate features that must be stringently managed to ensure industry survival and profitability. The production and delivery of goods and services to consumers require careful industry coordination with the diligent integration of numerous interdependent industry components. Commercial industry successes in growing world markets occur by aggressively capturing market share under increasingly competitive business circumstances. In competitive and growing world markets, goods and services must be mass-produced cheaply and efficiently, and then promptly delivered to meet existing consumer demands.

Food, health, and weight management industries exist to directly service human biologic operations. Human requirements for eating and maintaining health and appropriate weight for survival have provided industry with a wealth of opportunities to push humanity and commercial limits to profitably meet these needs. The bottom line for all commercial industry efforts that service humanity is industry viability and growth.

Therefore, *consumers beware,* as commercial industry comprises *financially motivated entities* that strategically invest capital, position labor, and influence individuals to maximize money flow back into the commercial entities.

The guiding institutional and business system behaviors that preserve the economic viability and growth of industries that humans establish and run substantially mirror primary "feed and breed with greed" principles governing individual human survival. Financially motivated commercial entities are built specifically to pull in consumers to drive up business profits. Consumers furnish the money that flows into and nourishes industry existence.

Ultimately, consumers are industry feed.

Industry promotes and rewards the sale of goods and services, pressuring sales associates to perform. More sales lead to higher industry profits and higher rewards for sales associates.

Unfortunately, commercial industry motives, goals, and incentives may not always be altruistic to humankind. Laws attempt to define the rules of commercial engagement for industry competition and temper unrestrained industry greed from creating illegal monopolies that exclusively corner markets to limit consumer choices. However, laws are not always written to protect consumer interests, and hired legal experts often find and exploit legal loopholes to benefit commercial industries financially at consumers' expense.

Industry profit earnings and business advantages are ultimately gained by skillfully exploiting the weaknesses and vulnerabilities of consumers, laws of industry and commerce, and industry competitors alike. Vulnerabilities, therefore, present industry with opportunities for exploitation and profitability.

2.1 COMPANY PARTY LINE

Catchy slogans selling individual company party lines to consumers abound within commercial food, health, and weight management industries. The company party line is the philosophical glue binding a business and aligning the efforts of the company to move in unison.

Party lines help create company brand loyalty.

Catchy slogans often express company party lines that supposedly reflect business philosophies but more often represent marketing ideals devised to push products and services. Business slogans are meant to become memorable, hollow reverberations permanently echoing within consumers' minds. For example, X-Company "Home-Cooked Freshness" may be an accurate business motto for a small company with timely local delivery of freshly made goods, but as the company grows to expand globally, the name becomes more of a recognizable company slogan. "Home-Cooked Freshness" then more aptly translates to reliable delivery of a consistent product quality, which requires prevention of product spoilage using artificial preservatives and complex industrial food processing techniques. Therefore, industrial "Home-Cooked Freshness" more accurately comes to reflect the maintenance of a consistent product with a long shelf life, allowing for national and international product distribution and storage for days, weeks, and longer.

Consequently, industry brand names, logos, and slogans are mechanisms serving to reinforce company identity and the party line. Company associates then retain their jobs and are rewarded for selling the company party line and increasing company profitability and growth.

2.2 SYSTEMS

Within civilizations, humans construct various institutional systems, including governments, religions, and commercial industries that elaborately control, direct, lead, restrict, and manipulate human interests and the natural, primal human instincts to feed and breed with greed. Thus, societal systems are instruments of humanity created for humans by humans, who are inherently programmed to survive by feeding and breeding with greed.

The life cycle of human-created systems mirrors the life cycle of human existence in progressing through inception, birth, infancy, growth requiring sustenance, reproduction into more and other systems, and eventual system death—with a goal common of humans and systems alike being to delay death. Systems continue to exist if life forces remain available to run system operations and eventually cease to exist when life forces running the systems die out.

Within societal, economic systems, businesses from various industries act and thrive interdependently. Individual businesses combine efforts and contribute to support economic systems collectively, like gears in a mechanical watch synchronously working to keep time.

Economic systems are built to achieve a common goal that provides an economic raison d'être, or reason for being, just as watches are made to tell time. The common all-encompassing goal of commercial industry within economic systems is for the system to survive and thrive, as revealed by various economic indicators, such as gross domestic product.

For example, complex societal systems have evolved to feed humanity. Feeding humanity is an enormous task demanding greatly coordinated efforts among many organizations and enterprises across various industries. Mass-scale production of commercial foods requires large numbers of industries to combine resources and accomplish numerous steps to produce the final food products sold to feed humanity. Raw food materials must be grown, harvested, processed, refined, and packaged, then distributed to society for consumption.

Societal movements to maintain the health and appropriate weight of individuals are additional examples of large-scale human endeavors that require servicing by multitudes of industries, which coincidentally profit from the failure of individuals to maintain health and appropriate weight. Likewise, pharmaceutical industry products to treat human ailments are eventually sold only after fulfillment of many prerequisites by diverse industry elements involving farming; animal procurement; scientific drug product development; animal and human testing; mass-scale product manufacturing, packaging, distribution, and delivery; and marketing, legal, and financial services.

All businesses working collaboratively within a system toward some common collective goal expect to earn a slice of the big financial pie by accomplishing their part to attain that goal. Ultimately, the goals of industry and economic systems are to survive and profit financially. Enormous systems are analogous to big fish that must continually eat smaller fish to survive and thrive. Consumers are ultimately the small fish feeding the big-fish industries. As large numbers of individual consumers consume commercial industry products and services, companies profit by feeding on the monies that consumers spend.

Just as company party lines are tools to motivate and guide workers toward working in concert to accomplish common goals, workers are the tools that ultimately execute industry goals to capture consumers and increase company market share. Consumers, in turn, become the tools manipulated to feed and sustain industry goals and profitability. Consequently, the successful economic survival of industry relies on the skillful manipulation of many tools, regardless of whether the underlying principles guiding that manipulation are intrinsically flawed or contrary to the appropriate attainment of individual and societal ideals benefiting all.

Enterprising companies ultimately survive and prosper by operating in creative ways to ensure viability under any circumstances. System existence depends on establishing complementary working relationships between interdependent participating system players, operators, and owners.

Successful system operations rely on designing intricate organizational structures with carefully crafted system rules that meticulously guide the undertakings and conduct of individual system components.

*The System Rule **is that systems make rules to keep the system viable and thriving.***

A corollary to the System Rule is that when uncertainties exist, and the consequences of pursuing any system course of action are controversial, unproven, or unknown, the system routinely chooses the most profitable course of action that primarily meets system needs and benefits system interests even at the expense of nonsystem entities.

Additionally, systems welcome and accommodate special circumstances that create default advantages favoring increased system activity, success, and prosperity. For example, health care industries are booming with growing societal obesity and associated eating-related disorders and consequences and fail to intervene at the source to terminate these system advantages.

Elaborate rules and guidelines streamline control of system players and operators to ensure that directives benefiting and generating revenue for the system are executed efficiently and at the lowest system costs. Authority, conformity, reward, and punishment are essential ingredients helping to reinforce successful system operations, while bureaucracy, red tape, misdirection, and dubious application of societal laws are all convenient tools utilized as necessary to accomplish system ends.

Systems provide incentives to spur system utilization, attract and retain vested players, and recruit talented operators that can capably meet player needs. System operators and players are encouraged to adopt mind-sets and behaviors best promoting system interests and successes and to influence and enlist others to think and do similarly.

Recruitment and consolidation of many individual human efforts lead to more formidable system power, control, and earnings, as demonstrated by established commercial monopolies.

Individuals working as system operators sacrifice personal time and energy in exchange for monetary pay that is readily spent elsewhere to support and sustain other similarly operating industry systems.

All-star participation is the foundation of successful systems.

Human-created systems, whether commercial, social, governmental, religious, entertainment, or criminal justice in nature, thrive best on all-star system membership and participation. All-stars are passionate participating system players and operators that best support and service system ends to ensure successful system survival and profitability, and consequently, successful systems work hard to procure and retain all-stars.

All-star operators skillfully run the systems, and all-star players heavily utilize and support the systems, with all system participants joining to perpetuate system successes.

Systems carefully select and enroll operator managers and associates, workers, and sometimes co-conspirators who can best work system angles and keep systems operating smoothly.

Devoted system operators driven by reward or profit incentives may even resort to aggressive sales tactics to promote system virtues to attract prospective members or increase system usage by players. System players may comfortably navigate and even exploit the system to derive personal benefits and rewards, and sometimes they may become trapped within the system without recourse or the ability to escape.

Some examples of industry systems that depend on all-star member operators and players to succeed include health care delivery systems that thrive financially on zealous health care providers and heavy health care utilizers; weight management systems that prosper under rising societal obesity rates to push weight management services on increasing numbers of individuals independently failing to maintain a healthy weight; purveyors of vitamin and health supplements who aggressively push artificial health products on individuals determined to improve personal health and well-being; and insurance carriers that play on consumer fears and uncertainties to sell insurance coverage plans to healthy individuals most fearing calamity and disaster and amenable to paying high insurance premiums without intending to utilize insurance benefits.

System existence requires membership and revenues.
All system players pay to play in the system.

Any money spent to profit a system essentially buys immediate membership into the system. Consumers spending money to join any commercial industry nutrition, health, or weight management system should be wary of underhanded system efforts to lock members in to profit the system at members' expense.

The **1% benefit/99% pay principle** summarizes the returns for commercial industry system membership and states that for many financially driven systems, only a minimal 1% of system members extract the bulk of system benefits and rewards generously paid for by the efforts of the remaining 99% of system participants.

Therefore, within economic systems, the vast majority of paying members subsidize the benefits reaped by a tiny minority of system participants in a kind of pyramid scheme.

The only honest and straightforward system that deals evenhandedly with all participating life-forms to allow all to have a fair chance to survive and thrive is the undisturbed natural earth ecosystem. The natural earth ecosystem exists genuinely, without the use of any advertising, marketing, lobbying, legislating, or peddling of influence to convince participants of system virtues and that system motives are fair, impartial, and legitimate.

On the other hand, financially motivated systems routinely manipulate the natural earth ecosystem with impunity for system profitability and gain, and then portray system efforts as being undertaken for the betterment of humanity and only for a relatively small price for humanity to pay.

2.3 COMMERCIALISM AND CONFUSION

In a commercial setting, everyone is a meal ticket for industry.

Industry growth and profitability are the primary objectives of commercial free-market enterprises, including those dealing with nutrition, health, and weight management.

When confusion reigns, profits rule.

Industry exploits consumer ignorance and confusion. The ability to control consumer chaos creates opportunities for the commercial industry.

Naive consumers who know less or are gullible are more vulnerable to having personal choices and actions commercially manipulated for industry gain. Hypnotic marketing overtures that sell an unrealistic health and longevity utopia more easily sucker misinformed consumers, who become led astray to purchase unnecessary, costly, and sometimes detrimental food and health items, generating large-scale industry profits in the process.

Fortunately, confusion and ignorance also present opportunities for learning.

Knowledge empowers, and awareness is the key to real health.

Possessing awareness and an understanding of basic food and health principles allows for more intelligent questions to be asked and increases the difficulty for industries to manipulate individual food and health decisions. Well-informed consumers are then more likely to make appropriate nutrition and health choices.

Living in a learning mode and seizing available opportunities to understand and optimally satisfy basic life needs as naturally meant will maximize health, well-being, and longevity for the least cost.

2.4 EXPERTS

*Expert **is a "relative" term.***

Humans routinely turn to experts to help guide personal decisions concerning food, nutrition, health, and weight management issues.

Experts are regarded as possessing considerable specialized knowledge and influence concerning matters of interest to individuals and various other entities.

Dedicating intellectual study and concentrating life experiences to understand specific matters in greater depth confer certain advantages over individuals less knowledgeable about those same matters. Therefore, an expert possesses more knowledge and expertise about particular topics than someone else who knows less or nothing at all about the same issues.

Knowledge is power.

Experts and expertise can be enlisted to help individuals and entities make better operational decisions and survival choices and to capitalize on special circumstances and industry and legal loopholes to gain some commercial advantage.

Problems arise when competing experts assert divergent views and present conflicting options concerning the optimal handling of specific issues. Experts can create confusion and generate considerable controversy by presenting adversarial opinions that are convincingly defended with supporting arguments, as curiously transpires within the food, health, nutrition, and weight management industries, especially when opposing views and commercial profit opportunities intimately intermingle.

Underhanded expert tactics can easily obfuscate pertinent controversial issues.

Experts can easily obscure and hide personal and system limitations in the knowledge and understanding surrounding specific subject matters by using complicated jargon with bewildering mechanistic, scientific, and technical language to justify their advice and recommendations. Unsavory experts may even deceptively muddle relevant points of interest or the importance of controversial issues to benefit commercial interests.

Given the immense complexity of biological life and life interactions and the vastness of the universe in which life exists, detailed knowledge of the elements of any life components is at best imperfect and incomplete and amenable to considerable misunderstanding and misinterpretation. Consequently, experts studying life and universal elements achieve various levels of understanding based on personal work and accumulated experiences and often adopt perspectives in accordance with the views of others doing similar projects and having like-minded attitudes and beliefs.

Experts are routinely hired to argue opinions and talk points that *talk up* and emphasize evidence supporting one side of a known story or perspective and *talk down* and criticize any contradictory findings. Unfortunately, unscrupulous experts willing to intentionally misuse their expertise for hire to profit financially and to promote some personal or system agenda at consumers' expense are readily available for commercial profit industries. Hired experts become the mouthpiece for corporate and commercial interests or to disseminate propaganda for special interest groups.

In opinion media news programming, political experts known as **pundits** are routinely employed to sway public opinion or confirm the political views and prejudices of their media-engaged target audiences. Experts are often under tremendous financial or system pressure to produce relevant opinions that address controversial issues of significant intellectual or economic impact. More directly, experts may be under duress to retain the pay and funding for their espoused expert opinions. Therefore, expert advice may not be entirely objective or unbiased and delivered without evidence of subtle or overt influences skewing rendered opinions.

Ideally, experts addressing any vital issues that impact society would clearly explain their understanding of the issues, support their knowledge with relevant facts, and qualify available facts with known limitations and any opposing perspectives. Furthermore, they would disclose the sources of funding they stand to gain, lose, or profit from with their adoption of any measures they present.

2.5 BIAS

Bias is the influence that impacts scientific inquiry, observations, and processing of data and information, intentionally or unintentionally skewing the results and interpretation of experimental work to favor personal, organizational, institutional, or system agendas. The human world would work better if all expert advice were for the sole purpose of maximally benefiting all humanity, particularly concerning food, health, nutrition, and weight management matters. Expert advice would be invaluable if it were delivered entirely without prejudice or underlying selfish motives. Unfortunately, designated experts wield enormous power to influence human behaviors and generate profits for commercial industries.

Commercial markets dictate that controlling consumers and securing industry advantages over competitors increase opportunities for industries to survive and profit commercially. The few win industry advantages by creatively utilizing all available tools to assert power over the many. Industry uses experts as leverage to steer the interests and behaviors of multitudes of uninformed, trusting, gullible, dependent, and vulnerable consumers for commercial purposes.

Therefore, experts are surrogate industry instruments to control consumers. Experts are humans programmed with the same underlying feed-and-breed-with-greed principles guiding individual survival for all humanity.

Human perceptions, opinions, and interests are subject to innumerable influences and manipulations and emerge in the context of belonging to systems and carrying out system demands. The perceptions and opinions of experts also become shaped and prejudiced through individual learning and personal experiences as well as by any surrounding environmental, social, and professional influences and pressures.

As for all members of humanity, numerous factors, including the need for personal gain, affirmation, and recognition and the opinions of other experts, affect and motivate the judgments and behaviors of experts. Therefore, science and health care experts are susceptible to being manipulated by various subtle and powerful lobbying forces, which may incorporate sophisticated marketing and brainwashing techniques and financial rewards to induce experts to carry out the specific agendas of profit-driven institutions.

Manipulation sometimes merely follows the rule of "Never bite the hand that feeds you."

Experts, politicians, and health care professionals who function at strategic points of industry profitability, and routinely make decisions and recommendations that significantly affect social spending and the financial interests and viability of commercial industries, are especially exposed and vulnerable to outside influences. Health care professionals are lynchpins leveraging enormous wealth opportunities for health care industry systems. Consequently, these pivotally positioned individuals become continuous targets for covert and overt industry influences, inducements, and control through all available means.

In the digital world, industries devise ever more sophisticated marketing strategies tailored for health care providers to influence clinical practice patterns insidiously and reap considerable profits. Advertisements that push pharmaceutical and health care products and services and peddle generous financial incentives and "honoraria" to entice health care professionals to participate in industry-sponsored studies and questionnaires permeate health care provider emails and social media applications; health-related educational services; mobile applications facilitating delivery of health care services to consumers; and electronic medical records services offered to health care providers for "free."

Commercial industry pressures and lobbying efforts can also influence expert definitions and representations of the actual scope of health conditions deserving of attention, intervention, and financial support from industry, professional organizations, and society.

Less subtle forms of expert bias that directly sell influence for personal and industry gain occur through the commercial endorsements, approval, and outright sale of specific products and services by health and fitness gurus, who profit by pitching health, fitness, dietary, comfort, and convenience retail products and services.

Experts who gain media celebrity status indirectly endorse industry interests through their commercial industry associations and by allowing their names to be identified with industry products and services. Subtly disguised commercial industry advertising and influence occur by using influential celebrity experts to recognize generous industry sponsorship of educational media delivered programming or scientific presentations on health-related topics at professional meetings and conferences.

Experts delivering educational media programming also influence consumers indirectly when paid commercials frequently interrupt programming to advertise multitudes of industry products and services to media-engaged consumers. The average consumer seeking expert guidance on commercial matters stands little chance to resist or oppose expertly delivered persuasion if industry manipulates experts to push its interests.

Average consumers are no match for experts who are educated or working at higher-order educational institutions, serving terms in public office, advising government, or are certified and backed by professional organizations, sometimes even being funded by industry or the experts themselves. An industry that has control of experts and other purveyors of influence and power has control of consumers.

Expert biases give real meaning to the saying that "money talks."

The adoption of policies by professional organizations that their experts must fully disclose at professional meetings and within scientific publications any financial associations and relationships with industry explicitly acknowledges that economic relationships and collaborative efforts existing between experts and commercial industries create conflicts of interest that may unduly influence, compromise, or bias their work and opinions.

2.6 RESEARCH

Experts attempt to enhance the predictability of outcomes associated with individual human behavioral choices and lifestyles and reduce the element that chance alone dictates what happens when decisions are made to behave selectively in specific ways.

Expert advice on food, health, and nutritional or weight management issues is typically distilled from and supported by experiences, observations, and knowledge acquired collectively through the collaborative efforts of various individuals and entities.

The undertaking by experts to gather and catalog vast amounts of experimental data to be shared formally for discussion, analyses, and application often follows professional, standard operating procedures structured to provide a common ground for all on which to consider and discuss the scientific work performed.

The collective understanding gained through the combined work of many experts then increases the accuracy of predicting consequences for pursuing various life choices and actions.

Scientific research, therefore, is an investigational search tool structured with standard operating procedures that provide a shared platform to consider and compare experimental work used to increase human understanding, improve human decisions, and support expert advice. *Research allows human existence and the observed and experienced universe and universal phenomena to be better understood and more amenable to human control.*

Research investigations follow systematic, scientifically established rules and protocols to search methodically for answers to relevant and thoughtful life queries. Formal research protocols increase the legitimacy of scientific observations and discoveries and theoretically allow independent workers, who perform separate investigations using published research methods, to reproduce and confirm experimental results and derive study conclusions.

Research helps experts to understand and control life circumstances and events that otherwise appear to occur randomly and unpredictably. In essence, research helps to create stories that put together acquired and accumulated scientific evidence, and known scientific understanding, to explain and predict life events—similarly to how crime scene investigation helps to explain criminal and motives to solve crimes and assist with crime prevention long after the crimes were committed.

Unfortunately, limitations accompany carrying out research work, since researchers often can only measure limited parameters of complex dynamic systems under restricted periods of observation, analogously to taking a still frame out of a small sector of a 360-degree panoramic movie.

Additionally, research isn't always performed purely to gain understanding or to find out the truth concerning how things work. Hardworking scientific investigators who hope to remain professionally viable and monetarily afloat are likely to pursue scientific interests that can be subsidized financially; they don't have the luxury to engage in scientific pursuits purely for fun or to explore the complexities of the world to satisfy their intellectual curiosity.

Some researchers may even accept compensation or are paid outright to produce scientific work and opinions that favor the self-serving interests of funding commercial industries and other entities. Consequently, research may well be performed to satisfy investigator and research sponsors' financial purposes and agendas, and possibly be used intentionally as a convenient commercial industry tool to manipulate the market decisions and behaviors of consumers.

To achieve research accomplishments, industry and experts often collaborate and perform work that frequently lacks transparency to preserve company and trade secrets and maintain a competitive industry edge surrounding completed research work. Entities performing research work may also intentionally obscure the real understanding, limitations, meaning, and impact of commercial products, services, and ideas being promoted and sold self-servingly to protect industry advantage and profitability, and only release the scope of scientific findings and information if compelled to by law.

In summary, various factors can influence scientific investigations:

1. investigator bias
2. investigator conflicts of interest
3. investigator funding
4. confounding errors, which are extraneous influences on scientific studies that research investigators fail to recognize, consider, or control in their experiments and that may significantly affect experimental results and study conclusions
5. logistic, time, sample size, and material limitations impacting the performance, execution, details, results, and significance of research work

Limitations affecting scientific studies that result in missing data may lead researchers to substitute unavailable experimental observations with estimations. **Extrapolation** estimates the apparent trend or direction of scientific findings, and **interpolation** is fill-in-the-blank guesswork for unavailable data; either approach may be applied to make up data to be incorporated into studies as necessary for analysis, along with actually obtained data, which in combination help investigators arrive at meaningful conclusions that later become employed to support expert advice and predictions and possibly to legislate societal policies.

Appropriately gathered research data may also be strategically manipulated statistically to enhance the importance of specific findings that support and strengthen arguments made for the relevance of scientific work performed.

The most creatively staged scenarios using only the very best illustrative examples of research work that persuasively promotes personal or organizational agendas serve as idealized platforms to present research observations and propositions. Even the most ostensibly objective scientific researchers have the potential for personal biases to influence the performance and presentation of their experimental work.

Publish or perish dictates survival in the research game, compelling scientists to perform research work acceptable for publication. *Unsurprisingly, scientists have been caught misrepresenting their research work and hacking online into peer review processes in journals so that submitted articles will be favorably received and accepted for journal publication.*

Research funding preferentially favors studies that may produce significant results that can generate revenues or cut costs. *Positive studies* that demonstrate scientifically predicted or financially profitable results are more likely to be published than *negative studies* that fail to show postulated research study effects or are unlikely to lead to financial gains.

Consumer demands for specific commercial products and services and their associated potential industry profitability are potent inducements spurring further scientific investigations of previously studied products and services that may have scientifically failed to demonstrate any meaningful human benefits. Scientific investigations failing to show any apparent human benefit or utility for factors studied, which may otherwise be of significant interest to commercial industries and society, are offered a second chance to be reconsidered within the context of secondary analytical studies that combine and scour research findings to glean any commercially marketable and societally applicable results. The data from research investigations that similarly examined specific scientific issues of interest but individually failed to demonstrate consistent, meaningful, or expected study outcomes could be combined and collectively subjected to additional rigorous scientific scrutiny.

Meta-analyses are investigations that mathematically scrutinize the combined data set, obtained from pooling a group of methodically similar research studies addressing a specific scientific quandary of interest, for any statistically meaningful or commercially useful findings and information. Studies included in a meta-analysis address a similar scientific question but are usually performed separately under different circumstances by various investigators employing distinct investigation techniques. Research meta-analyses lump many similar research studies together to increase the available data set and the power to tease out subtle and statistically relevant associations occurring between study interventions and observed treatment outcomes that otherwise may be too weak to detect within individual studies having limited data collection with small sample sizes and insufficient numbers of observations.

Hidden study relationships may only become evident or suggested by analyzing the pooled combination of studies that individually may have demonstrated inconclusive, minimal, or absent associations between study manipulations and obtained study results. Meta-analysis study results frequently only provide suggestive odds to favor or oppose research manipulations and pursue some course of action, with the odds being calculated through intensive mathematical analysis of the pooled combination of inconclusive and marginally conclusive study results. Within a meta-analysis, the complex factors affecting the relationships between manipulated study parameters and observed intervention effects are often unknown, incompletely understood, or unrecognized in the context of complicated biological systems.

Clinical research studying societally pertinent health, nutrition, and weight management matters frequently relies on meta-analyses to establish and drive home points of interest relevant to humanity and industry. Scientific study subjects selected from various geographic localities and socioeconomic groups that become lumped together in a meta-analysis may possess markedly different environmental and social influences that may significantly impact research findings derived from combining various studies, even those performed using similar research protocols.

Meta-analysis studies pooling research participants from diverse geographic zones and socioeconomic circumstances may draw conclusions for the combined samples that may not validly apply in a one-size-fits-all way for other, more homogeneous populations of individuals.

Additionally, combining studies individually performed during different time frames, under diverse circumstances, and by assorted investigators using distinct study protocols and techniques introduces numerous variables of uncertainty and confounding errors into the final meta-analysis conclusions.

Despite the numerous limitations affecting meta-analysis study results and conclusions, these statistical research tools are routinely employed to influence, persuade, and manipulate the perception and behaviors of consumers, health care providers, and scientists alike. The nebulous nature of meta-analysis study results ideally serves particularly to favor the self-serving financial agendas of commercial food, nutrition, health, and weight management industries standing to earn large-scale profits through any modality, which leverages consumer economic behaviors and choices involving complex, insufficiently understood human matters.

Findings from meta-analysis studies that might benefit commercial interests poised to score windfall profits also coincidentally promote the interests of meta-analysis study investigators who depend on industry funding and support to carry out their ongoing research work. Therefore, immensely complex human biological systems create tremendous challenges and obstacles for researchers to perform scientific studies that attempt to understand human life and interactions.

Consequently, given the enormous uncertainties and limitations affecting research work, conclusions reached from research efforts are applicable with greater certainty toward systems, populations, or individuals having characteristics more closely resembling those of research subjects selected for participation in research studies and may not at all apply to entities different from those chosen for study. Unfortunately, commercial industries broadly interpret and routinely generalize research study findings with impunity to manipulate consumer perceptions and push through agendas serving industry self-interests.

2.7 STATISTICS

Life certainty is uncertainty with probability estimates.

Life decisions are a game of chance guided by personal knowledge and experience and the advice of experts. Human life experiences can be studied systematically and analyzed mathematically to improve personal choices and actions under numerous life circumstances.

Statistics are mathematical tools that employ complex mathematical formulations to discover and compare differences between pursuing various courses of action in groups that are studied scientifically and, additionally, allow investigators to credibly advise or argue against choosing specific courses of action involving life decisions. Ultimately, statistics help humans better predict the possible consequences or outcomes of making certain life decisions and choices.

Food, nutrition, health, and weight management decisions typically depend on clinical research studies that employ statistics to legitimize and support expert recommendations for pursuing various decisional options. Statistics can also become a numbers game deliberately played to emphasize research findings that specifically promote industry agendas and influence and manipulate consumer choices benefiting commercial interests.

For example, research study effects can be reported numerically as either a percentage change or as an actual change, depending on the need to spotlight research findings when attempting to support scientific arguments and sway opinion. Therefore, if treatment A gives a 1% response rate while treatment B provides a 2% response rate within a study population, then treatment B can be represented as either being twice or 100% more effective than treatment A, even though both treatment effects are minimal within the studied populations.

Expensive research studies comparing various treatment options that offer industry substantial profit opportunities similarly often demonstrate only marginal treatment effects within study groups. Nevertheless, these marginal treatment effects become strongly highlighted and heavily supported by statistical data to promote the agendas of investigators and sources of research funding.

Additionally, the sample sizes for research studies to reliably detect the presence of a relevant and real treatment effect may be unattainable under practical life circumstances, which may limit data acquisition and consequently lead to incorrect interpretations of investigative findings—most notably observed when underpowered studies performed with insufficient samples of research subjects demonstrate only small treatment effects.

Statistical significance and **statistical relevance** are derived through rigorous mathematical analyses of research data and indicate the numerical probabilities or odds for research study observations to have occurred either incidentally by chance alone or directly due to research manipulations. The lower are the odds that research findings occurred incidentally by chance alone, the higher are the odds that research findings reflect true research effects as observed by manipulating study parameters.

For example, research outcomes are frequently assigned **p (probability) values** having numbers such as $p < 0.05$ or $p < 0.001$ to qualify research findings. The p-value indicates the probability or odds of research findings to have occurred by chance alone and not because of research manipulations. Consequently, for $p < 0.05$, the odds are less than 5 chances in 100, and for $p < 0.001$, the odds are less than 1 chance in 1,000 that study findings occurred incidentally by chance alone.

Statistical analyses of research data may alternatively examine study effects by mathematically comparing how study manipulations affect or move some average value or defined range of baseline values applying to undisturbed study elements or parameters. For instance, studies may compare the effects that various study manipulations have on shifting the 95% range of observed values for the undisturbed study elements, with the new 95% range of values obtained by manipulating study elements reflecting the presumed treatment effect of study manipulations.

Unfortunately, statistical significance does not necessarily elaborate any specific mechanism of action or provide explanations for encountered study observations and findings resulting from study manipulations, nor do statistically significant research findings necessarily explain actual interrelationships between studied research parameters or establish a cause and effect between study manipulations and observed study outcomes. Instead, statistical significance helps researchers formulate plausible scientific hypotheses and draw conclusions from associations discovered through their research work, which are often used by industry experts to provide professional advice, and which help guide subsequent research efforts and help obtain further research funding.

Industry expertly plays the *statistics game* to sensationalize research findings and deliberately manipulate humanity for industry purposes, best illustrated through the extensive use of statistics in politics. Industry frequently exploits statistical significance to promote industry agendas and interests.

Weak scientific studies demonstrating only statistically marginal positive results on issues relevant for industry purposes may be used to manipulate public perception and influence consumers by describing study findings using commercially familiar terminology such as "scientifically proven" or "large clinical trials show" or "statistically superior."

Drug companies routinely push statistically relevant research findings to promote widespread use of expensive, minimally effective pharmaceutical treatments for common, non-threatening health disorders, when less costly alternative health interventions, including behavioral modification, can easily suffice to accomplish similar clinical results at much lower consumer costs and risks.

The disconcerting side of statistical manipulations becomes apparent when research findings furthering commercial interests and industry profitability are deliberately highlighted and inflated, while negative or contrary study findings are minimized or suppressed and go unpublished, deceptively exaggerating the real benefits-over-costs comparisons available for truly informed scientific and consumer considerations and decision-making.

Why is it so difficult for individuals to achieve and maintain
optimal weight and health?
The simple answer is that commercial industry systems design challenges
predisposing individuals to fail in their weight management
and health maintenance efforts.
Consumers are more valuable to commercial industries when continually in

*need, struggling, and spending money to obtain personal satisfaction arti-
ficially through commercially sponsored means than they are when being
capable of satisfying individual needs naturally to secure gratification without commercial industry involvement.*

*Human struggles and failures with reliance on industry to provide an escape
from their predicaments create commercial industry profit opportunities.
Costs for some are earnings for others, and strife or conflict for the
many equals extreme wealth for the few.*

3 ADDICTIFICATION

Industry exists to supply consumer needs and demands commercially.

While basic human needs are relatively predictable and fixed, consumer demands change unexpectedly over time and are more difficult and challenging for commercial industries to anticipate and gauge.

All humans require food to exist and desire to live in good health. Proper nutrition and appropriate weight maintenance are cornerstones of healthy living for everyone.

Therefore, commercial industries opportunely profit by supplying and driving up consumer demands for products and services that favorably satisfy societal nutritional and weight management needs. The predictability of basic human pleasure-reward and survival feed-and-breed-with-greed programming opens numerous avenues for commercial industries to profit.

Profit-hungry corporate and commercial entities vying to control human interests bank on the premise that humans are optimistic gamblers driven by greed that take chances and strive for pleasure and vantage.

Industries assuredly guarantee themselves continuous streams of revenue by designing commercial products that service basic human survival needs to feed and breed but also coincidentally drive up human wants and desires for their designed products. Dopamine-based pleasure-reward programming is a valuable tool to train consumers and leverage consumer behaviors commercially for industry aims. Sales and promotional offers that solicit consumers to purchase commercial products and services substantially play the dopamine motivational reward system, especially when commercial wares providing pleasure-reward fixes are offered inexpensively or together with other incentives to potentiate dopamine motivational drives seeking to acquire the offered commercial pleasure-reward fixes.

Therefore, steering consumer interests and commercial drives are paramount for business enterprises to maintain profitability. **Addictification** is the deliberate implanting into brain software of commercial loops that stick body vehicle behaviors in mindless, unnecessary spending mode. Addictification is the creation of consumer *dependency* for commercial products and services of convenience, luxury, and pleasure, which become misconstrued as having the capacity to deliver happiness, satisfaction, health, or survival benefits or as being able to relieve unhappiness and suffering and help to cope with stress and predicaments.

Addictification reprograms primal human drives seeking indulgence, excess, and immediate gratification to trap consumers into costly, unproductive, and frequently harmful commercial behaviors that temporarily supply hedonistic wants and craves and relieve suffering and pain to become misperceived as necessary for daily existence. Therefore, addictification involves indoctrinating ritualistic purchases and regular consumption of particular commercial items that work on body vehicle hedonistic and pain-avoidance drives.

Typical addictification products include soda pop beverages; tasty chips or dip; convenient and easy-to-prepare processed food items; yummy candy bars; chocolates and sweets; special gum; fun, sugary cereals; delicious cookies and pastry goods; and favorite mouth-watering fast-food products easily obtained from drive-thru restaurants.

Consequently, *addictification* is the commercial entrapment of body vehicle behaviors to enslave the body vehicle life force energy physically in repetitive money-spending routines.

Possessing the capability to compel consumer behaviors with the perfect combination of biological and commercial market forces spells profitable success for business enterprise systems. Neglect to fulfill basic body vehicle survival needs appropriately creates a crater of unsatisfied needs vulnerable to being filled with commercial industry products and services that trigger addictification to increase wants and primal craves even further. The regular purchase of goods that predictably provide fleeting physical pleasures or relieve suffering short-term insidiously transforms into a self-perpetuating biological hook that needlessly and wastefully spends consumer money.

Addictification refocuses the body vehicle from engaging in meaningful life activities toward pursuing commercially promoted behaviors temporarily appeasing hedonistic pleasure-reward centers of the primal brain, while creating insatiable urges that are exceedingly profitable for industry to gratify repeatedly. Addictification slowly drains the body vehicle biological system of valuable personal resources, such as time, energy, and money, and derails naturally productive behaviors that optimize life quality inexpensively or for free. Therefore, consumers running on addictification programs unnecessarily spend time, energy, and money on commercial products and services that often compromise body vehicle health and function and foster dependence on retail industries.

Consequently, industry surreptitiously promotes consumer addictification whenever possible to deplete consumers of valuable personal resources while providing minimal human rewards in return, which are often only limited to deliver sensory pleasures and runaway escapes through oral taste bud titillation. Ultimately, addictification makes it easier to *suck the buck* out the wallet or purse to promote cash flow from consumers to commercial industry systems.

The trial-and-error mapping of physiologic brain activity is scientifically painstaking when carried out on laboratory animals and using various indirect human studies. Currently, scientific technologies directly image the brain in real time to divulge brain activities and communication pathways between different brain areas under various stimulating circumstances.

Brain-imaging technologies using functional **CAT** (computed axial tomography) and **MRI** (magnetic resonance imaging) scans anatomically map out brain centers involved with pleasure, pain, decision-making, and addiction and are available to confirm how brain pleasure-reward and addiction centers biologically excite through direct physical or chemical stimulation of body vehicle senses or manipulation of surrounding external environments to produce specific human experiences.

Functioning areas of the brain, including the pleasure-reward centers, work like motion detectors to turn on automatically when activated by appropriate stimuli. Commercial industries tap into neuroscientific understanding to create **neuromarketing,** which uses technological advancements, such as functional brain imaging and measurement of evoked brain waves, as tools to characterize and exploit consumer behaviors.

Functional MRI and CAT brain imaging can be purposefully applied to guide the design of manipulative advertising campaigns and to engineer unregulated "food" products, which strategically stimulate addictification brain centers to influence and control the behavioral and emotional responses of unsuspecting consumers subconsciously.

Technology assistance allows industry to target the vulnerabilities and weaknesses inherent within human survival programming to create powerful inducements that reprogram executive brain functions into sustained commercial behaviors. Commercial forces engage society on various levels to drive human lives into addictification routines for commercial profit, and then devise elaborate industry systems to support and promote human addictification and all the ensuing fallout, profiting industry.

Individuals and societal, governmental, and industrial systems sharing in the revenues, fees, and taxes generated through human addictification, approvingly endorse, facilitate, and advance addictification behaviors. Addictification itself then reliably serves to retain human membership within profiteering addictification systems, surreptitiously imposing exorbitant costs on unsuspecting member participants and society.

3.1 BEHAVIORAL INFLUENCE

In a commercially designed world, industry manufactures artificial realities that express the corporate and commercial thinking that best manipulates mass perception and controls human behaviors to increase commercial activities and commercial profits. Advertising and marketing enterprises embark on sophisticated campaigns to insidiously or overtly manipulate consumer decisions and behaviors that accomplish industry directives and allow commercial entities to thrive financially.

Enormous industry profit opportunities especially exist in controlling and driving consumer retail behaviors involving weight management, nutrition, and health. Industry uses various media to brainwash and program consumers to carry out commercial agendas. Conditioned consumers then mindlessly engage programmed behaviors in response to appropriate industry triggers. That regular purchase of coffee, donuts, fast foods, sweets, treats, snacks, and many other specific commercial industry products and services may well be the mindless execution of commercially programmed behaviors.

It is tempting to speculate whether the English parting salutation "goodbye" really means "good buy" and has been industry contrived to encourage individuals subliminally with every opportunity to purchase retail goods and services.

3.1.1 Conditioned Responses

Some of the more difficult life challenges humans face are to change or extinguish ingrained personal habits and social or ethnic customs and norms particularly concerning dietary choices, which are learned at home or indoctrinated through repetitive behaviors, especially if those habits, customs, and norms continue to manifest under the same extraneous circumstances, influences, and cues. Success in changing ingrained individual behaviors depends on altering or reducing the external cues and environmental triggers that promote the programmed behaviors and then finding alternative, more suitable routines that can substitute for and reprogram repetitive behaviors.

3.1.1.1 Pavlov's Dogs

In a famous behavioral experiment performed in the late 1800s, Dr. Ivan Pavlov paired the sound of a ringing bell with the delivery of food to dogs, which caused the dogs to salivate, and eventually trained or conditioned the dogs to automatically salivate solely at the sound of the ringing bell. Similar tendencies for biological conditioning have been demonstrated in humans, showing that specific human biologic responses can be activated predictably under appropriate circumstances and cues with training, which is one reason why food commercials typically advertise heavily during mealtimes, when the stomach is growling and ready for food.

Additionally, human emotions can also be trained to occur predictably by associating objects and circumstances with specific emotional responses and then reintroducing those objects and conditions later to reelicit those same emotional reactions. Processed food products with heavily concentrated sugar and fat produce pleasure when consumed, so that later sightings of these food products create anticipation for the foods to generate similar pleasurable experiences upon consumption, consequently inducing people to purchase the foods. Thus, humans can be trained or conditioned to behave biologically and react emotionally in specific ways on command.

The addictification industry works similarly to the principles established by Dr. Pavlov to condition and groom consumers into executing automated commercial behavioral routines upon specific cues presented at opportune moments. Consumer addictification routines likewise activate on command to engage consumer spending rituals that reap industry substantial monetary earnings. Ideas implanted covertly into primed consumers lie dormant, awaiting trigger words, circumstances, and situations that spring commercial behaviors into action, analogously to how specific commands engage hypnotic suggestions to control hypnotized subjects. Similarly, addictification biologically redirects the body vehicle under a designed set of circumstances to impulsively and automatically execute expected commercial behaviors that satisfy industry objectives. Therefore, addictification reprograms human behavioral circuits to entrench behaviors that commercially "salivate" on command in response to market triggers to activate desires to purchase and consume industry goods, which ultimately serves to turn the wheels of industry.

Undoubtedly, many experience strong emotions and perhaps salivate uncontrollably with mouth-watering desires to purchase and eat food products at iconic global fast-food industry outlets upon seeing the advertising logo and markings. Behavioral programming tying into general customs, social norms, everyday habits, personal routines, and commonly experienced circumstances facilitates and deeply ingrains addictification.

3.1.2 Thought Influence and Control

Thought influence and control target **pleasure, convenience, greed, pain,** and **fear** as the main forces to drive human behaviors, especially when human ignorance, misinformation, and blind obedience prevail.

Thought influence and control are implemented strategically through various channels:

1. education
2. expert advice
3. media programming
4. social and public opinion
5. peer and family pressures
6. religious doctrines in faith and worship institutions
7. governmental and organizational rules, laws, and restrictions
8. oppression
9. punishment

Sinister, self-serving intentions to control and manipulate human behaviors and thinking hide more readily by assimilating into established organizational systems, which conveniently have built-in controls of humanity with rules of order and governance, to hijack readied participants who collectively obey, trust, depend on, and enforce rules within their organizational structures.

The use of motivational fear to create the notion that behavioral delays or inaction will lead to missed opportunities, loss of benefits, retribution, group exclusion, penalties, punishment, pain, and other unwanted negative consequences is another effective strategy to control human behaviors. The doubts and uncertainties that individuals possess provide innumerable opportunities for systems to exploit and manipulate human interests and actions. Subtle human manipulation also occurs by playing on greed through industry incentives that entice consumers into commercial rituals that gradually foster dependency on industry products and services.

Industry cleverly devises commercial rules and restrictions to spur consumers into addictification routines. Advertising offers that strictly limit the purchase quantity of specified items to only a few create false scarcity to hurry consumers into buying products and services, thereby maximizing consumer exposures to offers that promote addictification. Similarly, promotional offers may be time-limited to pressure consumers to buy. For example, a food establishment may offer "For one week only, drive through and purchase a donut and coffee for only $2 and get a second donut for free" to indoctrinate a consumer ritual of driving through for coffee and a donut daily, which generates profits well beyond the original time period of the sales offer.

3.2 ADDICTIFICATION INDUSTRY

The increasing complexity of modern life is becoming progressively more demanding to navigate and unpleasantly challenges human survival to create extreme stresses from which humans seek to run away, escape, and break free and use any available means to cope.

Addictification industries are in the business of providing temporary *runaway escapes* that help humanity cope with life stresses. The sale of convenient stress escapes and coping options deliberately aims to sow dependency in the vulnerable and unwary to relieve personal suffering through commercial means.

Addictification industries embed a commercial hook through human lives into the wallet or purse to extract money and make an economic "killing" selling addictification products and services to humanity. "Birds of a feather" addictification industries supply

1. commercially processed and refined food products
2. alcohol
3. tobacco and other nicotine products, including e-cigarettes
4. pornography
5. various recreational and illicit drugs
6. gambling opportunities

Addictification industry birds of a feather "stick" together, regularly combining to "stick it" to humanity jointly.

Addictification industries appeal to the higher-order brain to seduce the intellect to initially try and then mindlessly get hooked on repeatedly buying their commercial products and services without restraint. Marketing schemes associate acquisition and use of addictification products and services with clever depictions of human belonging, companionship, bonding, accomplishment, and nurturing or flat-out promise immediate gratification of primary human drives to seek pleasure or relief from pain.

The repetitive use of addictification industry products and services that stimulate and temporarily appease primal survival drives to feed, breed, seek pleasure, and reduce stress, boredom, suffering, and pain conditions human behaviors to seek to reproduce these experiences compulsively. Industry exists to *feed the needs* of humanity, whereby humanity regularly confuses its own needs, wants, and craves.

Many of the commercial wants and craves of humanity are created intentionally through the concerted efforts of addictification industries, which readily supply human desires for money to generate human meal tickets that feed industry profits. Addictification industries condition individuals to pay industry a monetary charge in exchange for the commercial delivery of a temporary sensory or emotional charge, which reinforces payers to continue doing the same thing repeatedly and indefinitely.

Creating and supplying consumer wants and craves stringently adheres to the **business principle** that *if a profitable activity is not illegal or considered immoral and generates revenues, then that activity is a good business practice to carry out* regardless of any ensuing costs and consequences to individuals and society. The troubling reality is that addictification industries not only operate to control and manipulate human behaviors but also use their amassed corporate earnings and accumulated wealth to influence human interests and further industry self-interests by powerfully leveraging important legislative and health care decisions. The enabling of insatiable human wants and craves through addictification industry products and services commercially locks in consumers into growing industry profitability. Therefore, addictification industries commercially marshal that vulnerable and unsuspecting mass portion of humanity that will incontestably fund commercial industry profits.

Classic addictification industry outlet traps are gas station mini-marts and free-standing convenience stores ubiquitously dotting neighborhood landscapes and existing within commercial strip malls. The addictification industry traps almost exclusively sell tobacco and nicotine products, alcohol, lottery tickets, candy, processed and refined snack food items, pornographic magazines, a few beauty and personal hygiene products, and sometimes an occasional banana as an afterthought of health.

3.3 TARGET DEMOGRAPHICS

You are being studied.

Commercial industries could not thrive without knowing the segments of consumer populations interested in and purchasing their products and services. All commercial industries appeal to *target consumer audiences* to sell their industry wares. Consequently, industry carefully studies everything possible concerning consumers and consumer behaviors and influences.

Copious amounts of information concerning consumer wants, desires, needs, aspirations, preferences, and fears are collected and amassed using marketing questionnaires, focus groups, online internet and social media applications, testing of volunteer and paid subjects, and scientific experimentation and behavioral observations and then are meticulously compiled and statistically analyzed to ascertain commercial human drives.

All identifying individual, societal group, and population-based information and statistical data, known as **demographics,** are correlated with the signature interests, characteristics, needs, and wants of targeted segments of studied consumer populations to identify and expose behavioral patterns amenable to commercial exploitation. Data concerning consumer age, gender, race, religion, ethnicity, occupation, political party affiliation, socioeconomic status, and health help industry create predictive models of commercial human behaviors and controlling influences, which are employed to gauge consumer demands more accurately for available or prospective commercial industry products and services.

Consumers are sometimes offered nonexistent ghost products and services through electronic media modalities to test consumer demand for potential products and services being considered for development and better assess the economic feasibility of creating and mass-producing such products and services for actual commercial market availability. Industry learns what specific interests drive consumer commercial behaviors and precisely which human characteristics and qualities to manipulate commercially for industry purposes. Identification of the individual and group triggers, preferences, and habits for spending money increases consumer predictability to better match consumers with commercial product lines that correspond with individual and group wants, enhancing the likelihood that consumers will buy commercial products.

Sophisticated **artificial intelligence (AI)** computing programs embedded within media device applications rapidly analyze the individual consumer preferences of media device users, allowing dynamic tailoring of more directed marketing strategies to sell commercial industry wares and service lines to specific consumer populations. Modern modalities that employ target demographics to collect vast amounts of consumer information, which becomes readily available for industry to sell or dynamically tailor advertisements to meet individual consumer preferences, include internet search engines, online social media applications, and numerous other computer, television, and cellular smartphone applications. Email service providers even permit third parties to access and scan email accounts and messages for key words and personal data which then are sold to other third parties to target advertisements to email users.

Individualized target demographics occur with every online click of the mouse navigating the internet and making selections on cell phone media applications. Tracking "cookies" on search engines trace, record, and indefinitely store online choices and divulged individual likes and dislikes in the cloud for analysis and demographic scrutiny to understand user habits and preferences and predict the next consumer commercial move to turn a profit for industry. User choices are then sold to commercial interests to target consumer segments selectively with specific commercial products and services.

Computer IP addresses and cell phone numbers carry unique identifiers that allow profiling of electronic device app users for **hyperselective marketing,** which uses **online behavioral advertising** to target the app user's commercial interests.

Internet and smartphone app designers specifically create **click bait** to entice users to make choices that expose personal interests and preferences, which facilitate directed marketing and financially reward app designers and advertisers successfully uncovering consumer desires. Therefore, knowledge of consumer characteristics, interests, and commercial preferences allows mobile targeting of product and service lines to best match individual consumer needs, utilization, biases, and purchasing patterns dynamically with every available opportunity and permits fluid adjustment of sales and marketing strategies to increase industry sales and profit margins.

Interactive electronic media modalities perfect profiling of individuals to better snare unsuspecting consumer victims.

Genetic testing, performed by scientists and clinicians for research and medical purposes and sold commercially to the public sector to help discover ancestral origins and create a family tree, is providing fertile grounds to identify and locate individuals with specific health disorders who commercial industries can target to sell disease-specific interventions.

Consumers are continuously "made" through targeted marketing strategies.
Target demographics help industry craft the best lures to bait and hook consumers commercially.

Without awareness and a healthy life philosophy, consumer resistance collapses against sophisticated commercial industry strategies, tactics, and techniques that trap consumers into addictification.

More insidiously, corporate and commercial interests increasingly use AI with big data-mining software to ascertain fundamental human interests, behaviors, and influences.

Augmented reality (AR) and **virtual reality (VR)** technologies can then simulate human qualities and artificially stage physical constructs within electronic paradigms that appeal to the likes and dislikes revealed by unwary, naive, and vulnerable online individuals to control their behaviors covertly.

3.4 INDUSTRY WORD GAMES

Commercial industry word games transform consumer perceptions into market connections.

3.4.1 Words Are Tools

Words can be used to inform, persuade, guide, lead, shape, mold, program, manipulate, and control humans. Political correctness exemplifies how words are used to control human behaviors.

Political correctness prohibits and omits the usage of select words during social discourse involving any discussions of certain restricted topics and sensitive societal issues. Offenders who break the rules of political correctness risk social rebuke, castigation, condemnation, shunning, and punishment for their transgressions.

The commercial nutrition, health, and weight management industries likewise rely heavily on manipulating words to achieve industry purposes. Commercial industries, experts, and sales personnel all seek to benefit and profit from the skillful manipulation of communication through spoken, written, depicted, and portrayed language forms.

Some industry-created words and phrases that are unique, catchy, and powerfully persuasive in connecting specific commercial products to consumer consciousness become **money terms,** which are legally copyrighted and branded into trademarks to provide select companies exclusive rights to use and restrict other commercial entities from using these terms.

Individuals trained in human psychology and other behavioral health disciplines who are not actively practicing clinically to provide behavioral health counseling become useful industry resources for devising effective word strategies that influence consumer commercial behaviors.

3.4.2 Industry Is about Consumer Control for Money

Advertising messages that deliver cleverly phrased words dispatched with the appropriate visual imagery and auditory cues surreptitiously influence human behaviors like hypnotic suggestions to promote mindless consumer spending for commercial items. When consumers transfer money to industry without much thought, the opportunity exists for consumers to step back and consider whether spending is voluntary, deliberate, and performed with awareness or is being executed ritually, automatically, under the surreptitious control of implanted mind malware which is driving body vehicle behaviors involuntarily.

3.4.3 Food Word Games

*Industry creates and sells words to manipulate and steer consumer
purchase instincts and commercial behaviors.*

Nutritional words that subliminally direct consumer choices and steer consumers
toward or away from food products include calorie, cholesterol, fat, fiber, sodium,
salt, trans fats, high fructose corn syrup, fresh, gluten, natural, artisan, real, organic,
whole foods, gourmet, home-made, original, and lean, especially when combined
correctly with directional words, such as all, no, low, high, and free.

Consumers regularly invest in words when satisfying nutritional needs through
commercial food manufacturers rather than through available natural whole earth
foods delivered word-free. For example, consumers are more likely to buy products advertised as no or low salt, low or no fat, gluten free, no high fructose corn
syrup, high fiber, all natural, and no artificial than to purchase items advertised
as high salt, high fat, low fiber, or all artificial.

Industry also uses the latest consumer and social **buzzwords** relating to
health and human concerns and societal fads in progress to entice and promote
consumer commercial behaviors on a more personal level. Industry gets personal
to increase the likelihood for commercial behaviors to ingrain into deeply rooted
habits perpetuated indefinitely, while consumers are misled to believe that their
individual retail choices are being made intentionally.

Manufacturers may even include human uniqueness and connectivity terms
and add personal sayings on packaging labels and cans to attach consumers
emotionally to their commercial products.

Industry word games play consumers for profit.

Some examples of catchy and trendy subliminal, commercial plays on words
include "Drink Responsibly"; "Know When to Say When"; "'Fresh' Lunchmeat";
EggBeaters®; ReaLemon®; LeanCuisine®; HealthyChoice®; Nature's Own®; "All Natural"; and "Made with All Natural."

Industry word games employ fake or **pseudo-authoritative endorsements**
to persuade consumers that specific commercial products or services have been
officially designated to be best in their category and that choosing these products
confers unique advantages or inclusion into select groups, as indicated by the
following:

1. Most doctors recommend . . .
2. The number 1 recommended . . .
3. The number 1 chosen . . .
4. The number 1 preferred . . .
5. The winner in a national survey . . .

6. In a national study, most households prefer . . .
7. Official sponsor of the . . .
8. Research studies show . . .

There are more word games. For example, "Great Cola Taste" advertises that the particular cola product delivers an exceptional sensory taste experience, and "Oven Baked Family Time" markets that food product use enhances family gathering opportunities, with both commercial strategies promising special returns for product purchase. Not many commercial ideas selling carrots or broccoli could supplant such powerful manufactured food product associations and imagery.

Familiar sports and entertainment celebrities commonly endorse commercial products and services to misdirect consumers to imitate them through **what do I know mind control**. This approach enlists the celebrities to promote the commercial products and services authoritatively, anticipating that consumers will follow their lead. Celebrities having mass consumer appeal and influence reach the pinnacle of commercial, economic success when recruited by industries to represent commercial wares.

3.5 ADDICTIFICATION FOOD INDUSTRY

The addictification food industry seductively procures cozy relationships with consumers and then craftily employs misdirection, illusion, and deception to drive consumer commercial behaviors. Addictification food industries sell tasty flavors over substance since tasty flavors are cheaper and more profitable to create, mass-produce, and market compared to healthy, natural-tasting whole foods, which have limited availability, spoil easier, and are more expensive to grow, harvest, distribute, and sell.

Gateway foods in the form of tasty candy, chips, soda pop, cereals, pastries, bread, pasta, and various other processed and refined snack and convenience foods facilitate consumer food addictifications. The addictification food industry resorts to all the sophisticated tricks of the commercial industry trade, including the use of restrictive nutritional directives and complicated rules, to manipulate consumer food choices and herd consumers commercially to generate industry profits.

Addictification food industry advertising strategies use memorable word games and seductively embed commercial products within inviting vignettes to link products to enjoyable human experiences, desirable life circumstances, and admirable human qualities. Directional phrasing, such as "low salt," "low fat," and "gluten free," on food packaging delivers cues appealing to preconditioned consumer mind-sets to germinate commercially implanted behavioral programs.

Marketing strategies heavily advertise **brand names** to increase and strengthen consumer familiarity with product names and distinctive identifying package markings, and they innovatively connect specific commercial products with everyday human activities and experiences to enhance consumer recognition of products at every available commercial opportunity. For example, strategic marketing campaigns may connect using products with human uniqueness or the exhilarating feeling of riding a roller coaster. Clever industry illusions intentionally bait commercial product hooks to capture consumers, who are the big game.

Industry trains the brain to go with the show and trust the products that one doesn't know.

Product brand names may last indefinitely, but specific product formulations may be modified whenever without notifying consumers. Many universally recognizable food and beverage industry products are made using secret formulas that are amenable to proprietary revision at any time to incorporate new food engineering ideas and production innovations or to accommodate changing societal fads and taste preferences.

Basic nonproprietary natural whole foods having generic names, such as strawberries, bananas, berries, lettuce, peas, chicken, and lamb, cannot compete commercially against packaged brand-name addictification food products, which are heavily marketed by internationally recognizable food industry giants that present persuasive messages to steer consumers to buy their commercial products and often sweeten sales overtures with tempting sales offers.

Coupons and special-deal offers for commercial products and services are consumer bait that play on human greed, which seeks more for less or for free. Addictification food industry deal offers are designed specifically to capture consumer prey hook, line, and sinker.

Offers appeal immediately to the "thoughtful," intellectual, higher-order brain to purchase addictification food products, which, when ingested, access the "reactive" primitive brain to unleash primal feeding craves predisposing to addictification dependency.

Special offers for addictification products appear to be great deals at first but become expensive on numerous accounts later with the establishment of addictification, which contributes to costly health deterioration. Ultimately, sophisticated commercial mind control techniques tempt consumers into trying addictification products and services. Once established, addictification creates dependent customers with a mind out of control that easily caves in to primal impulses and craves to seek addictification industry items repeatedly. Investment costs for addictification product development, marketing, advertisements, and delivery are a mere pittance compared to the massive profits subsequently generated through unrestrained consumer consumption and spending on addictification products.

Addictification industries endeavor to feed vulnerable victims into their commercial systems in any way possible by hook or by crook.

3.6 SURVIVAL UNDER COMMERCIAL MARKET ADDICTIFICATION PRESSURES

Can humankind successfully exist without relying on commercial industries to sell fast foods and processed and refined addictification food products prepackaged in containers to subjugate human behaviors for profit?

Yes, the answer is seemingly obvious.

Microbes, insects, animals, and humans have survived together for millions of years through billions of complete life cycles without the existence of commercial enterprises.

More pertinently, why bother to care for the body vehicle maximally naturally?

The answer is that commercial industry systems exist to profit at the lowest industry expense and work to provide consumers the least for the highest possible cost. By optimizing body vehicle maintenance naturally, one can relish knowing that body vehicle care is carried out correctly at the highest level without any shortcuts benefiting outside entities at personal expense.

Ultimately, the best helping hands are at the end of one's arms. No one shovels anything into the mouth without the full consent of the brain and cooperation of those helping hands. The commitment to use those helping hands correctly to take the utmost care of the body vehicle naturally maximizes life quality to allow successful accomplishment of individual life potential.

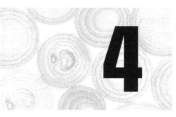

4 RESCUE INDUSTRY

Letting the body vehicle break can make one go broke.
A broken body vehicle is a ready source of revenue for commercial
interests.

The **rescue industry** comprehensively encompasses all entities that commercially provide products and services ostensibly and purportedly to maintain, enhance, and restore human health, well-being, and longevity and consists of various commercial segments:

1. **Medical:** comprising doctors, nurses, and other traditionally licensed health practitioners who directly or indirectly provide human health care and restoration
2. **Pharmaceutical:** manufacturing and supplying chemical and biological substances and products to artificially modify, restore, and sustain body vehicle physiologic functions
3. **Herbal:** offering nonprescription plant-based biologic agents for the restoration and maintenance of health.
4. **Vitamin/supplement:** artificially manufacturing and distributing biologically vital micronutrients required for human survival.
5. **Probiotic/prebiotic:** producing and supplying commercial products that incorporate various microorganisms and their products and microorganism modifying substances to influence human health and function.
6. **Ancillary:** constituting large systems of individuals who support medical industries to allow implementation of prescribed and advised health care interventions.
7. **Alternative and complementary:** utilizing and providing human health interventions other than scientifically established and endorsed traditional mainstream health care options.

The vast consortium of rescue industry entities competitively vies for consumer spending by selling products and services that target various aspects of the human life cycle, including health, nutrition, illness, disease, aging, weight management, fitness, sexual potency, vigor, and stamina.

In addition, the rescue industry encompasses not only traditionally licensed and regulated commercial health entities and nontraditional health care provider services but also all indirect health-related enterprises, such as blender vendors, fitness centers, exercise equipment dealers, health spas, personal trainers, weight management food delivery services, specialty health food stores, colonic cleansing businesses, and other businesses selling health-related products and services.

The public has dependently entrusted commercial rescue industry elements with the enormous responsibility of maintaining and restoring human health. Unfortunately, despite any existing rescue industry good intentions to maintain, promote, and restore human health, rescue industry endeavors are significantly constrained by various extraneous factors and routinely driven by financial interests.

Scientific research and understanding that conclusively explain human biological and behavioral complexities in a world abounding with innumerable undefined social and environmental influences and interactions are frequently limited or absent. Obstacles that restrict the scientific capacity to characterize and understand complex human behaviors and biology and to implement acquired scientific knowledge also impede rescue industry efforts to promote truly optimal human health and well-being.

When technical, logistic, and financial limitations reduce scientific understanding of complicated living systems and hinder the applicability of fundamental biological concepts to benefit human health, rescue industry efforts risk being diverted by commercial interests toward more profitable, easily implemented, and scientifically unproven health rescue options unrestricted by law.

Shortcomings in consumer knowledge concerning health matters provide unprincipled health care professionals fertile opportunities to compromise health care delivery efforts when profit generation supersedes professional obligations to provide consumers with the best health care. The delivery of tempered holistic health care is also jeopardized when more profitable commercial rescue industry interventions that indifferently manipulate the body vehicle like an inanimate object are selected as the preferred means to address human health needs.

Rescue industry work is continually subjected to commercial influences arising through industry sponsorship of preferred projects, governmental funding of rescue work favoring commercial interests, and rescue industry worker ambitions, who strive to profit financially through commercial industry support.

Commercial influences serve industry interests at consumers' expense when funding induces researchers to select commercially backed projects preferentially and decline to pursue alternative health investigations that reduce or limit commercial industry profitability and lower consumer costs at industry expense.

Rescue industry workers indebted to commercial interests risk becoming stewards of industry who powerfully influence consumer markets to profit the enterprises financing rescue work efforts. Rescue industry providers are also strategically positioned as ideal conduits for industry who can channel costly health care into perpetuity, as occurs when health care providers continually refill expensive prescription medications without much thought.

Financial interests compromise the level and quality of rescue work when the objectivity necessary to tailor work efforts to satisfy the needs of individuals and society most appropriately becomes undermined.

Therefore, excessive and exclusive consumer dependence on commercial rescue industry systems to deliver health is by default subjected to the numerous limitations and compromising circumstances that affect rescue industry efforts to make societies truly healthier.

Societal, economic pressures and financial shortages that negatively impact health care revenues and affordability also unfavorably transform the attitudes and motivations surrounding health care delivery and utilization. Rescue industry providers expecting to be fairly compensated for delivered health care from available health care monies, reduce times committed to meet consumer health care needs to compensate for falling health care revenues.

Increasing economic and time constraints pressure health care delivery efforts to shift from empowering and motivating individuals to protect their own health and prevent disease naturally, toward performing expensive diagnostic tests and prescribing high-priced pharmaceuticals, which are misperceived as adequately replacing thoughtful health care interactions between health care providers and consumers when time becomes limited.

Furthermore, busier individuals are more likely to sacrifice their obligations to maintain health by correcting adverse personal behaviors and lifestyles leading to illness and health deterioration, and then surrender personal control over health matters and health maintenance into the possession of profit-driven commercial elements.

Time-pressured consumers expecting to achieve health quickly by substituting chemicals for healthy living are vulnerable to industry brainwashing that pushes adoption of artificial commercial conveniences as replacements for personal responsibilities to choose healthier.

Profit-driven commercial industries promote consumer misconceptions that incompatible health behaviors can be successfully carried out simultaneously. Thus, the rescue industry becomes a convenient *crutch* for health care consumers to compensate for individual failures to meet personal responsibilities to care for and maintain the body vehicle in an optimal state of health naturally.

The practice of medicine and delivery of health care services demand adequate time to provide cures, relief, and comfort as necessary for human ailments and suffering. Time and effort are required to understand and characterize individual human illnesses and suffering and help individuals correct any physical, emotional, and social circumstances and behaviors contributing to their health disrepair.

Progressive shortening of health care visits to accommodate economic and time constraints reduces available opportunities to address pertinent issues affecting individual health matters thoroughly. When health care reimbursements and revenue collections fall, and administrative and professional health care delivery costs rise, abbreviating health care visits to increase the daily number of reimbursable contacts attempts to compensate for growing health care practice financial shortfalls.

Health care business operations must meet fixed medical practice expenses to remain economically viable and often depend on delivering a certain amount of health care to meet those expense obligations with reimbursements that are limited and fixed by third-party payers. When reimbursements drop by 15%, then 15% more, health care delivery must be squeezed into the same amount of available health care delivery time to make up for reduced practice revenues and cover the fixed costs of delivering health care.

Following successive rounds of health care reimbursement cuts, reduction cycles for health care delivery times spiral even more tightly, attempting to cover the rising costs of doing business within competitive commercially driven markets.

Additionally, just as the cost of living escalates over time, business expenses also rise progressively, particularly within health care sectors having to absorb the costs of uncompensated health care delivery, exerting even greater financial and time pressures on practices to make up monetary shortfalls.

Increasingly, many of the growing financial and time demands levied on health care delivery entities are of an administrative and regulatory nature not directly involving health care delivery to consumers, and, therefore, are not financially compensated for by payers. The health care industry system factors that dramatically contribute to the growing costs of health care delivery include the requirements that health care delivery practices record all health care encounters in **electronic health records** (EHR); invoice and code all delivered health care services meticulously in detail; precertify ordered health care interventions and medication prescriptions on a regular basis; and appeal increasing third-party denials for approval and payment of health care services expeditiously.

The cumbersome nature of documenting and inputting complex human health care encounters into complicated and inflexible electronic medical record systems consumes time and inordinately increases the costs of delivering health care and, additionally, robs opportunities for fruitful interactions between health care recipients and providers.

Additionally, the increased demands placed on health care providers to manage the EHR and carry out administrative duties reduce the available time and opportunities for providers to communicate directly with each other to discuss and coordinate health care activities involving mutual patients. Human thinking, information gathering and processing, and interpersonal interactions have minimum time requirements for effective execution and completion. Complex health care–related activities and procedures likewise demand minimum times to accomplish correctly and safely.

Limits exist as to how fast health care can be delivered to avoid omitting crucial information and services and committing reckless mistakes that adversely affect health care delivery quality and safety. Consequently, when health care delivery is compressed into less time to compensate for health care practice financial shortfalls, and portions of health care delivery times are redirected to complete administrative tasks unrelated to health care, then the times available to adequately address consumer health care matters and concerns and to educate consumers on pertinent health issues impacting their health are short-changed to deprive opportunities for improving health outcomes.

The general demands of health care and the acuity and complexity of patient health care needs intensify in modern societies living under more complicated circumstances and progressively toxic environments. Less time spent to address increasingly complicated health matters impacted by complex extraneous influences as medical options multiply ultimately costs consumers and society more.

Communication efforts between health care providers and recipients, which can effectively reduce health care delivery costs, suffer when curtailed by abbreviated health care encounter times. Shorter and more hurried professional health care encounters accommodating economic time constraints become more defensive minded, technically oriented, and costlier overall. Uncertainties generated by less thoughtful health care interactions facilitate ordering of expensive healthcare testing and medical specialty consultations to screen for less likely health conditions that predispose to high professional liabilities if missed.

One common health care delivery measure evolving to compensate for rising health care delivery costs and falling reimbursements is to employ lower-tier trained **physician extenders,** such as **nurse practitioners** and **physician assistants,** to provide primary health care services to patients.

Conveniently, physician extenders free up physician providers to manage group conducted healthcare delivery efforts and to perform more specialized professional health care services, such as surgeries and other technical procedures, that are reimbursed higher and raise declining practice revenues back up.

In busy modern societies, deft pharmaceutical and technical manipulations of the body vehicle increasingly substitute for sound medical advice generated through thoughtful discourse between physicians and patients and replace the healing power inherent within direct interpersonal interactions. Occasionally, high-tech professional manipulations cause unintended medication side effects and procedural complications requiring additional costly interventions to correct fallout from failed chemical and mechanical health care delivery. Therefore, physicians experiencing economic time pressures may forgo providing valuable counseling and health care education to patients and resort to using costly medications and technical interventions to address human health disorders, which otherwise may resolve entirely and only require additional time and reassurance with careful monitoring.

Under economic time pressures, practicing "medicine" risks progressing into a self-perpetuated commercial enterprise directed toward generating rescue industry revenues using medications, diagnostic testing, procedures, and devices to deliver health care, rather than growing toward the thoughtful promotion of health, with the MD degree being reduced to symbolize "More Drugs," "More Diagnostics," and "More Devices" to the satisfaction of profiting pharmaceutical, medical testing, and health care device industries.

To this effect, modern health care visits increasingly dispatch consumers with orders to buy medicines, complete tests, use medical devices, undergo technical procedures, and participate in special therapies that raise individual and societal costs, while sacrificing the appropriate patient education necessary to promote personal health care responsibilities and improve the understanding of simple and inexpensive health care strategies that restore and protect health naturally and reduce the need for rescue industry interventions.

More routinely, individuals suffering from health problems who turn to "medicine" or "alternative medicine" providers for help receive "medicine" or "health supplements" for health complaints and are scheduled for return visits to refill "medicines" or "health supplements," establishing dependency rituals that marry health care visits with pharmaceutical interventions.

The best medical advice health care consumers can expect to obtain with condensed health care delivery encounters is to "take and refill prescribed medicines, complete ordered tests and interventions, and return for follow-up office visits soon."

Rescue industry providers, whose primary objective for delivering health care is to raise practice revenues and deliver more reimbursable health care at the expense of performing quality professional work optimizing consumer health, benefit financially from practicing a "give-and-go," revolving door–style of health care delivery.

In all fairness, the rescue industry is not entirely responsible for the shortcomings and current plight of the modern health care delivery system. Health care encounters are a collaborative effort between participating providers and health care consumers, who function interdependently within the rescue industry matrix and often mutually agree to compromise on health care delivery choices.

Rather than adopt courses of action requiring the discipline to make behavioral and lifestyle modifications that can reverse and correct personal maladies and illnesses, health care consumers often choose convenient, **quick-fix** solutions employing expensive pharmaceuticals and technical interventions that only slow or temporarily stabilize health deterioration rather than fully meeting complex health needs.

Societal acceptance of convenient health care solutions that only temporarily appease complex health care needs fosters dependence for addressing health issues on the rescue industry, leading to repeated health care visits with runaway spending on health care services and pharmaceutical products to produce expensive, self-sustaining rescue industry profitability and consumer losses.

To break the binding chains of rescue industry dependency, consumers need to expect and demand levels of professional attention at the time of health care encounters that thoroughly address personal health needs.

The vital elements that make healthcare encounters more effective include meaningful health education of patients to promote genuine health understanding and the formulation of intelligent health care strategies to maximize health safely at the lowest cost.

Regardless of time constraints and existing payment agreements made between health care providers, payers, and consumers, temporary, quick-fix health care solutions that placate busy provider and consumer schedules but ineffectively address the actual sources of health problems are without real benefit.

On the other hand, health care consumers must be agreeable and willing to carry out their part of the health initiative bargain, which is to implement and execute the behavioral and lifestyle strategies collaboratively devised with providers that optimize and defend personal health at the lowest individual and societal costs.

4.1 DEPENDIFICATION

Dependification is the establishment of excessive and costly consumer reliance on commercial rescue industry options to meet individual health and survival needs.

Consumers who lack health understanding and possess unwarranted worries for developing adverse health consequences by pursuing health-related behaviors apart from conventional commercial rescue industry health care directives are vulnerable to becoming locked perpetually into commercially driven health care rituals.

Commercial industries inseminate fear and uncertainties into consumers to effectively impound health decisions for ransom. Health care consumers held hostage by health and survival fears and doubting their own capacities to achieve and maintain health independent of industry involvement are ripe for the rescue industry to extract exorbitant health care costs.

Industry expertly plays consumer health and survival fears and uncertainties to profit commercially by inflating consumer risks for developing certain health issues while exaggerating consumer benefits of utilizing commercial interventions to address personal health matters. Two profitable means for the rescue industry to push health care products onto consumers include endorsing scientifically unfounded consumer health behaviors, such as taking high doses of numerous vitamins and health supplements, and furthering unwarranted concerns that relate especially to a fear of germs.

Additionally, industry capitalizes on consumer concerns to magnify any dangers for experiencing adverse consequences by not playing according to rescue industry rules and recommendations, while minimizing the risks of using rescue industry interventions.

Consumer fears and uncertainties conveniently help industry reinforce and drive rescue industry–supported health care behaviors and deter consumer behaviors contrary to rescue industry approval. The threat of adverse outcomes is sufficient to dissuade many from not complying with industry advice to pursue alternative health care strategies unendorsed by industry.

Therefore, industry tactically manipulates consumer health concerns to condition consumers into dependification, or dependence on the commercial rescue industry to fill consumer health-related needs. Dependification then predictably feeds rescue industry profits as consumers rely entirely on the rescue industry for health care.

Rescue industry entities profiting through consumer dependification welcome commercially devised health care strategies and guidelines compelling consumers to depend on industry for meeting individual health care needs. Medical and pharmaceutical dependification materialize when consumers unrealistically expect rescue industry interventions and pills to possess exceptional capabilities to correct any health problems.

Dependification occurs more readily when consumers believe that available rescue industry health care options can adequately recoup health and lifetime lost to unhealthy behaviors and lifestyles. Failure to understand and appreciate the extent to which behavioral choices and lifestyles impact personal health and refusal to accept that appropriate behavioral choices and lifestyles can lead to lasting health and longevity without requiring commercial rescue industry involvement are ingredients that help rescue industry dependification to become established. Ultimately, dependification plays health care consumers on the short end of a high-cost, low-health yield health care game.

The following two scenarios provide limited examples to illustrate circumstances predisposing health care consumers to rescue industry dependification.

1. An obese diabetic with high blood pressure and elevated cholesterol levels making a brief health care office visit is vaguely advised to lose weight and continue all prescribed medications, "beautifully" controlling blood pressure, sugar, and cholesterol levels, while his underlying sedentary lifestyle with excessive consumption of convenient, fast foods and other addictification food industry products is not explicitly addressed and continues unabated.

Real "health" caring would identify and address the individual shortcomings and predispositions directly interfering with achieving true health. Then, intensive health care education with counseling and support would guide the individual through the appropriate steps to modify adverse health behaviors and reduce the need for pharmaceutical treatments and dependence on the rescue industry.

2. A stressed-out individual living in an emotionally turbulent household filled with familial discord, who is overwhelmed by multiple unmet personal, social, and financial obligations and responsibilities, and experiences difficulties simplifying his own life complexities to feel anxious and depressed and have insomnia, is prescribed various pharmaceuticals to treat anxiety, depression, and insomnia, which are then continued indefinitely to artificially balance behavioral health dysfunctions and enable artificial coping with the numerous unaddressed personal challenges of daily living.

Optimal health care would direct efforts toward identifying factors contributing to behavioral health dysfunction and would provide the support to promote a positive mindset and the health care education with intensive counseling to teach the appropriate skills necessary for sorting out, prioritizing, and constructively dealing with encountered stresses of daily living.

Suffering individuals would be taught powerful cognitive behavioral health techniques that could beneficially modify personal predicaments and life circumstances to reduce behavioral stresses, suffering, and excessive dependency on the rescue industry.

Unfortunately, the stark reality is that addictification and rescue industries, instead, regularly join forces to exploit and capitalize on vulnerable consumers' dependence on industry, who become the feed sustaining profitable commercial industry systems.

Governmental initiatives have established **meaningful use** decrees for health care delivery, which mandate rescue industry entities to use EHR ostensibly to push for safer, more efficient, and higher-quality health care services and to better coordinate health care services, engage patients and family members with health care matters, collect health care delivery data, and ultimately improve societal health. EHR are instead becoming elaborate invoicing systems to bill health care delivery activities more precisely and allow detailed and comprehensive input of health care activities to justify requested reimbursements for documented services.

Use of EHR allows for more effective invoicing of health care activities to access the bureaucratic money envelope and warrant payments for delivered health care services but does not necessarily improve health care activities. For rescue industry system opportunists, EHR computer programs conveniently provide billable cut-and-paste health care documentation without requiring that any actual or additional health care services be delivered.

Health care delivery entities accept governmentally mandated meaningful use as a challenge to push more health care services through and deliver commercial health care more profitably, rather than as an opportunity to promote real preventative health care measures to eliminate health care redundancy and reduce consumer dependency on rescue industry products and services.

In the end, *meaningful health care use is still health care use,* and more suitable health-driven approaches would target improving societal choices and lifestyles to defend health and prevent health loss, leading to costly rescue health care and human suffering.

4.2 RESCUE INDUSTRY BAIL-OUT PLAN

Within the commercial scheme of preserving human life and function, health care is a euphemism for recovery of body vehicle health using commercially profitable repairs and interventions that attempt to correct body vehicle deterioration and damages at a monetary cost to individuals and society.

Healthy, optimally functioning body vehicles have no requirement for rescue industry repairs and interventions. Consequently, the rescue industry profits by selling body vehicle repair and damage control and not health, chiefly by merchandising options to fix and restore broken and malfunctioning body vehicles often in disrepair through personal neglect or abuse with toxic behaviors and lifestyles.

Commercial rescue industry health care options are **bail-out plans,** which conveniently serve as behavioral compromises that partly compensate for body vehicle abuse, neglect, and incorrect care occurring through injurious behaviors and maladaptive lifestyles. Rescue industry bail-out plans insufficiently restore or prevent progressive loss of body vehicle function and well-being when body vehicle abuse, neglect, and incorrect care continue. Individuals solely can proactively change toxic behaviors and lifestyles that lead to body vehicle injury, deterioration, and demise. Simple and free proactive behaviors can completely satisfy basic health maintenance needs of the body vehicle to protect against the premature shortening of body vehicle functioning and life-span better than any commercial rescue industry options can.

Rescue industry profitability depends on consumers to adopt convenient, commercially sponsored health care behaviors as substitutes for naturally healthy body vehicle routines. The rescue industry undermines natural consumer fulfillment of essential health maintenance obligations by supporting consumer beliefs that commercial options sufficiently fulfill personal health needs more quickly, simply, and conveniently and are preferable to not following any health routines at all.

The rescue industry promotes consumer reliance on commercial options that provide individuals an escape from the responsibility to fulfill personal health maintenance appropriately, by catering to consumer misperceptions that rescue industry options effectively cancel out the consequences of adverse health behaviors to produce beneficial health outcomes.

Rescue bail-out and cancellation of unhealthy behaviors *falsely* implies that

UNHEALTHY BEHAVIORS + RESCUE BAIL-OUT
= BENEFICIAL HEALTH OUTCOMES
and
UNHEALTHY BEHAVIORS + RESCUE BAIL-OUT
≠ *HARMFUL HEALTH OUTCOMES*

Commercial industry products and services poorly compensate for ongoing adverse health behaviors.

Any harmful stresses on the body vehicle system result in some injury and deterioration, which provoke body vehicle survival responses into action to recover body vehicle integrity and reestablish a healthy body vehicle balance. Body vehicle biological responses attempting to repair the body vehicle and restore lost health often independently produce adverse health effects, leading to short- and long-term health consequences. Additionally, rescue industry interventions can unintentionally cause detrimental side effects and even death.

The rescue industry profits by selling consumers the notion that well-being is achievable commercially without the investment of personal effort into health maintenance and the discontinuation of unhealthy behaviors and lifestyles. Addictification and rescue industries combine efforts to profit selectively at the expense of many and sacrifice societal health to create industry wealth as per the 1% benefit/99% pay principle.

Basically, unhealthy behaviors and lifestyles lead to undesirable health and survival outcomes as expressed by the adverse health behaviors outcome principle.

An adverse health behaviors outcome *correctly* asserts that

ADVERSE HEALTH BEHAVIORS + HEALTHY BEHAVIORS
= ADVERSE HEALTH OUTCOMES
and
ADVERSE HEALTH BEHAVIORS + HEALTHY BEHAVIORS
≠ *BENEFICIAL HEALTH OUTCOMES*

For example, no amount of exercise, relaxation, meditation, eating a pure diet with all-natural whole foods, drinking clean water, and living an otherwise pristine lifestyle would adequately offset the toxicity caused by regularly ingesting a small amount of arsenic or taking some other poison daily.

Various immediate and long-term adverse health effects similarly follow repeated behaviors detrimental to body vehicle well-being. Consequently, it is insufficient to do what is not good enough for the body vehicle system, and the body vehicle should not be expected to work optimally without working optimally for the body vehicle.

Therefore, foods need to be "healthy" rather than "healthier," "lean" not "leaner," et cetera.

Payments to the rescue industry for bail-outs that attempt to buy back lifetime lost to addictification and other unhealthy behaviors and lifestyles purchase commercial industry illusions selling inferior ways to live healthy and longer. "An ounce of prevention is worth a pound of cure," said Benjamin Franklin.

Thoughtfulness saves in many ways.

Thoughtfulness is free and unlimited. Health-minded thoughtfulness is an ally against unnecessary spending for costly commercial health care services and products and avoidable suffering. Rather than "trying" to get healthy, be healthy.

5 FUELING DISORDERS

Human illnesses are commonly the preventable outcomes and the expensive fallout from body vehicle deterioration and disrepair resulting from nutritional, physical, and social body vehicle neglect; inappropriate and inadequate body vehicle maintenance; and inadvertent, unrecognized, and intentional body vehicle abuse, toxicity, and poisoning.

Human fueling disorders particularly result from supplying body vehicle energy and nutritional needs improperly.

Concentrated, processed and refined nutrients laced with synthetic and artificially added substances are substantially responsible for causing much of the human illnesses, health-related suffering, and avoidable expenses in modern industrial societies. Industrially processed and refined food products having artificially added ingredients deliver concentrated nutrients in unnatural quantities, composition, and proportions beyond immediate body vehicle nutritional needs and biological handling capacities and introduce foreign, nonnutritive chemicals that require expeditious removal from the body vehicle system.

The functional existence and life-span of the body vehicle are negatively impacted when body vehicle physiologic capabilities to assimilate the delivery of excess biomolecules safely are repeatedly overwhelmed to challenge the limits of protective body vehicle detoxification processes. The sustained delivery of excessive, highly processed and refined body vehicle fuels and additive chemical food ingredients into the body vehicle induces dramatic structural and functional changes in the cellular microbiology of all exposed body vehicle cells.

Prolonged exposure to excessive levels of processed and refined fuels and nutrients and artificial chemicals deleteriously affects numerous body vehicle components.

Excessive fueling harms body vehicle cells composing the gut and digestive system, forming blood vessels and nerve circuits connecting the digestive system and brain, making up the immune system of defense, and constituting the brain and other body vehicle organs. Adverse physiologic effects induced by excessive nutrients and nonnutritive chemicals impair body vehicle function and promote the premature breakdown of body vehicle components under usually tolerable wear and tear daily life stresses, shortening cellular and overall body vehicle survival.

Fueling disorders include, but are not limited to,

1. obesity
2. hypertension
3. diabetes
4. high cholesterol
5. gout
6. gallstones
7. diverticulosis and hemorrhoids
8. GERD with acid reflux, and eosinophilic esophagitis
9. irritable bowel syndrome
10. chronic diarrhea and constipation
11. excessive gas and chronic bloating
12. celiac disease (gluten intolerance)
13. heart attack
14. stroke
15. cancer
16. degenerative arthritis
17. sleep apnea
18. fatty liver
19. aging and dementia
20. various rheumatic and autoimmune disorders, including systemic lupus, rheumatoid arthritis, psoriasis, multiple sclerosis, and autoimmune liver disease
21. inflammatory bowel conditions, such as Crohn's disease and ulcerative colitis
22. acne
23. depression, anxiety, hyperactivity, and various other behavioral health conditions

and so on, and so on.

The incidence and prevalence of many of the listed fueling disorders are skyrocketing in modern, Westernized societies that increasingly subsist on modern diets and progressively consume processed and refined food products.

5.1 ILLNESS IS EXPENSIVE SUFFERING

Human illness is an individual, family, community, and societal affair, exerting costs on afflicted individuals, loved ones, and society alike.

Illness costs are varied and broadly encompass numerous elements, including personal and family time commitments, health care expenses, lost individual and societal productivity, as well as raised taxes and insurance rates to cover the expenses of increasing societal health care needs and utilization. Growing demand for and overutilization of health care services additionally lead to health care rationing, which may deny dependent consumers access to needed health care services when availability is limited.

Therefore, learning to keep the body vehicle healthy through appropriate behaviors and lifestyle choices, and steering the body vehicle away from toxicities, reduces risks for developing illnesses that lead to expensive suffering for all.

5.2 HUMAN ILLNESS IS BIG BUSINESS

Food addictifications and resultant fueling disorders ultimately support and fuel rescue industry existence. Rescue industry systems ensure their own profitability by being silently complicit with addictification food industry efforts to control consumer nutritional behaviors and spending. Consequently, addictification food industries create unhealthy food products consumed by humanity, and the rescue industry profitably cleans up mass-scale health fallouts from human consumption of harmful food products.

Therefore, commercial industries cultivate and farm consumers to labor and spend earnings to support industry on various levels. Commercial market forces work on and not for consumers, continually squeezing consumers to generate business profits sustaining industry viability and growth. Consumer health is routinely trapped in a vicious tug-of-war between addictification and rescue industries, each aggressively vying for every shred of consumer spending. The volume of customers served, units of product sold, and the extent of services delivered express the work accomplishments of commercial industries to amass and relegate consumers to become industry feed.

Hospitals and health care clinics thrive being human body vehicle repair factories and shops that charge exorbitant premiums to provide health care services that attempt to reverse established illnesses and suffering and restore health frequently lost through addictification behaviors. Health care entities advertise to attract clients by boasting accomplishments such as the number of patients treated, the range of health care product lines offered, and track records for delivering health care services. Addictification and rescue industries commercially thrive symbiotically with rescue industry personnel, providing rescue bail-outs for addictification-induced illnesses. This symbiotic industry relationship ensures that both vested enterprises continue to partake in the spoils of their collective efforts, ultimately victimizing consumers, who are vulnerably trapped funding addictification and rescue industry profits.

It is no coincidence that escalating human illnesses and the rising costs of health care parallel the continual growth and soaring profitability of commercial food and rescue industries.

5.3 CANCER

Cancer, which develops as an unfortunate consequence involving a complex interplay between numerous health influences that include genetics, aging, environmental factors, nutritional choices, personal neglect of body vehicle maintenance, and intentional or inadvertent ingestion of toxic chemicals and other poisonous substances, is big business for rescue and addictification industries combined. Capitalizing on a tragic diagnosis of cancer makes dollars and sense for commercial industries. For the rescue industry and the scientific community, cancer cells are considered opponents in the cancer-fighting game, which understandably has toxic effects and is enormously expensive to humans.

Rogue cancer cells strive to gain unfair survival advantage over other body vehicle cells without playing cooperatively to benefit the entire body vehicle system. Attempts to target and kill primitively functioning cancer cells often fail because cancer cells are a part and carry the signature DNA of individuals in which the cancer develops. Consequently, cancer cells are programmed to exhibit those same basic survival tendencies inherent to all body vehicle cells and undergo mutational changes to escape the pressure of attempts at killing them.

With every diagnosis of cancer, industry strikes a mini mother lode of profitability at the expense of individuals with cancer and society. Fear, uncertainty, and hope drive people living with cancer to bargain desperately and accept almost anything to reverse the plight of their cancer diagnosis and obtain a reprieve from their dire predicament. Cancer creates numerous unwelcome expenditures requiring the sacrifice of personal and family time, money, and many other resources for diagnosed individuals and their associated families and opens up many vulnerabilities to commercial interests selling industry rescue bail-out options. Health care consultations, professional office visits, hospitalizations, laboratory testing, radiographic studies, surgeries, and treatments such as chemo and radiation therapy are all rescue industry services that individuals newly diagnosed with cancer and society will have to finance.

Companies that sell specialty health food products, miracle health cures, vitamins, health supplements, ancillary health care, and numerous other health-related services collectively join in to profit from diagnosed catastrophic health conditions such as cancer. Commercial industries even target patient advocacy websites for individuals suffering from cancer and other serious health disorders to advertise specialty wares, drug products, pertinent health care industry developments, and health care web links, which commercially influence consumer choices to increase industry profitability when consumer vulnerability for disease-specific industry products and services is highest.

Collectively, consumers and society spend enormously more revenue treating and living with cancer and other serious health conditions than would ever be spent on interventions to prevent debilitating health conditions such as cancer from developing in the first place.

Genuine societal prevention directed health efforts would translate into substantially reduced health care spending, undoubtedly to result in the not-so-unwelcome closure of many businesses and industries feeding and thriving off human illnesses and health predicaments.

Various charitable organizations established to solicit donations to fund human disease and cancer research often ironically exist through the creation, backing, guidance, and funding of commercial industries that directly profit from human diseases such as cancer. Charitable funding to finance expensive disease treatments and research work to discover disease cures pays for intercessions that happen after diseases develop when rescue industries financially benefit most from monies paid for services rendered.

Directing scientific efforts, societal attention, and charitable and governmental funding toward preventing cancer and other human diseases would likely greatly reduce health care expenditures and human suffering, especially since factors such as pollution, tobacco, alcohol, and processed and refined food and beverage products and their chemical additives are known to cause and contribute toward the development of cancer and numerous other human diseases and are amenable to targeting for alteration. Therefore, rather than allowing cancer to develop and then working to cure cancer and risk eliminating individuals with cancer, preventing cancer by eliminating the factors leading to cancer formation seems like a much more reasonable, practical, and less expensive health strategy for individuals and society to pursue.

5.4 TOBACCO AND ALCOHOL

The **World Health Organization (WHO) International Agency for Research on Cancer (IARC)** designates tobacco and alcohol products as **Class 1 carcinogens** that have been scientifically determined to cause and increase the risk for cancer in humans in many different body vehicle organ systems, and yet curiously both alcohol and tobacco are governmentally supported, controlled, and sanctioned for human use and regulated to generate tax revenues. Profit-driven industries selling tobacco duped the public and health professionals concerning tobacco product safety for many years before tobacco was finally deservedly proven to be and ultimately labeled the human poison that it indeed is.

More recently, tobacco industries have focused intently on disseminating the use of e-cigarettes to vulnerable tobacco users in an attempt to capture as much market share as possible, before time and independent non-industry-sponsored research studies can uncover all associated health hazards resulting from e-cigarette usage, which may persuade governmental bodies to clamp down and strongly regulate or even prohibit this new line of tobacco industry profitability.

Additionally, research studies have surfaced to support the regular intake of one or two mainly red wine alcohol beverages daily, suggesting that drinking alcohol may provide humans with some health benefits particularly involving the cardiovascular system. Consequently, "one drink a day is OK" has been eagerly adopted and recommended even by health care providers as an acceptable routine in the armamentarium of healthy daily living.

Common sense would declare that recommending any Class 1 carcinogen for regular human consumption to achieve health benefits is inconsistent and incompatible with correct and appropriate health advice. However, consider the alcohol industry profitability generated through the consumption of one glass of wine daily by a limited segment of the U.S. population.

Only one 6-ounce glass of wine consumed daily equals approximately one 750 ML or 26-ounce bottle of wine consumed every four days to total roughly 90 bottles of wine consumed per 365-day year. If the average cost for a bottle of wine is $10, then drinking 90 bottles of wine spends approximately $900 yearly. If 1 million individuals or approximately only 1 in 320 inhabitants living in a U.S. population of 320 million drank one glass of wine daily, then alcohol industry earnings would approximate $1 billion ($900 million) per year.

Consider the additional profits that the alcohol industry earns from a U.S. population estimated to be at least 10% alcoholic (32 million), who uncontrollably drink substantially more alcohol than one glass of wine daily throughout the entire year.

Therefore, alcohol industry financial incentives associated with convincing health care providers and the public that consuming the Class 1 carcinogen alcohol daily is beneficial to body vehicle health are easy to appreciate.

The total cancer-producing effects and overall health care expenses associated with regular daily consumption of various Class 1 carcinogens, such as alcohol, especially in combination taken throughout the lifetime of many individuals, generate massive costs to society. Alcohol in particular not only causes cancer but also when consumed excessively can directly injure many body vehicle tissues and organ systems, including the gut membranes, liver, pancreas, heart, muscles, bone marrow, blood cells, nerves, and brain, to cause permanent, irreversible physiologic impairments. Alcohol consumption additionally contributes to obesity and social problems. Furthermore, regular alcohol consumption over many years, even at moderate levels consisting of a couple of beverages daily, has been determined in clinical studies to shorten human lives, and the earlier that regular alcohol use initiates, the greater lifetimes shorten.

Societal alcohol consumption has been estimated to be responsible for hundreds of billions of dollars or more spent yearly for health care and other economic cost burdens imposed on individuals and society. *Back in 2006,* financial estimates for the economic burden to U.S. society from alcohol misuse–related problems alone exceeded $200 billion.

Societal, economic costs from alcohol use are analogous to stock market profitability, whereby financial losers far outnumber winners. In the case of societal alcohol use, a few predominant industries selectively siphon alcohol-related money flow to profit financially, while the bulk of society pays dearly to finance those industry profits. Consequently, creative "research statistics" from "experts" should help clarify the alcohol "health" quandary to guide future strategies that address regular alcohol consumption as related to societal health.

Although, since mass alcohol consumption predictably delivers a profit windfall for addictification and rescue industries, creates many societal job opportunities surrounding alcohol product use, and generates tax revenues, alcohol consumption is unlikely to be discouraged by industry, society, or the government anytime soon.

Similar potential mass-scale industry profitability applies to recommendations made by the rescue industry for the wholesale use of statin medications by society to combat elevated blood cholesterol levels artificially in individuals often caught within the clutches of the addictification food industry. Unsurprisingly, recommendations for widespread use of statin medications in society have financially benefited both the rescue and addictification industries combined. With statins, individuals ostensibly can pay less attention to eating healthy and eat what they like whenever, since statins can artificially improve blood cholesterol numbers despite unhealthy diets.

More recently, marijuana has slithered into the mainstream of societal acceptance. Previously, marijuana was illegal to use and considered dangerous to health and society but now is approved as a medicinal agent and has been decriminalized or legalized for recreational use in many states to generate tax revenues to fund social programs and state payrolls and decrease the cost burdens of enforcing laws prohibiting marijuana use. The marijuana industry is now maneuvering strategically to win over consumer approval and quickly introduce marijuana into the mainstream of commercial acceptance and use by riding the addictification food industry coattails of success.

The addictification food industry has gained such deep footholds within the minds and consciousness of consumers that the marijuana industry has packaged edible marijuana products in addictification food industry *look-alike wrappers*. Addictification food industry look-alike wrapper designs have been diabolically created by marijuana sellers to disarm wary consumers and rapidly create mass appeal for marijuana products to make quick inroads into profitable mainstream commercial industry markets.

Societies hooked on specific addictification food industry products and deeply connected to brand-name commercial foods having distinctive and easily identifiable food packaging designs are vulnerable to being tricked into trying out new commercial products delivered in look-alike wrapper designs. Consequently, marijuana Munchy Way product wrappings resemble those of Milky Way bars, marijuana Oeo covers copy Oreo cookie wrappers, and so on, to deliver edible marijuana products enticingly in packaging carrying strikingly similar cover designs found on mainstream mass consumed addictification food items.

Marijuana marketing strategies incorporate look-alike design packaging to mimic common commercially processed and refined food products with established household names not only to deliberately mislead consumers into buying the products but also to obfuscate the safety of marijuana products and lower barriers for consumer initiation and societal spread of marijuana product use.

The marijuana industry has also commercially exploited human survival breeding instincts to gain openings into commercial markets. Marijuana advertisements in magazines have sex appeal. Sexuality captivates attention and creates human vulnerability.

Marijuana advertisements also cleverly pitch human freedom of thought and expression and champion the decisiveness to be different, along with sexuality to lure potential "recreational" marijuana users into trying highly potent industrially created versions of psycho-active marijuana plants and concocted marijuana plant derivatives, ultimately to procure human addictification for marijuana use.

Given the profound and pervasive societal penetration of alcohol, tobacco, and addictification food industry products, and the mass dependency on the rescue industry to salvage society from addictification fallout, the actual societal, economic burden from addictification and rescue dependification can only be surmised.

The tragic reality surrounding arguments that advance revenue generation as being a societal benefit of selling commercial services and products that prey on human vulnerabilities is that governments can justify legalizing just about anything, which biologically enslaves human behaviors to generate public revenues.

Addictification industries propose that any negative fallout and societal costs associated with the mass consumption of toxic substances will be more than offset by tax revenues collected through legalization and regular use of harmful elements, and that generated monies will be available to subsidize many essential societal projects and services.

Unfortunately, many of the schemes implemented to increase tax revenues by enslaving vulnerable humans through addictification are **high-interest payday loans** made entirely at the expense of society, which initially derives tax revenues for societal services but later pays high-interest penalties to fund the societal costs of addictification and rescue bail-out dependification.

5.5 RISK AND PREVENTION

Disease prevention is about body vehicle *preservation* and *defense* against loss of intrinsic body vehicle health. Consequently, *prevention is proactive* and requires implementing behaviors and lifestyles that preserve and defend personal health. Appropriate body vehicle maintenance serves as the foundation to retain body vehicle health and prevent body vehicle illnesses, disease, and premature demise.

Health risk is the *potential for body vehicle compromise* through specific choices, actions, or genetic determinants. Risk factors for compromising body vehicle health and survival and for developing certain disease states may be overt, subtle, or only scientifically ascertained.

Scientific studies identify patterns of human behaviors and circumstances that increase the odds for specific body vehicle compromises and breakdowns to emerge. Therefore, *health risk factors are predispositions for body vehicle health disrepair or premature death to occur.*

When individual risk factors for developing a disease state combine, the overall risk or odds that the disease will occur are far higher than the total risk derived by just adding together the individual risks or odds for the illness to happen from each risk factor. For example, combining three separate risk factors for developing a health condition may not add up to merely increase the overall risk for an illness to develop times three $(1+1+1\neq3)$ but may instead multiply the odds for that disease process to present times nine $(1+1+1=9)$.

Consequently, consider the astronomically elevated risk or odds of developing cardiovascular disease or cancer in individuals possessing many risk factors, each of which individually increases the chances for these disorders to unfold. The cumulative odds and total risks for a heart attack, stroke, cancer, and death to occur in obese smokers with high blood pressure and diabetes, who drink alcohol excessively and consume too many calories from processed and refined food products, approach certainty in that health and survival will be undermined prematurely by a heart attack, stroke, cancer, or death.

By eliminating the main risk factors, such as smoking and excessive consumption of alcohol and processed and refined food calories that predispose to numerous disease states, the risks to develop secondary adverse health conditions, such as obesity, diabetes, high blood pressure, and cancer, dramatically decline or disappear entirely to significantly reduce the overall chances of succumbing prematurely to catastrophic illnesses. Behavioral and lifestyle modification of risks categorically work to achieve health and longevity better than using artificial interventions with expensive rescue industry antidotes and bail-out options that partly compensate for high-risk behaviors and lifestyles and that only forestall the inevitable consequences of high-risk routines and activities.

Individuals and society would benefit immensely by joining forces and working together to prevent disease development altogether with all the attendant costs and suffering. The rescue industry opportunely feeds and financially thrives on the fallout and plight of human self-neglect and self-abuse, which secondarily lead to dependency on rescue bail-out interventions to compensate for human illnesses as individuals and society desperately fight to salvage crumbling health.

Disease and illness interventions are damage control measures implemented to mitigate the fallout from behavioral, genetic, environmental, and social factors that cause physical and mental body vehicle compromise, deterioration, and suffering. *Health rescue is reactive,* demanding costly measures that attempt to recover and restore lost health. A preventative health strategy eliminates the opportunity and need for the rescue industry to intervene and mend compromised health or to slow health decline.

Illness interventions occur late during disease activation when diseases are already established and progressing. Secondary health interventions are analogous to attempts at restoring a broken heirloom vase to the original form, while primary prevention efforts focus on taking the appropriate precautionary measures to guard against vase breakage to preserve the vase in original form. Primary health prevention efforts require thoughtful and inexpensive behavioral and lifestyle modifications to optimize and preserve health before diseases activate.

Profiteering rescue industries have no motives to promote real primary health prevention and change consumer misperceptions that primary health prevention efforts are labor intensive, boring, unfashionable, and ineffective compared to more convenient, quicker, and generally applied commercial industry–backed preventative health options. The adage "an ounce of prevention is worth a pound of cure" unfortunately is uselessly unprofitable for commercial health care delivery systems, since that pound of cure is the bread and butter that profitably feeds and sustains health care industry system interests. Consequently, health care delivery systems have no real financial incentives to teach and promote real disease prevention to health care consumers and society.

> *Profit-driven health care systems seek to maximize the profitable delivery of health care.*

Commercial health care industry–sponsored prevention primarily directs efforts toward detecting established diseases earlier, restoring already lost health, and slowing deterioration of irreversibly failing health rather than toward intervening preemptively to eliminate unhealthy and detrimental elements from human lives that harm individuals and society and lead to illnesses and disease states with exorbitant attendant costs and suffering. Industry earns big money when societal disease prevention efforts involve expensive commercial testing to discover silent and dormant disease states and uncover illness predispositions on large segments of the population, which often result in more testing, interventions, and expensive monitoring following any adverse health discoveries made through "preventative" testing.

Disease prevention efforts that interpose expensive rescue industry interventions to reduce disease progression after health disorders and illnesses materialize greatly increase health care costs to society. Established disease states additionally risk compromising the health status of individuals further through unexpected procedural complications resulting from testing and treatments; through erroneous, false-positive test results leading to more rescue industry interventions; and through false-negative test results which provide a false sense of security to curtail necessary health evaluations prematurely. Societally adopted preventative health strategies using colonoscopy to prevent and find colon cancer, mammograms to detect silent breast cancer, and PSA blood testing to expose hidden prostate cancer are some examples of measures attempting to uncover underlying diseases earlier to increase the chances to cure or prevent progression of established disease processes. Therefore, commercial rescue industry preventative health strategies systematically search for active disease states as opposed to preventing diseases from developing in the first place.

Upon disease discovery, the health care delivery system switches on to intervene and work aggressively to implement all available health care product lines as expeditiously and as profitably as possible to concerned individuals afflicted with ominous health findings. Early detection "preventative" health care efforts are highly costly to society when applied carte blanche to entire populations and unfortunately not infrequently produce inconclusive or erroneous test results in substantial numbers of individuals, precipitating additional clinical evaluations that cost individuals and society even more on many separate accounts.

Unfortunately, health care consumers assume the risks and costs associated with any diagnostic and therapeutic interventions carried out to evaluate or restore health or to prevent disease progression.

False-positive and inconclusive test results resulting from preventative testing applied to human populations on larger scales lead to numerous subsequent evaluations and interventions that further increase societal health care expenditures and individual suffering, while false-negative test results may undermine the motivation for individuals to change behaviors and lifestyles affecting health adversely.

The scientific evaluation of health benefits provided through appropriate nutrition and the pursuit of healthy behaviors and lifestyles without reliance on commercial industry involvement is unlikely to gain widespread industry support, since industries fund research projects expecting to profit from research findings that support industry interests.

Additionally, studies comparing healthy eating and lifestyles with using commercial rescue industry interventions to achieve health would likely expose the enormous compromises, financial wastes, and squandering of valuable human resources costing society immensely, which result from depending on profit-driven commercial industries to help individuals and society attain any meaningful long-term health benefits. Whereas health care industries profit when consumers spend money to recover and restore lost health, consumer conservatism to defend and preserve health naturally reduces consumer health care spending to decrease commercial health care industry profits. Therefore, commercial health care industry profitability increases when health care consumers are commercially active spending more money for health-related matters, which further incentivizes industry to promote more of the same activities.

Consequently, commercial industries encourage **addition therapy,** which encourages consumers to layer and combine multiple commercial-grade health care maintenance options to compensate for behavioral and lifestyle indiscretions that compromise health and lead to detrimental health consequences. **Subtraction therapy,** which eliminates the adverse behaviors and lifestyles compromising and deteriorating health and discontinues commercial products that artificially compensate for correctable harmful health behaviors and lifestyles, counters the preferred standard of care for commercial health care industries, which profit by promoting the continuous consumption of industry wares.

For health care consumers, compensatory commercial products only increase the potential for developing costly adverse side effects from using these products. Complete disease prevention through appropriate behavioral, lifestyle, and nutritional choices is consistently the true, correct, and least expensive maneuver to perform with every opportunity that arises to preserve and defend health.

Unfortunately, real prevention efforts often encounter commercial industry resistance, since true prevention efforts are not lucrative for-profit industries that count on risk behaviors and lifestyles to produce costly attendant adverse health consequences requiring rescue industry bail-outs. The main costs to individuals for executing prevention efforts that preserve and defend health, and consequently lower lifetime health care expenses and suffering, are in committing time and energy to choose and behave appropriately to meet the basic body vehicle needs that essentially prevent diseases altogether.

An aggressive societal focus on changing mind-sets, behaviors, and lifestyles that predispose to cancer and other major diseases would markedly lower the risks for individuals to develop cancer and other preventable diseases. Preventing human illnesses from occurring altogether would seriously threaten the livelihood and existence of many addictification and rescue industry businesses, but would greatly reduce overall societal expenditures and lead to economic savings that can fund many other services benefiting societal health.

Consequently, since commercial addictification and rescue industries survive and thrive by profiting from every available opportunity at consumer expense, these industries, and their motivations should be approached with skepticism and wariness.

Individuals should experience more "wait a second" moments, pausing to question more and become better informed concerning any intended purchases of commercial food and health industry products and services before spending hard-earned money. The commercial rescue industry deftly minimizes the importance of consumer expenses to obtain health care, which are **economic side effects** that often become the final straw breaking the financial backs of individuals, families, and society, depending on industry rescue to address unfortunate and often preventable human health problems.

Therefore, addictification and rescue industries depend on repeat consumer business generated through addictification and rescue dependification and work to hook consumers on commercial products and services sold as serving the best interests of consumers and society.

Addictification and rescue industries could not survive without money continuously pouring in to pay for industry products and services. Commercial addictification and rescue dependification introduce more easily into consumer routines by insidiously piggybacking industry offerings onto basic body vehicle survival needs and drives.

Tobacco and other inhaled industry products hijack breathing; alcohol, sports, and rehydration beverages saddle onto water requirements; processed and refined foods ride the need to eat; pharmaceutical sedatives and energy boosters hook onto the demands for rest or to maintain wakefulness; pain medications fasten onto the drive to eliminate suffering; exercise facilities and analgesics accompany the necessity for movement; and pornography industries link into human drives for procreation and connection. Guilty feelings then often follow personal failures to satisfy basic body vehicle needs healthily, which creates additional opportunities for commercial industries to sell products and services to help individuals cope with guilt and remedy other health fallout from poor behavioral choices.

6 MONEY AND TIME

Most are likely to be familiar with the universal business concept that **time is money.**

The most formidable challenge humans face is to make the best use of individual lifetime, a non-renewable, finite, and continuously diminishing resource and commodity. The incessant competitive human drive to obtain, accomplish, and learn ahead of the pack illustrates an innate recognition for lifetime limitations and time-limited life opportunities.

Human weaknesses such as cheating and taking shortcuts to get something for nothing, for less effort, or in less time indirectly acknowledge lifetime limitations to secure time-limited opportunities. Commercial industries are forever competing to own and control consumer time and money. Commercial sales that offer more sooner, faster, and for less are typical time inducements to entice time-conscious consumers similarly to how carrots are dangled in front of donkeys to motivate their behavior. Individuals or entities seeking to cheat themselves and others to save time can easily find accommodating commercial enterprises willing to help with the cheating for the right price.

6.1 MONEY IS LIFETIME

Whereas money can accumulate, individual lifetime progressively dwindles to be lost permanently. Lifetime continuously burns away merely by existing and burns away faster through unhealthy living. Spent lifetime is irreplaceably gone forever.

Working to earn money expends lifetime, with the money earned economically capturing some of the lifetime sacrificed to make money. Working harder and longer to earn money transfers more valuable lifetime into money. The portion of lifetime expended working and partially stored in money is available to spend later elsewhere possibly to employ others to complete work tasks that might otherwise needlessly waste more personal lifetime, which makes money a desirable force to possess.

Spending money represents spending stored lifetime, with the value of money spent reflecting the lifetime value sacrificed earning that money. Therefore, **money is lifetime.**

Respect for the value of money respects the value of the lifetime that humans sacrifice to earn money. Human existence is also energy dependent and driven by energy transactions. Money value indirectly stores life energy since money can be transacted to buy food to energize the body vehicle and power physical existence to carry out life activities.

Money is also routinely used to purchase labor energy to accomplish work projects. Consequently, having money equates to possessing energy and lifetime reserves.

Lifetime value is regularly exchanged to pay for services and to obtain physical material goods. The lifetime value spent directly on physical material possessions or **durable goods** only partly reflects the actual lifetime expenditures paid to exist within human societies. The aggregate face value of material possessions excludes the lifetime value spent for **consumable goods,** such as food, medications, health supplements, and supplies for the home or office, and any monetary gifts or personal, professional, and societal services purchased, or taxes and fees paid for purchased goods and services.

Actual lifetime expenditures necessary to meet basic food, shelter, and clothing survival needs are relatively minimal compared to usual lifetime expenditures to purchase all other economic goods and services, which often levy additional lifetime expenditures to pay for any taxes, bank loan and credit card interest, and insurance coverages on made purchases. The value of each commercially obtained item and service also incidentally embodies some portion of lifetime value sacrificed by others to design, construct, and deliver or provide those items and services, which coincidentally may be devalued through depreciation and reduced consumer demand. Ideally, the value of any purchased items or services should be well worth the value of the lifetime sacrificed to make the purchases.

A telling question to ask oneself to better appreciate the value of monetary decisions is whether a *lifetime* expenditure adds real lifetime value to own existence. Spending lifetime judiciously to preserve and defend health, prevent disease, and increase time efficiency to ensure, enhance, and extend individual survival and slow lifetime losses reduces the frivolous expenditures of a precious, limited, and irreplaceable human commodity.

Humanity lifetimes are *currency* for industry profitability. Human lifetimes and life force energies are financially engineered to profit industry commercially, and become industry owned and controlled through human addictification and dependification. If any residual life force energy exists within a body vehicle, then there also exist opportunities and potential for industry to profit economically from that life force energy during any remaining body vehicle lifetime.

Industry captures body vehicle life force energies and lifetime through employment or by extracting money either directly from individuals or indirectly from third-party entities that make payments on behalf of individuals. Ultimately, human life force energies and lifetimes are vital ingredients necessary to create, run, and sustain commercial industry systems.

Industry also works on owning future lifetime. Credit industries sell and profit from consumer debt and run sophisticated marketing campaigns to encourage individuals to take on financial indebtedness to achieve high credit scores. Consequently, credit score advertising pitches glamorize and sell debt to humans.

Credit purchases leverage currently available and future consumer lifetime of enough value to allow consumers to possess commercial products and services immediately and defer repayment of creditors for goods purchased for later with interest. Therefore, credit purchases buy debt to be repaid later at higher rates with future lifetime.

Human oblivion to lifetime commitments made is a foe to humanity and friend to industry. Excessive consumption of health care services and products can drain current and future lifetimes rapidly, and mortgage lifetime commitments beyond the lifetime availability to repay accumulated health care debt obligations. A lifetime mortgaged to exceed any reasonable ability to repay debt obligations is a *leveraged human existence* that is gainfully owned, controlled, and traded by industries like a commodity, annuity, or stock investment.

Addictification and rescue industries can milk and possess all immediately available and future lifetime when poor nutritional, behavioral, and lifestyle choices lead to expensive illnesses and suffering to create massive debt obligations. Ultimately, addictification and dependification siphon off body vehicle life energies and permanently bleed away lifetime.

The actual economic costs to consumers for making poor nutritional, behavioral, and lifestyle choices are losses of lifetime that compound quickly, especially when present lifetime expenses add to future lifetime expenditures to pay for higher health care utilization and reduce the lifetime available to earn a living and accomplish other productive human endeavors.

Lifetime balance sheets that compare the lifetime benefits consumers derive with the costs of invested lifetime reflect the lifetime value consumers earn to interact commercially with industry. Most consumers are likely to accept paying industry a fair price for the actual value of benefits received. Consumers benefit most when the costs of lifetime invested are minimal while lifetime returns are maximal, whereas industry conversely benefits by extracting maximal consumer lifetime for the lowest industry costs. Unfortunately, balance sheets tallying the value to consumers of encounters with addictification and dependification industries show massive industry profits with limited and insufficient returns for consumer lifetime invested.

In comparison, lifetime expenditures for simple, naturally healthy behaviors and lifestyles that eliminate commercial industry involvement weigh balance sheets heavily in favor of consumers and return maximal consumer benefits at the lowest consumer lifetime investments.

An example that illustrates consumer spending of lifetime to heavily benefit industry at consumer expense considers consumer costs associated with a well-characterized addictification behavior such as smoking tobacco. When individuals suck on cigarettes, the cigarettes suck lifetime and money out of individuals and society to benefit industry exclusively. Use of tobacco products leads to many direct and indirect lifetime costs to users and society arising from tobacco addictification and rescue bail-out and dependification:

1. the costs to purchase toxic tobacco products
2. reduced physical capabilities and survival of tobacco users translating to lower lifetime productivity and earnings
3. monetary and time costs for health care, hospitalizations, and medications assessed to individuals, families, and society to evaluate, treat, and monitor tobacco-caused health impairments, including emphysema, bronchitis, cancer, stroke, and heart attack
4. increased taxes and other societal costs ironically levied on all to pay for the economic repercussions of health care burdens resulting from a toxic and self-destructive human activity that is governmentally approved and regulated to reap tax dollars to pay for various societal services
5. the cost of smoking cessation aids, medications, and counseling sessions
6. the costs of addressing health burdens that develop in individuals exposed to second- and third-hand tobacco smoke effects
7. many other unlisted costs that could fill volumes

Parallel cost burden analyses apply for other addictification activities that lead to mass societal health problems, including consumption of addictification food industry products which produce fueling disorders such as obesity and other health disorders requiring rescue industry intervention, as illustrated by the following:

1. the costs to purchase often expensive, unhealthy, and lower-quality food products that deliver excessive sugar, fat, salt, and chemical additives toxic to humans
2. reduced physical function and survival of individuals developing obesity and compromised health status from unhealthy diets to reduce lifetime productivity and earnings
3. monetary and time costs for health care, hospitalizations, and medications assessed to individuals, families, and society for evaluating, treating, and monitoring processed food–caused health disorders, including obesity, diabetes, hypertension, elevated blood cholesterol, gout, arthritis, cancer, stroke, heart attack, and autoimmune conditions
4. increased taxes and other societal costs ironically levied on all to pay for the economic repercussions of the health care burdens resulting from a governmentally approved, regulated, and often promoted self-destructive activity such as consumption of exces-

sive processed and refined food products that reap tax dollars to pay for various societal services

5. the costs of weight loss aids, medications, and counseling sessions

6. health burden costs to all having to navigate through food industry offerings limited to unhealthy food products that are artificially laced with various chemicals to promote addictification in susceptible individuals

7. innumerable other unlisted costs that could fill volumes

Spending any money or lifetime on addictification products and services that compromise health, cause illness, and mortgage future lifetime only profits the addictification and rescue industries combined, while costing individuals and society a great deal without providing consumers with any good lifetime returns.

Consequently, consumer costs profit industry as follows:

Consumer Costs = Industry Earnings
Whereby
Costs = Lifetime Expenses and Suffering
So that
Consumer Lifetime Expenses and Suffering = Industry Earnings

Reducing and eliminating unnecessary lifetime costs by refraining from engaging in unhealthy behaviors and lifestyles and commercial activities that expensively burn away valuable lifetime and lead to suffering are consistently the most desirable savings strategies to pursue to reduce consumer lifetime costs.

Lifetime investments in proper nutrition and healthy behaviors and lifestyles preventatively lower risks for developing illness and suffering to decrease immediate and future lifetime expenditures. Therefore, spend lifetime value thoughtfully and judiciously. Lifetime spent on healthy activities makes for healthier, longer, more satisfying, and less expensive life existences benefiting individuals and society alike.

Understandably, society punishes offenders committing crimes and offenses against humanity to pay society back financially and by doing time, since murder, kidnapping, robbery, theft, and extortion undeservedly and unjustifiably seize the life, possessions, money, or time of individuals directly or indirectly to rob humans of lifetime. Ironically, addictification and dependification industries surreptitiously capture and confine human lifetime to undermine productive human existences and profit at the expense of humanity without punishment and with the acceptance of society.

6.2 FEEDERS

Feeding and breeding humans create, staff, and run commercial industry systems. Industry forces and motivations are patterned according to human survival drives and instincts. Industries feed and breed economically to grow and thrive in commercialized societies. Addictification and dependification industry feeders consume human lifetime to survive.

Businesses likewise commercially feed and breed with greed, when run by individuals who preferentially feed their self-interests while compromising their responsibilities to provide professional services and products in the best interests of paying consumers. Therefore, the maxim "buyer beware" suitably applies to all commercial transactions, including those taking place with the rescue industry.

Money or lifetime exchanging hands demands wariness and vigilance for opportunists, deception, and greedy feeders. Professional degrees and organizational certifications and affiliations represent stamps of approval created by industry for industry system members to promote industry interests and industry-approved activities.

Commercial industry systems, including the rescue industry, create official certifying bodies that privilege system members to work under system backing and advertise certified achievements performing system supported activities. Official certifications, recognition, and endorsements can also conveniently obfuscate underhanded business motives steering trusting consumers for business industry gain.

Professional and governmental rules and regulations that direct industry activities often only serve to provide basic guidelines to ensure minimum negotiated standards of work quality and safety, offering a limited measure of consumer protection, while not significantly interfering with industry potential to profit financially.

All humans are feeders to various extents, but greedy and cheating feeders exploit human vulnerabilities and weaknesses to gain an unfair advantage and benefit at the expense of others.

Unfair advantage may be overt, such as by cutting the quality of work performed, or subtle, such as using specialized training to manipulate others for personal and financial gain.

Greedy and cheating feeders exist abundantly within all money-making industries and enterprises. Cheating feeders misleadingly substitute quantity for quality when selling more earns more revenues. Providing substandard products and services with a hoodwink and a smile to trusting consumers occurs too often in all aspects of the business world where money exchanges hands.

Generic techniques utilized by unsavory commercial entities and individuals to squeeze revenues out from work efforts and monetary investments include misrepresenting actual work performed for charges rendered; cutting expected quality of workmanship and craftwork for payments received; and reducing the intensity of work efforts and duration of interactions with clients to increase the number of contacts and interventions completed within available revenue-generating time slots.

Likewise, within the rescue industry, mounting economic and legal pressures and increasing societal health care demands drive deceptive rescue industry business practices to seek profitable opportunities despite unfavorable societal circumstances.

Declining governmental and third-party insurance reimbursements for rescue care, and rising practice costs to deliver health care push industry feeders to implement creative business survival strategies to secure higher earnings.

The condition that rescue industry reimbursements are based on documented and invoiced work activities can be abused to report more reimbursable activities to increase revenues. Third-party payers attempt to limit health care work invoicing and reimbursements by bundling together various health care work–related activities and paying less for the bundled work than would be paid for each service performed in combination.

Computerized documentation systems and invoicing can also be manipulated to skew the reporting of the actual quality, intensity, and duration of health care work provided to extract higher payments. Industry feeders misrepresenting professional work efforts play on system vulnerabilities and consumer trust, ignorance, and naïveté to direct an undeserved share of health care payments to themselves while providing consumers and taxpayers less than paid for and expected.

Rescue industry opportunists exploit human fear, uncertainties, weaknesses, and growing expectations for better health in modern societies to steer health care consumers readily into unnecessary dependification on commercial rescue industry products and services. Unwary consumers are trapped more easily into playing high-cost rescue industry dependification games that exact a high price for playing.

Health care consumer complacency; ignorance concerning personal health matters; denial or acceptance of own health plight; desensitization to individual and societal economic costs of health care delivery; and conformity with rescue industry rules and authority are some mechanisms that facilitate unnecessary consumer rescue industry dependification.

Unscrupulous rescue industry feeders resort to various tactics and strategies to raise declining revenues back up. Opportunists exploit health care delivery systems and trusting, dependent, and unwary health care consumers in numerous ways, including by

1. misapplying complicated health care guidelines to run tests and administer treatments that clinical circumstances do not clearly indicate
2. scheduling excessive professional health care visits and services unnecessarily

3. selling unproven, nonessential, and controversial health care goods and services, including high-priced vitamins, health supplements, and ineffective ancillary health treatments to increase practice revenues

4. gratuitously shortening and hurrying professional work efforts and then attributing insufficient health care delivery to declining reimbursements for professional services rendered

5. using automated EHR cut-and-paste health care encounter documentation programs to inflate the level, degree, and extent of health care services provided during visits, by combining documentation from numerous preceding health care encounters to generate the impression that complicated health matters are being addressed using complex health care measures[3]

6. performing suboptimal examinations, evaluations, and procedures beneath expected levels of professional workmanship necessary to address complex health matters correctly

7. reflexively prescribing medications, ordering expensive testing, and performing procedures to address consumer health concerns rather than providing attentive, professional health care that individualizes and directly addresses consumer health needs and concerns

8. providing suboptimal and inadequate health care leading to repeated office visits and hospitalizations for unresolved and poorly managed health conditions

9. failing to adequately and appropriately inform, teach, and reassure health care consumers concerning individual health issues and health care options at professional visits

10. collaborating with hospital administrators, commercial health care facilities, medical suppliers, and insurance providers in elaborate schemes that impact health care utilization and professional reimbursements at consumer and taxpayer expense

Consequently, greedy and cheating industry feeders take advantage of the vulnerably unsuspecting, unaware, and uninformed to steal away and feast on any of their available lifetime.

Slick industry operators then employ ambitious clerical staff as unwitting accessories to scour records and meticulously document support for submitted invoices billing payers for any reimbursable services.

---

3. Cut-and-paste documentation not only predisposes to misrepresentation of work efforts but may also compromise the exercise of thoughtful consideration to deliver more appropriate health care. In the modern era of electronic documentation and invoicing of health care delivery, professional activities using an EHR, virtual cut-and-paste health care delivery that never actually took place is fast becoming a modality for opportunists to squeeze out additional revenues at consumer and societal expense.

If paperwork and formal documentation genuinely reflected benchmark achievements indicating a job well done, then parents would be inclined to routinely itemize and document all parental work efforts undertaken at every aspect of their children's development, care, and upbringing.

Instead, increasing and onerous health care provider documentation requirements reflect growing distrust of unrestrained and questionable rescue industry health care spending of dwindling consumer dollars at economically unsustainable levels.

Societies running out of money for health care are battling to reduce exorbitant health care costs and prevent unnecessary health care delivery by demanding extensive provider documentation to justify advised and performed health care work. Meanwhile, health insurance industry payers perch on the alert to swoop down and scoop up any health care delivery savings as payments for administrative efforts to shuttle around consumer health care dollars.

Health care industry payers routinely proclaim that reduced health care payouts equal consumer savings, even though payers channel health care savings to fund insurance industry profits and not to increase provider reimbursements or reduce insurance premiums, copays, and deductibles or medication expenses.

Ironically, health care savings regularly translate into rising consumer costs and decreasing provider reimbursements, with payers asserting that consumers are receiving better health care spending more money.

Continually rising health care costs create a vicious cycle of consumer and rescue industry economic pressures demanding additional compensatory cost containment measures to accommodate growing rescue industry financial shortfalls. Ultimately, health care consumers end up paying progressively more for health care services while being ever more short-changed receiving "health care."

The stark reality is that in the commercial world industry systems feed competitively on customers to thrive and remain viable financially. Consequently, any available life force and lifetime are fair game for commercial snaring to profit industry. Hungry industries ultimately consume customers sacrificing one lifetime moment or dollar at a time to sustain bottom-line industry profits. Unfortunately, industry feeders that game health care systems to profit unfairly at the expense of humanity detrimentally spiral human existence downward to poison life quality for all.

6.3 ECONOMIC NUTS & BOLTS OF THE HEALTH CARE RESCUE INDUSTRY SYSTEM

Rescue industry systems exist to deliver health care and must deliver health care to exist.

The rescue industry occupies the commercially enviable position of having a ready supply of dependent consumers hoping to achieve and sustain health scurry frantically into the rescue industry clutches. Addictification industry efforts, governmental mandates, and health care insurance industry decrees and restrictions also conveniently sweep health care consumers into the rescue industry fold.

Rescue industry systems are commercial entities devised, built, organized, and maintained to economically survive and thrive by supplying and maximizing the sale and delivery of health care products and services to individuals and society. In many states, health care institutions are legislatively endorsed to set up monopolizing local or regional health care systems through governmentally mandated **Certificates of Need (CON).** A CON grants selective health care facilities and institutions exclusive rights to deliver specific health care services within geographically designated localities, giving CON-holding entities special economic privileges that provide market advantages over competitors.

In the 1970s, the U.S. federal government tied health care funding and payments to a mandate requiring health care delivery enterprises to obtain a CON before building or establishing health care facilities to deliver health care services to consumers. The mandate intended to even out health care delivery across geographic areas to prevent health care services from concentrating exclusively within more profitable health care delivery zones.

In 1987, the U.S. federal mandate for obtaining a CON was repealed, although many states have been slow to reverse their individual mandates so that most states continue to require that health care institutions obtain a CON before building health care facilities or expanding health care delivery services.

CONs stymie health care competition within demarcated geographic zones and can disincentivize CON-holding institutions to deliver innovative and inexpensive health care delivery to consumers. Having a CON equates to possessing a politically legislated golden ticket that essentially permits a health care business entity exclusive access to health care consumers living within a geographic area without contention from similar market competitors.

Given the high desirability to own a CON-approved facility, securing legislative approval for a CON from governmental agencies may involve using aggressive, high-pressure lobbying efforts, underhanded influences, and sophisticated pay-to-play schemes, tactics not uncommonly employed in political maneuvering as exposed during the bitter political fighting in the 2016 U.S. presidential campaign.

Since a CON essentially knocks out the free-market competition in CON-bounded health care delivery zones, CON-possessing facilities can considerably ratchet up charges for health care services provided through CON-approved facilities to greatly increase health care delivery costs to individuals, society, and third-party payers.

Additionally, with absent market competition, there is minimal incentive for CON-holding entities to negotiate and accept lower service rates and facility fees for services provided.

For example, whereas the professional fee charged by providers to perform a simple medical procedure, such as a colonoscopy, may be several hundred dollars with the actual reimbursement significantly reduced by third-party payers, a CON-holding medical facility separately charges thousands of dollars strictly for the use of procedural equipment and a procedure room staffed with a couple of supporting health care workers for the provider to accomplish the procedure.

Additionally, patient monitoring at the CON-holding facility during recovery following the procedure may incur another few thousand dollars or more in fees, which is billed separately from any additional charges imposed for extra equipment and supplies used to perform the procedure or during the postprocedural recovery period, for laboratory processing and examination of specimens, and for medications given before, during, or after completion of the procedure, which in all may total many thousands of dollars.

A non-CON facility would not be entitled to receive the same reimbursements despite incurring comparable bottom-line costs to carry out the same procedures by the same providers using essentially the same equipment, level of skilled workers and nursing staff, anesthesia recovery services, and supplies. At non-CON facilities, the entire procedural experience might be paid through third-party payers at a flat rate often amounting to a small fraction of the total reimbursements otherwise paid to CON facilities for carrying out the procedure.

Similar elements apply when comparing charges and reimbursements at CON and non-CON facilities for the performance of various other clinical services, such as laboratory tests or X-rays. CON facilities may charge consumers and third-party payers several hundred dollars for blood tests or X-rays costing pennies to several dollars to process, while similar testing offered through independent non-CON laboratory and X-ray facilities may be priced at a fraction of the cost charged by CON facilities.

CON-holding health care institutions can also coercively pressure health care practitioners geographically dependent on using the CON-holding facilities to administer professional health care services to their patients. Independent health care practitioners are limited in challenging CON institutions owning local or regional health care monopolies on any matters of disagreement since CON institutions exclusively control the availability of health care resources, such as facilities, equipment, and staff, necessary for practitioners to deliver professional services to their geographically bounded consumers. Consequently, practitioners dependent on CON facilities must abide by CON institutional edicts or lose the option of using the CON facilities to provide their professional services to patients.

However, within unrestricted free markets offering various alternative health care resources, practitioners have greater options for delivering health care to their patients, and third-party payers and practitioners can negotiate more equitable rates to provide health care services to consumers, who then also have numerous health care alternatives.

A more significant problem develops when CON-holding facilities string together to form large conglomerates that sew up economic control of broad geographic zones. Competitive free-market enterprises that increase health care options and lower health care costs to consumers often conspicuously vanish when commercial health care delivery systems unite to deliver health care on larger scales. Larger-scale CON-holding conglomerates economically limit health care delivery options more extensively on greater levels to forcibly dictate health care delivery costs without contention to dependent consumers and third-party payers locked into health care delivery service zones without reasonable alternatives. CON conglomerates that charge exorbitant rates for health care delivery hamper access to affordable health care and corner consumers into having to purchase high-cost insurance coverages allowing access to available health care, which otherwise costs uninsured or out-of-network individuals prohibitively expensive full list prices.

A substantial portion of health care costs to individuals and society can be attributed to pharmaceutical expenses and to less-negotiable institutional charges for the use of health care facilities, equipment, staff, and the performance of technical services, while any medications administered within health care institutions are further marked up above the already exorbitant rates charged by drug companies and pharmacies. Periodic health care visits are individually costly, while monthly medication expenses and regular blood and other technological testing amount to an annuity paid to the rescue industry.

In short, health care "delivery" systems function like well-oiled machines that are strategically geared to *maximally extract lifetime* by collecting monetary payments for attempting to restore lost health and slow the premature shortening of human lives. Sources that financially reimburse health care delivery systems for provided services include contracted commercial businesses, governmental social health care agencies, and consumers who pay directly out-of-pocket or through insurance intermediaries.

Financial rewards then become distributed among all vested entities sharing in health care delivery responsibilities.

Intermediaries such as health care insurance companies, which manage the consumer money flow that ultimately pays for health care delivery, expect to profit handsomely for their administrative efforts. Health care insurance intermediaries collect and distribute health care funds to spread the individual risks for incurring health care expenses among many health care consumers, and in return help themselves to a hefty slice of the health care monetary pie to manage the costs of assuming the financial risks to cover health care delivery expenses.

Insurance industries angle at every opportunity to profit plying their trade and routinely sell fear and uncertainty to ratchet up health care insurance demand in consumers, who hope to avoid financial ruin paying exorbitant list prices to repair lost health. Profiteering health care delivery financiers, such as insurance intermediaries, orchestrate elaborate *keep-the-money schemes* to profit at health care consumer and provider expense.

Examples of tactics that health care insurance intermediaries creatively use to secure their own profitability include

1. progressively increasing insurance premiums charged to consumers and other payers to manage and assume the financial risks of disbursing health care payments to health care providing entities

2. raising insurance deductibles and copays to shift payment responsibilities for health care services progressively onto premium paying health care consumers

3. reducing health care delivery payments to contracted health care providers and institutions to ensure that insurance intermediaries retain greater percentages of consumer paid premiums

4. bundling together multiple individual health care services that providers deliver and then reimbursing bundled services with single reduced payments that substantially undercut the combined costs of individually provided services (the two or more for the price of one game plan)

5. creating *red tape impediments* and *delay-of-game strategies* that employ encumbering requests for insurance authorization, precertification, and approval for prescribed medications, testing, treatments, and other services that insurance intermediaries reimburse, and which threaten insurance profitability

6. creating out-of-network, uncovered, lower-tier, and preferred lists for health care services, products, and providers to limit insurance intermediary profit losses

7. routinely denying approvals and payments to delay permission and reimbursements for health care services, and then requiring that consumers appeal denials expeditiously within limited time frames to secure health care benefits, while the insuring intermediaries continue to collect premiums without suffering any economic costs or reprisal to themselves

For consumers, health care insurance companies function as societally sanctioned gambling institutions siphoning off health care delivery funds paid with consumer *lifetime.*

Insurance systems essentially manage health care delivery slot machines that are endlessly played by many insured lives repetitively feeding insurance company "slots" with relatively smaller insurance premiums, while expecting to "cash out" and leverage much larger health care expense payouts in the event of suffering catastrophic illnesses.

Prohibitively costly health care services and exorbitant medication prices force individuals without recourse to purchase expensive health care insurance coverages to access necessary but otherwise unaffordable health care, which, despite being partly covered financially by insurance policies, remains unaffordable to most health care recipients.

As health care delivery costs escalate while societal financial resources plummet, health care, rescue industry systems devise enterprising strategies to maintain commercial profitability. Health care payers contract providers through various payer product lines that reimburse providers for delivered health care services under an assortment of financial schemes. Contracted providers commonly agree to accept reduced payments for rendered services in return for receiving in-network or preferred status designations, which result in bonus payments and preferential steering of insured lives to the providers that can save money for the industry by delivering health care services more cheaply.

The usual objectives of rescue industry system payer and provider collaborations under various health care delivery schemes are to *beat the system* and *get the money* from any available sources disbursing health care funds and maximally profit operating health care delivery enterprises. The core principle guiding commercial rescue industry strategies and health care activities is to gain a financial advantage in the marketplace. Ironically, health care providers agreeing to lose practice revenues by delivering cheaper health care to individual insured members expect to make up revenue losses by providing higher volumes of discounted health care to greater numbers of consumers. Health care delivery systems also trim redundant and non-revenue-generating health care services to the bone to retrieve any vestiges of potential financial profitability for rendering health care services. Thus, receiving true "health" care within sharply streamlined and financially driven health care delivery systems that routinely drive up profits at consumer expense becomes purely coincidental.

Health care industry product lines partnering health care providers and payers that are available to consumers exist under various names with acronyms such as IPA (Independent Physicians Association), HMO (Health Maintenance Organization), ACO (Accountable Care Organization), PPO (Preferred Provider Organization), MIPS (Merit-Based Incentive Payment System), or are simple economic marriages between hospital or health care network entities and health care providers, which sometimes expand into regional or national health care delivery system corporations.

The simplest payer and contracted provider health care delivery enterprise is a PPO (Preferred Provider Organization), whereby participating providers deliver health care services to PPO insured members at a discount, expecting that revenue losses for delivering health care services cheaper to individual members can be reconciled by delivering higher volumes of health care to PPO members steered through insurance carriers to the "preferred" providers.

A payer and contracted provider collaboration assessing greater financial accountability on providers is an HMO (Health Maintenance Organization).

Within an HMO, providers receive fixed monthly stipends from payers per assigned insured member, regardless of the number of HMO member office visits or the intensity of administered health care, with the aim of lowering average health care delivery expenses per assigned HMO group member, when compared to industry benchmarks or health care delivery costs accrued by similarly contracted providers caring for other groups of insured HMO lives.

HMO providers responsible to care for assigned groups of HMO members are typically generalist physicians, who are strategically positioned as **gatekeepers** expected to prevent HMO revenue losses by restricting HMO members access to health care services that are HMO unapproved, identified as "experimental," out of the HMO network, or deemed medically unnecessary by the gatekeeper.

HMO payers penalize provider gatekeepers failing to lower health care delivery costs by reducing provider stipends for assigned HMO members. Contracted HMO providers become the gatekeepers of insurance industry cash flow and profitability.

ACOs (Accountable Care Organizations) are health care delivery networks that partner groups of health care providers with or without hospital systems, which then contract with governmental and other third-party payers to deliver more "economical" health care to a large group of insured members, and results in the payment of financial bonuses or higher reimbursements from payers to the ACO for delivering less costly health care to the designated group of insured members.

An ACO typically provides health care for a large block of Medicare beneficiaries often numbering in the thousands in return for splitting with governmental payers any monetary savings achieved reducing health care expenses to the selected group of insured individuals, as determined by comparing the costs to care for the designated groups during current and previous fiscal years. The ACO can earn even higher financial rewards by entering into **at-risk contracts** with payers, which financially penalize the ACO with revenue loses when the ACO fails to meet negotiated savings goals for their designated groups of insured lives. Unfortunately, ACO health care delivery cost savings are typically eaten up by the ACO as revenue bonuses and not transferred back to cover or reduce the health care expenses of the insured beneficiaries.

Therefore, the ACO is essentially a population scale HMO that financially rewards health care delivery networks for lowering health care costs to payers and economically penalizes health care networks failing to meet contracted cost reductions. The **diagnostic intensity** or number of health care diagnoses attributed to the insured members assigned under an ACO network impact payer reimbursements, with higher reimbursements provided by payers for sicker patient groups having more complex health conditions, which may incentivize ACO reporting of diagnoses to maximize payments for assigned patient groups while reducing ACO incentives to correct health conditions associated with higher payer reimbursements.

Additionally, unlike for an HMO, Medicare beneficiaries assigned under the care of an ACO may not always be informed of, entirely aware of, or appreciate the implications of their ACO participation.

Medicare beneficiaries may be induced to participate as members of an ACO network by being advised that the ACO health care team will deliver higher-quality and more coordinated health care at the right time when needed, without being informed that the ACO provider team is financially incentivized to profit by rationing, limiting, or withholding care to participants or that the team may incur financial penalties and lose significant revenues if health care costs caring for designated member groups fail to meet prenegotiated benchmarks.

An IPA (Independent Physicians Association) contracts with payers to receive large lump sum payments to administer health care services comprehensively to insured member groups; then subcontracts with various specialty health care providers, who agree to accept reduced rates to provide health care services in exchange for receiving exclusive access to insured members and possibly a share of any residual IPA profits, generated by lowering the costs to deliver health care to insured members.

MIPS (Merit-Based Incentive Payment System) is a proposed Medicare health care delivery product slated to roll out to society some time in 2019 that incorporates health condition–specific bundled payments. Under MIPS, individual health care providers can earn more revenue by meeting specific cost containment targets for groups of Medicare patients lumped under their health care delivery umbrella. If providers working under MIPS fail to reach their financial cost-savings target goals, they would have to repay Medicare with monetary penalties. Thus, MIPS is another health care delivery scheme that fits into a long list of health care delivery products, whereby health care providers gamble to earn more health care revenues by reducing health care delivery costs usually at health care consumer expense.

Large groups of insured members covered under various health care payer plans are fast becoming commodities traded like pork bellies and bushels of corn that provide health care industry systems with profit opportunities, which emerge by gambling that health care services can be delivered cheaper to the insured member groups. Rescue industry system operators paid to increase health care delivery profit margins regularly devise strategies that measure the "quality" of health care delivery based on generating revenues and not necessarily on improving the health of insured members. Revenue-driven health care delivery schemes incentivize and reward health care networks and providers to restrict and reduce the delivery of health care services rather than to increase human health.

Health care providers practice continuously under pressure to reduce risks and vulnerabilities delivering health care, which arise through practice omissions or the commission of medical and surgical complications that produce professional liabilities or through revenue losses that jeopardize the financial viability of professional practices.

Increasingly, industry benchmarks judging the quality of health care work assess whether providers are successfully meeting their contractual obligations to reduce health care delivery costs.

Economically driven health care reimbursement strategies place health care providers *at-risk* not only for professional liabilities but also for revenue losses and insolvency when providers fail to reduce health care costs to meet profit-driven industry established financial objectives. Commercial health care payers increasingly expect that health care delivery to large pools of consumers strictly abide by commercial rescue industry system rules and guidelines. Consumers and providers who fail to address health care matters conforming to industry directives risk penalization through raised premiums, denied care, and reduced reimbursements.

The ultimate goals of health care payer and provider collaborations are to increase industry profitability through stringent, across-the-board cost-cutting measures that deliver cheaper and less health care to consumers. Under strategies that financially incentivize provider groups to reduce health care delivery expenses, incurring excessive costs to provide specialized health care services to one or a few health care recipients can serve as the death knell squashing provider group expectations for profitability, which consequently serves to deter provision of specialized health care services to insured members.

When financial objectives are the priority in delivering health care on mass scales health care is provided using a blunt instrument, since personalized health care interventions incorporating specialized and expensive cutting-edge maneuvers benefiting only a few are routinely denied due to cost.

Therefore, emerging health care delivery concepts such as **precision medicine,** which *individualize, customize, and personalize* health care, are *contradictory* to health care delivery strategies that economically lump together large groups of health care consumers, and then financially reward or penalize providers based on successes and failures in achieving economic cost containment goals in delivering health care to the group of insured members as a whole. Contracted health care providers must essentially short-change health care delivery in some way, at the consumer's expense, to profit industry.

Despite numerous opportunities for health care delivery systems to adopt strategies that promote genuinely healthy behaviors and lifestyles benefiting all in many ways, efforts substantially focus on optimizing profitable opportunities to pitch and sell more health care products and services to consumers already victimized by addictification and rescue dependification. Rarely do cost-savings measures direct efforts primarily toward providing consumers with the health education and services that preserve health and altogether prevent the development of illnesses and diseases to stem the rising tide of societal health care needs.

Health care delivery strategies, instead, attempt to boost the efficiency, lower the costs, and raise the profitability of pushing health care onto consumers. Governmental efforts to resolve societal health care delivery predicaments and shortcomings focus predominantly on increasing access to and expanding financial coverage for pared-down health care services lacking cutting-edge interventions and on improving health care delivery outcomes, meaning that individuals must first become patients to then qualify for available "health" care.

Corporate invasion into human health needs has created business-minded health care delivery entities principally concerned with doing what profitably benefits the entities themselves and not necessarily what preserves human health and benefits humankind. Revenue-hungry health care delivery entities swallow up independent medical practitioners and physician groups to territorially expand financial control of health care delivery to consumers. Then corporate interests work to raise consumer demand for and increase the supply and delivery of commercial health care to maximize health care profitability.

As health care delivery systems progressively corporatize, consumer health is no longer the main focus of health care delivery strategies. **Corporatization** redirects health care from preserving human health and using highly skilled health experts to individualize professional attention to consumers, to the delivery of health care services and products on larger scales, applying business productivity principles, models, and quotas to increase business efficiency and reduce expenses to make health care delivery activities more profitable.

Corporatization makes economic productivity, and the profitability of health care delivery entities the primary goals of health care delivery and abandons unprofitable efforts that focus on meeting the societal needs and challenges enabling individuals to remain healthy and achieve true health. Corporatized health care delivery forces providers and consumers to conform to economic standards and pressures imposed by business-minded entities.

Financially engineered health care delivery that is driven by monetary objectives, which obey sophisticated mathematical computations to reduce the costs and raise the productivity of delivering health care to satisfy financial goals, forfeits individualized health care.

Additionally, corporatized health care delivery entities more easily succumb to financial pressures to become more competitive, territorial, and adversarial to gain economic advantages and protect corporate interests, viability, and profitability, leading to deterioration of health care provider camaraderie, collegiality, and collaborations necessary for maximizing health and well-being for all humanity.

Health care recipients require sufficient time with health care professionals to understand pertinent health information and advice correctly to carry out tasks relevant for achieving true personal health. Commercial maneuvers that financially discount health care services pressure providers to shorten interactive times with patients and increase the number of health care visits to compensate for discount losses, which invariably leads to the herding of consumers through rescue industry pipelines like heads of cattle are herded through stockyards for consumption.

All fixed health care practice expenses for insurance, office labor, rent, equipment purchases and maintenance, supplies, administrative record management, and professional accounting and legal services continue to rise even in difficult economic times and ultimately become passed on to health care consumers in one way or another. As third-party reimbursements for health care services decline or fail to keep up with rising costs, and payers restrict providers from raising professional fees to compensate for revenue losses, health care practices implement typical business survival strategies to raise falling revenues.

Since most health care practice revenues are generated from payments for provided health care services, business survival strategies predominantly involve increasing billable services and billings per available health care delivery service times. Conventional methods employed to offset falling health care practice revenues are to shorten professional health care visits to schedule more patients, deliver higher reimbursed procedures, perform more ancillary services, and use lower-paid auxiliary providers to deliver health care services.

Time and economic constraints in technologically driven and pharmaceutically oriented health care systems sacrifice opportunities for consumers to interact with experienced physician health care providers to discuss relevant health matters and factors impacting personal health. Economically pressured health care delivery reduces time, intensity, and quality of interactive face-to-face health care encounters, limiting chances for consumers to address complex sources of health disrepair directly with higher-level trained health care professionals and promoting quicker dispatch of consumers from professional appointments with medication prescriptions and orders for testing, specialty consultations, and other costly interventions.

In rushed health care delivery settings, physician health care providers spend progressively less time with health care recipients; nurse practitioners and physician assistants increasingly administer primary health care services; medication prescriptions conveniently serve to address individual health problems and complaints, and expensive testing and procedures readily substitute for thoughtful human interactions to diagnose and treat human ailments.

Stressing safety and quality while the volume and speed of pared-down health care delivery escalate are analogous to equipping a stripped-down nitro fuel powered race car driving recklessly fast with a seat belt to protect occupants against accidents and injury.

Economically time-compressed health care encounters risk lowering the quality and safety of health care delivery when hurried health care addressing complex health matters omits critical health information and increases the chances for making crucial mistakes to compromise health care. Therefore, business-focused benchmarks for health care delivery predispose to hurried professional interactions that risk compromising the quality and safety of health care delivery encounters.

Recommending that health care recipients make appropriate behavioral and lifestyle changes that can inexpensively correct health problems at lower levels of personal risk, unfortunately, fails to generate the high-volume revenue streams necessary to fund bloated rescue industry system financial needs. Human greed leveraging the business decisions of profiteering health care delivery entities can further compromise the quality of delivered health care.

Rationing health care delivery to conserve and redistribute limited health care services and resources to more recipients is another mechanism to ensure higher rescue industry profitability. The health care consumers most affected by rationing are incidentally those dependently utilizing rationed health care services, who coincidentally are individuals with health care needs that most reduce health care industry profitability.

The health care industry is progressively disengaging from health care consumers by restricting and rationing health care resources, increasing health care delivery costs, and decreasing provider time commitments to interact with and educate health care recipients directly and, unsurprisingly, is losing public credibility and trust as societal health deteriorates while consumers pay rising and unaffordable costs to receive ineffectual health care.

The loss of health care industry credibility has increasingly predisposed health care providers to be pushed around, dictated to, and controlled by various commercial entities managing health care money flow and profiting at the ultimate expense of health care recipients, whom health care providers supposedly are entrusted to protect.

6.4 ONE HAND WASHES THE OTHER

6.4.1 Profitable Marriages of Convenience

Hospitals that hold a certificate of need and professionally licensed health care providers frequently join forces to enter economic marriages of convenience and enjoy geographic exclusivity in delivering health care services and product lines to geographically corralled health care consumers. Health care delivery entities align expecting to support and promote each other's economic interests within restricted geographic domains so that all parties signing on to work together mutually profit.

Licensed health care providers apply for "medical staff privileges" at specific hospitals or health care facilities to practice their medical specialties and provide professional health care services to patient populations dependent on using the health care institutions within their health care delivery zones. Once part of the medical staff, the most active and vested practitioners at the institutions may be selected or offered the opportunity to represent the special interests of other institutional staff members and, additionally, may be appointed by hospital administrators to serve on special committees or to act as department administrative heads to oversee institutional activities surrounding their areas of medical specialization.

Medical staff selected to represent the interests of their medical specialties monitor the professional activities of similar specialty staff members within the institution. Heads of medical specialty departments commonly are also charged to serve on hospital executive committees comprising the hospital CEO and other hospital corporate members to ensure successful hospital operations and profitability. Executive committees then ensure the smooth delivery of institutional, health care services and product lines, enforce staff and institutional compliance and conformity with professional and governmental health care delivery standards and regulations, and assure fulfillment of any institutional certifying and inspection agency requirements.

Medical staff members who head committees receive compensation for time served to provide professional expertise to optimize the delivery of health care services, keep medical specialty provider troops in line, and safeguard the profitability of the hospital and other providers utilizing health care facility services. Hospital executive committees leverage conformity of hospital staff members using legally orchestrated rules titled **medical staff bylaws,** which must be agreed to and abided by staff members granted permission to use hospital facilities to practice professionally.

Executive committees punish staff members who do not comply with institutional rules by imposing economic fines, restricting staff member privileges to practice within facilities, or enacting sanctions that may threaten staff member professional ability to practice their medical trade. Medical staff executive committees also sanction and approve institutional health care delivery protocols and guidelines that streamline institutional health care delivery by automatically imposing health care delivery regimens on consumers presenting to the institution with specific health care needs.

Noteworthy is that the principal activities of hospital staff members responsible for institutional health care operations are not concerned with reducing consumer dependence on health care delivery or on finding natural, inexpensive, and noncommercial ways for individuals to improve and optimize personal health without having to rely on health care delivery systems and institutions for assistance.

Health care institution executive committees inhabit the apex of rescue industry system supply and demand economics and, therefore, attend to developing strategies to increase the supply and delivery of and demand for and access to institutional health care services and products. Institutional health care committees are responsible for devising strategies that lower institutional costs and liabilities; maximize the speed, safety, and efficiency of health care delivery; create new health care services and product lines, and attract health care consumers to utilize institutional facilities for personal health care needs. Therefore, operators running health care delivery institutions and systems focus on establishing system rules and member compliance to ensure that institutional delivery of health care to consumers remains profitable.

6.4.2 Protocols and Guidelines for Health Care Delivery

Protocols within the rescue industry are predetermined sets of health care delivery actions devised to be implemented rapidly automatically on health care consumers, who present to health care institutions with specific health criteria and complaints. Protocol health care is increasing in the modern era of fast-paced health care delivery and rising consumer expectations for immediately responsive and flawless health care.

Protocols play the odds and attempt to gain a head start in identifying and treating suspected illnesses by quickly running numerous medical tests and simultaneously initiating various medical treatments. When protocols are enacted, whole batteries of expensive diagnostic and therapeutic maneuvers are carried out on health care consumers satisfying criteria established for protocol implementation. Protocols allow for mass processing and throughput of health care consumers presenting to health care institutions for medical help.

For example, presenting with a fever, high pulse rate, and low blood pressure to a health care facility may activate an infection protocol that automatically leads to starting intravenous fluids; performing a chest X-ray to check for a pneumonia; obtaining a urine sample to screen for a urinary tract infection; drawing blood cultures to test for microorganisms in the blood; and taking blood samples to measure blood counts, clotting factors, chemistries, oxygen and pH levels, and possibly other biological markers to examine for body vehicle system disturbances associated with an infection.

Protocols immediately cover all health care delivery bases preemptively at once to address common, usually severe health disturbances treated at health care facilities, presumably to improve the quality, efficiency, and safety of health care delivery. Unsurprisingly, the typical health disorders targeted with protocols are the more common health conditions, such as heart attacks, strokes, pneumonia, heart failure, and severe infections, that ironically are carefully audited by health care payers and certifying agencies.

Health care delivery protocols allow physician and nonphysician health care providers to conveniently implement comprehensive autopilot health care strategies with minimal effort and forethought, while ensuring that ordered health care activities satisfy monitored health care payer standards and quality metrics used for institutional comparisons and to determine levels of reimbursements. Protocol-delivered health care can drive up health care costs immensely when applied with minimal restraint on larger scales, especially when some automatic health care maneuvers may be unnecessary under presenting health circumstances and may not offer health or survival benefits compared to the thoughtful application of health care delivery strategies by experienced health care professionals.

While health care protocols increase the efficiency and decrease the delays in administering health care services in busy health care settings, protocol health care further limits health care professional time commitments to individualize health care delivery thoughtfully and reduces opportunities for direct interpersonal health care interactions that positively influence individual and societal health.

Activated protocols may also lead to unnecessary costs or even affect health care recipients detrimentally when health care management has not been contemplated carefully.

Unfortunately, the potential threat of malpractice litigation for adverse health care outcomes associated with failure to implement institutionally devised protocols additionally reinforces the application of profitable autopilot health care delivery strategies.

With growing health care delivery liabilities, protocol health care defensively serves to divert implications that any adverse health care delivery outcomes might have been due to inadequate, substandard, or omitted health care delivery practices.

Guidelines in health care are general rules derived through consensus among health care experts that provide recommendations to evaluate, monitor, and treat specific health conditions more effectively as determined by health care experiences on larger scales, which are to be applied proactively as *one-size-fits-all* to segments of health care recipients experiencing similar health conditions. Health care delivery guidelines selectively channel provider activities and resources toward implementing preferred health care strategies, considered by experts in their fields to benefit individuals suffering from certain health problems. Guidelines also conveniently help steer health care activities by less experienced and less knowledgeable health care practitioners, allowing health care to be practiced more uniformly by all providers at some minimum standard of care established by professional health care organizations and licensing bodies.

Health care industry standards of care set by professional health care organizations frequently become quality measures used to grade and compare health care delivery across various health care institutions and professional practices. Some of the more notable health care delivery guidelines provide specific recommendations to treat high blood pressure, diabetes, blood cholesterol, heart failure, pneumonia, and other health problems in affected individuals; to use aspirin and statin anticholesterol agents to lower risks for heart attack and stroke in vulnerable populations; and to detect silent colon, prostate, and breast cancer.

Protocols and guidelines are industry tools for delivering commercial health care more efficiently and profitably on a mass scale and keep both health care providers and consumers busy focusing on and attending to rescue industry system directives and health care strategies.

Health care providers failing to practice according to rescue industry guidelines and protocols risk suffering liability or being disciplined. Institutional health care committees establish chains of command to ensure medical staff compliance with forged health care delivery protocols and guidelines. Health care institutions monitoring practicing staff providers enforce strict adherence to established protocols and guidelines by using punitive measures that threaten employment, practice revenues, or legal liability for noncompliance.

The rescue industry implicitly enlists the assistance of the legal system and counterpart attorney professionals to threaten liability for any failed health care, which helps motivate providers to diligently carry out devised protocols and guidelines to keep rescue industry entities protected, working, and benefiting financially. The legal system also profits by litigating health care delivery complications that may occur following, deviating from, or failing to implement established health care delivery protocols and guidelines.

Ironically, enormously costly autopilot commercial health care delivery that increases individual and societal debt without benefiting or improving health or survival is not considered malpractice or negligent. Certifying health care agencies and licensing bodies also regularly support protocol- and guideline-directed health care delivery strategies believed to enhance the quality and safety and lower the costs of delivering health care.

Health care institutions additionally develop and implement protocols and guidelines to ensure the fulfillment of health care delivery standards of accreditation for payer-monitored health disorders. Consequently, protocols and guidelines conveniently enforce the delivery of health care services and products as designed by the commercial rescue industry system.

On the other side, health care payers create **care-pathways** modeled according to health care delivery protocols and guidelines that *predetermine health care delivery strategies,* which consumers and providers must follow or risk losing the privilege to receive access to health care benefits and payments. Health care institutions that comply with national regulatory and insurance industry benchmarks for quality health care delivery, which commonly include maintaining proficiency in adhering to protocols and guidelines, become certified, recognized selectively, and rewarded with increased payer reimbursements. Additionally, health care payers steer insured members to preferred health care institutions satisfying rescue industry quality metrics that often include protocol and guideline adherence, further reinforcing autopilot health care that profitably drives health care delivery activities.

Therefore, reimbursement pressures and the fear of litigation and punishment for noncompliance with established health care delivery norms and standards compel provider and institutional adherence to care-pathways, protocols, and guidelines, especially for health conditions scrutinized and audited under quality metrics established by health care monitoring entities. Unfortunately, autopilot commercial health care that ostensibly improves the quality and safety of health care outcomes scrutinized by payers as health care costs skyrocket economically burdens consumers having limited opportunities to have health care needs efficiently addressed on an individualized basis. All-encompassing autopilot health care delivery, designed as one-size-fits-all to conform to payer care-pathways and meet professional health care organization and payer quality metrics, further contradict the intent of **precision medicine,** which aims to individualize health care delivery for all.

Economically motivated autopilot universal health care delivery applied selectively to commercially tracked health conditions obscures the actual quality of health care delivered by institutions, which otherwise may perform deficiently throughout the health care continuum and fail to provide real health benefits to individuals and society. Consequently, the routine use of protocols and guidelines by rescue industry entities is associated with numerous limitations, can hide the true realities of health care delivery, and predisposes to misuse and misapplication by less experienced and apathetic health care providers and by profit-driven entities.

6.4.3 Health Care Delivery System Producers

Health care institutions carefully monitor and measure the billable work output and productivity of staff health care providers. Some of the work parameters recorded for staff health care providers within health care institutions include the length of stay for admitted patients, number of hospital procedures performed, quantity and type of diagnostic tests and therapeutic interventions ordered, ancillary services requested, and medications prescribed.

Productivity measures for providers ensure efficient institutional health care delivery at the lowest facility costs, maximizing revenues and profitability from reimbursements and avoiding payer financial penalties for unnecessary, excessive, or drawn-out health care delivery.

Therefore, health care delivery systems focus on delivering large volumes of health care products and services efficiently to maximize institutional profit margins.

Hospital staff providers who consistently achieve high work productivities generating profitable cash flow for institutional coffers may be selectively recognized for their loyal efforts and possibly be appointed with pay to direct committees with like-minded staff, which work jointly to streamline institutional health care delivery and to design work performance models for fellow staff to follow.

Productivity-driven systems value health care delivery processes based on their potential to generate institutional revenues and not necessarily on their propensity to produce real societal health or enlighten dependent health care recipients on how to avoid having to spend any personal lifetime receiving expensive commercial health care products and services. The health care system focus on productivity shifts the health care mission from attending to the actual health needs of individuals to the minding of economically profitable industry processes and bottom lines, consequently to negatively impact the pursuit for genuine health and life satisfaction for health care consumers.

Rescue industry systems have become economic tools operating to maximally extract human *lifetime* by scouring all options to reap available revenues due from third-party health care payers and health care consumers for any delivered services and product lines. Very few earnest attempts in the grand health care delivery scheme exist to completely shut down the swelling pipeline of human health disorders and thwart the burgeoning flow of illness-driven consumption of health care.

If rescue industry systems were actual instruments of health forged to care for individual and societal well-being, these systems would aggressively pursue eradication of the root causes of human health suffering and expenses, often constituting the health-undermining activities of profit-driven addictification industries, which tactically institute and strategically disseminate human addictification to achieve their own commercial, economic successes.

The fundamental objectives of a caring health system are to implement interventional strategies that defend and preserve human health and entirely prevent human illnesses and diseases from occurring.

The primary goals of a genuine health-driven system are to have fewer patients and to lower the societal need for expensive health care services and products, and not to have more health care providers and to increase the delivery of health care services and products to all.

Instead, modern health care delivery systems are essentially **sickcare delivery systems** that depend on human sicknesses to drive the delivery and consumption of commercial health care products and services. Sickcare delivery systems then devise numerous rules with complicated checks and balances to create a commercial union with consumers that will last indefinitely and ensure commercially profitable health care delivery to individuals and society both in sickness and in health.

Health care professionals entrusted to be guardians of human health take on roles to restore lost health and deliver health care products and services to consumers to profit from sickcare delivery. Sickcare interventions work not only to eradicate existing disease and help individuals recover lost health but also to seek and uncover silent or dormant disease states and disease predispositions to create even more profitable opportunities for sickcare delivery.

Therefore, the sickcare industry acts on a "sick" premise rather than working for health, and individuals must become "sick" to participate in system "health" care.

Many disease cures in modern medicine result from studying illnesses and then intervening to interrupt or reverse the natural course of identified disease processes or predispositions. Within the sickcare system, the rescue industry idly stands by witnessing progressive societal health demise from human addictification only to intervene too late at a high price for humanity to pay.

The rescue industry has been complicit with addictification industry efforts by remaining silent, patiently waiting for a turn to profit from the fallout of societal health indiscretions, and then opportunistically jumping onto the commercial gravy train to capture its portion of profitability by offering repairs for preventable human deterioration that traps individuals into dependification.

Commercial rescue care patches up and dispatches health care consumers to continue fighting and getting harmed in the addictification game, similarly to how boxing corner cut men patch up hurt boxers between rounds before approvingly shoving the boxers back into the ring to fight and suffer through another punishing round of beatings generating revenues for the sports industry.

Dwindling societal revenues that cause rising economic pressures and commercial industry demands for profitability have disturbed altruistic rescue industry intentions, responsibilities, and goals, and redirected rescue industry efforts toward focusing on healing and recovering lost human health rather than on protecting and defending human health from being lost in the first place.

"Health" care efforts are deteriorating into managing human illnesses, while prevention efforts transform into controlling established illnesses to keep expenses from skyrocketing out of control to threaten the profitability of providing commercial health care.

Therefore, caring health systems value defending and preserving physical and mental health, whereas sickcare systems value profitable delivery of "health" care as in the governmentally legislated MACRA (Medicare Access and CHIP Reauthorization Act) program: whereby "performance" in 2017 determines "reimbursement" for 2019 in a sophisticated play by the rules to get paid better scheme for "health" care providers.

Consequently, "health" care delivery systems have mutated into illness management systems driven, sustained, and dependent on profitably selling health recovery and restoration, and limiting the consequences of already established human health disorders.

In sickcare delivery systems, the "Sick" premise is that real health and wellness are less profitable for rescue industries than sicknesses for which industries can sell revenue-generating interventions, treatments, and cures.

Sickcare delivery keeps health care consumers playing the rescue industry game and spinning the wheels of health care consumption driving industry profitability.

Sickcare systems regularly employ human affirmation, using praise such as "you are a good patient," and "did a great job with your tests or taking your medicines," as a tool to reinforce illness behaviors and essentially encourage health care consumers to remain patients depending on the system, rather than working to make health care consumers understand that human illnesses, testing, and artificial interventions and treatments are expensive, can reduce life quality, and are potentially life-threatening.

Sickcare systems incentivize and pay providers to manage illnesses expertly and essentially *maintain sickness* perpetually by rewarding for illness intensity and the complexity of health care services delivered; whereby reimbursements increase for higher levels and loads of illnesses in designated groups of insured members and more complicated and demanding procedures performed, effectively to reduce incentives for the rescue industry to reverse underlying sicknesses.

Medicare Relative Value Units (RVUs) are one sickcare system reward metric that specifically scales governmental reimbursements progressively upwards commensurate with the intensity and complexity of health care services and procedures provided. RVUs are higher for more technically difficult procedures and for more complex health impairments demanding more time and work energy to manage. The EHR then serves as a convenient tool for providers to itemize the levels and extent of illnesses addressed and procedures performed for billing purposes to increase payer reimbursements.

Clearly, preventing sicknesses altogether would likely put many industries and providers profiting from treating human illnesses out of business but would create healthier and more productive societies that suffer and spend less to exist and could accomplish more for all.

Therefore, human illnesses that compromise life quality and threaten survival create victims vulnerable to commercial rescue industry forces looking to profit from unfortunate human predicaments.

The rescue industry has failed to work earnestly for humanity to sever the links between human health disorders and the powerful commercial forces that are substantially responsible for creating those disorders. Genuinely caring health systems value preserving physical and mental health and work predominantly on promoting healthier societal behaviors and lifestyles to prevent human diseases and illnesses from occurring altogether.

Since industry systems can commercially manipulate and train humanity to consume unhealthy processed foods, alcohol, and tobacco products, and engage in various behaviors and lifestyles detrimental to human health and survival, ample opportunities exist for caring health-directed enterprises to effectively teach and train humanity how to live healthier to defend and preserve personal health.

The education of society to increase health awareness and understanding, and intensive lobbying of lawmakers and the public to create hostile economic and societal environments for addictification industries that thrive financially at the expense of humanity, would be prime objectives for caring health systems.

The selling of health care products and services that only slow or postpone inevitable health demise from unhealthy behaviors and lifestyles that lead to widespread economic fallout in society would be of low priority for genuinely caring health systems. Unfortunately, commercial rescue industry systems have instead evolved to maximally captivate and retain dependent health care consumers within complicated multispecialty health care delivery schemes.

GPS-like health care delivery navigators, sometimes described as **Human Trafficking Clinical Ambassadors,** are created to meticulously escort consumers through elaborate health care delivery mazes to guarantee that profitable health care is expeditiously completed as ordered by providers. The escorting services of health care navigators then combine with health care delivery protocols, guidelines, and directives and the skillful manipulation of health care consumer fears and uncertainties to maximize societal health care consumption profiting industry.

Inflating the benefits of following commercial health care delivery options and magnifying the risks of noncomplying with health care industry advice, additionally serve to promote health care consumer compliance with devised commercial health care industry directives. Finally, meticulous invoicing of provider and institutional health care activities with supporting documentation conforming to bureaucratically established guidelines secures payer reimbursements to fuel the rescue industry machines expertly extracting diminishing human *lifetime.*

6.4.4 Incentives, Kickbacks, and Health Care Delivery Monopolies

The recognition that self-serving health care provider motives and outside economic influences interfere with the unbiased and professionally appropriate delivery of necessary health care to recipients has existed since the inception of the physician Hippocratic Oath in ancient times. Societal concerns for medical industry **conflicts of interest** from self-referrals have led US lawmakers to legislate health care delivery antikickback laws called **STARK LAWS.** These laws are established to prevent licensed medical practitioners from self-referring to medical and laboratory entities in which they or any family members own or have any financial or economic interests or stakes.

Additional legislated efforts known as **sunshine laws** confront the influence of health care providers with graft provided by financially benefiting commercial rescue industry elements. Sunshine laws expose remuneration, "honoraria," and "gratuitous" gifts from commercial drug and medical devise industries to health care providers.

The reasoning behind sunshine laws is that commercial rescue industry gifts of money and objects of economic value to providers taint provider behaviors against the best interests of health care consumers who depend on health care providers and industry to address personal health needs.

Ironically, although legal restrictions prohibit physicians from referring health care work to facilities in which they or family members have financial interests to prevent conflicts of interest, health care systems increasingly hire physicians to leverage system profitability from health care provided to consumers. Private health care delivery systems are reacting to mounting financial pressures from commercial market forces that threaten business solvency and viability by buying up medical practices and hiring physicians as employees to make them system owned and controlled and steer consumers into their health care networks to increase institutional revenues. Hired hospital staff physicians generate millions of dollars in revenues yearly for their employer health care institutions by performing surgical procedures, requesting ancillary services and interventions, ordering laboratory and radiology studies, and prescribing medications through employer institutions.

Hospitals and health care delivery networks that own medical practices and employ practitioners enjoy the financial benefits of having employee ordered health care work conducted substantially through employer facilities, which then can charge a premium to deliver necessary health care services. Health care institutions incentivize employee providers to increase work output by rewarding workhorse providers exceeding productivity goals with perks and bonuses, and special appointments to select committees providing extra pay. Motivated health care provider employees keep health care maximally flowing through employer health care delivery systems.

Physician-owned medical specialty practices hoping to avoid the fate of being swallowed up and bought out by institutional health care delivery networks also join forces and merge to geographically form into mega health care delivery practices, which are intent on gaining stronger market positions and attaining greater financial bargaining power in progressively difficult economic times.

Insurance companies then buy the mega-sized medical practices to control health care delivery at the very core of health care expenditures and ensure corporate industry profitability entirely at consumer expense.

Likewise, independent hospitals progressively join forces and band together to territorially monopolize delivery of health care and engineer control of health care consumers, strengthening market financial bargaining power to circumvent any reductions in reimbursements contemplated by payers.

The profit-driven conglomeration of health care systems and providers into geographic and functional monopolies limits consumer health care choices and access to more economically favorable health care delivery options to hold large segments of society financially captive.

Contrary to the claims of providing higher-quality, more efficient, and lower-cost health care, health care system monopolies reduce market competition to constrain health care delivery and restrict consumer health care options and mobility, raising the costs of health care without consumer recourse. Health care delivery monopolies can extract higher payments for the same, or even lower-quality health care work when market competition is absent. Health care consumers are commonly labeled as clients and customers as if they deliberately choose to utilize specific health care services and facilities within specific health care systems and health care delivery zones.

Commercial health care systems also mislead consumers to believe that seeking health care equates to shopping intentionally to spend discretionary income judiciously on optional commercial industry services and merchandise such as entertainment, dining, sporting events, or fashion items and accessories. The need for urgent or expeditious medical or surgical attention, transportation limitations, existing occupational and familial demands and scheduling conflicts, and numerous other personal difficulties curtail health care consumer options and access to more distant health care delivery alternatives.

Additionally, health care consumers are frequently forced to receive health care services from providers and institutions on their insurance plans and where insurance preferred or assigned health care providers have staff privileges to practice. Health care delivery charges and the reimbursements negotiated with third-party payers to ensure profitability coincidentally are generally unavailable for health care consumers to review and help financially guide those seeking more affordable health care options. The actual costs to consumers for health care services lack transparency, and when available are often more complicated to read, evaluate, and understand than a legislative bill riding through congress attempting to gain bipartisan congressional approval.

Merging health care system entities and established health care system conglomerates routinely adopt cozy corporate names to assimilate within local or regional communities, gain favor with health care consumer populations, and disguise business driven aims for economic profitability.

Corporate and institutional labels name the locality of service, espouse a religious affiliation, or convey some higher-order institutional mission emphasizing human mercy, advocacy, or dignity as sales tactics to attract health care consumers into profit-driven health care delivery operations. Health care entities then work rigorously to retain customers using services by providing for all active and potential consumer health care needs; which may even include offering programs that teach how to accept and live with illness, rather than on how to live healthier and become liberated from depending for health care on commercial systems that trap individuals into paying exorbitant rates for health care services.

Ultimately, monopolizing health care delivery that restricts consumer choices form under the legislative approval and oversight of policymakers who work to benefit health care providing entities preferentially at consumer expense.

Legislating bodies and health care policymakers routinely tailor societal health care delivery options to cater to the needs, directives, and lobbying influence of powerful conglomerate health care systems and corporate entities. Employers, health care delivery system institutions and networks, and various other commercial entities negotiate and contract with commercial and governmental health care payers to dictate consumer health care utilization, by designating preferred health care delivery providers and networks and restricting utilization of out-of-network health care, whose costs for usage are deliberately made prohibitively expensive to deter consumer use.

The rising costs of health care are always passed on to consumers, who are churned by all health care delivery entities to shoulder the financial burdens and pay through any means for increased health care costs and any institutionally expected health care delivery profits.

Health care consumer options to receive health care administered apart from mega health care delivery circumstances are disappearing.

Within mega health care delivery practices where time is money, and ordering tests and group specialty consultations and performing procedures increase profitability and gauge practice productivity, personalized health care interactions devoting adequate professional time to health care recipients to promote health understanding and advance preventative health care strategies become neglected or entirely abandoned.

On larger scales whereby health care is administered through assembly-line clinic type settings, common ailments are more likely to be categorized to trigger knee-jerk health care responses, which implement care protocols and initiate pharmaceutical treatments sooner to reduce health care provider effort and interaction times and profitably increase consumer throughput, while consumer costs rise, and consumer health concerns are addressed insufficiently. Automated health care delivery that sacrifices interpersonal health care interactions to compensate for declining practice revenues further compromises opportunities for health care providers to dispense less costly expert advice and individualize professional interventions to meet consumer health care needs simply and inexpensively.

Growing time and economic limitations pressure health care providers valuing high-tech procedural and pharmaceutical health care to change roles from promoting health to implementing fast-track health care services and products more readily. Take-it-or-leave-it health care delivery machines patterned after large-scale commercial utility industries provide one-size-fits-all health care progressively to become an unaffordable societal health care delivery norm without alternative consumer options or recourse.

The health care insurance industry erects additional impediments to thwart insured members from rightfully accessing their purchased and expected health care benefits. Health insurance administrative bottlenecks encumber approvals for health care services and reimbursements to hinder consumers from recouping tightly held insurance industry revenues siphoned off to manage consumer and societal health care money flow.

Widespread societal, economic pressures and shortfalls produce additional restraints that choke off consumer access to alternative options for managing personal health problems. Progressively, health care consumers encounter more difficulties in acquiring health care benefits, receive less health care for monies spent to service personal health matters, and have less recourse when experiencing problems attempting to address individual health care needs.

Health care systems driven to increase business profits work to restrict health care delivery and access and improve the efficiency of health care delivery rather than to promote the appropriate behaviors and lifestyles to keep consumers healthy and eliminate consumer need for expensive health care services and products.

Universal healthy living to achieve true societal health and decrease or elim-inate societal needs for commercial health care delivery would be financially disastrous for the rescue industry and prompt many rescue and insurance industry businesses to go bankrupt and defunct.

Strategies that aggressively conserve health and inexpensively prevent body vehicle disrepair and disease to preserve body vehicle function for long-term use are inconsistent with the goals of commercially driven market societies, in which convenience objectives and escalating mass consumption of throwaway commercial products and services replace health conservatism.

An additional element that places health care consumers squarely behind the eight-ball of health care delivery is that of the government backing of a health care system which appears unsustainable and risks collapse under tremendously accumulating societal debt as gauged through numerous foretelling economic indicators.

The welcoming and support of addictification behaviors that reap substantial tax revenues, which are more than consumed by the expenses resulting from societal health demise, misdirects and derails true societal health efforts while significantly escalating already burgeoning societal debt.

The rescue industry has been the beneficiary of the perfect storm of opportuni-ties that have sustained rescue industry growth and economic successes. Factors benefiting the rescue industry include

1. *addictification,* promoted through governmental legislation of policies and tax incentives that commercially favor addictifica-tion industry practices
2. *governmental support* of misdirected societal health strategies and goals, with legislated appropriations repeatedly endorsing and sustaining failing rescue industry system efforts
3. *victimization of consumers* trapped between commercial addicti-fication schemes and rescue bail-out dependification

The rescue industry is uniquely situated to prevent the unfortunate health demise of individuals and society suffering from the fallout of frequently preventable body vehicle health predicaments.

Unfortunately, rescue industry hierarchies that govern and direct rescue industry work efforts use their power and political influence to lobby and fight battles prin-cipally to raise reimbursements for conducting business as usual under the same old failing health care strategies, thereby leveraging available health opportunities and revenues to benefit industry as opposed to helping society achieve true health. Then, rank-and-file rescue industry providers are motivated and charged through rescue industry incentives, directives, and sanctions to follow hierarchy-devised edicts to ensure smooth and profitable health care system operations across all rescue industry service lines.

Health care delivery systems incentivize provider participation to drive health care delivery down the usual failed course by making higher reimbursements to keep doing the "same old" a bonus of health care quality benchmarking programs. Consequently, providers who deliver health care meeting the standards and fulfilling the quality metrics devised by commercial rescue industry entities are rewarded with more money.

> *Genuinely healthy individuals do not require health repair and have limited needs for health care services and products.*

Health care providers receive no financial rewards from healthy consumers who fail to utilize health care products and services to generate industry revenues from health care activities. Consequently, dependent health care consumers expecting health from rescue industry efforts are steered instead into increasingly complicated rescue industry mazes, which ensure implementation of all rescue industry directives precisely as planned by revenue-hungry systems.

Some health care consumers even become inescapably trapped within rescue industry health care mazes to depend on receiving health care services continually and achieve unfortunate distinctions of being known within the rescue industry as **frequent flyers.** Frequent utilizers of rescue industry system services and products become captive addressing unresolvable health problems continually within a health care system that applies health care delivery paradigms perpetually feeding rescue industry profitability but offering no real solutions and opportunities for escape from personal health predicaments.

Profitable health care occurs by finding and treating diseases and disease predispositions and by creating unattainable health challenges and ideals that hired rescue industry experts convincingly push onto consumers to pursue commercially. The rescue industry would even be inclined to find disease in beauty if delivering health care attempting to make beauty more beautiful was profitable.

Consequently, rather than principally promoting healthful behaviors and life-styles to increase individual and societal health, rescue industries self-servingly direct efforts, power, and influence to advance industry devised ideals and raise provider reimbursements for services rendered to assure business survival and profitability. Therefore, rather than caring for and protecting societal health assertively through intensive health education and aggressive illness prevention, the health care delivery system instead focuses on efficiently maximizing the spread and penetration of health care products and services to consumers to benefit industry.

Health care delivery systems financially thrive working like damage control hazmat crews to salvage irresponsibly and carelessly contaminated and damaged body vehicles, frequently to intervene too late to restore lost health from self-inflicted human illnesses.

Inpatient hospitalizations in particular often reflect the failure of outpatient health care to keep consumers from developing illnesses and compromised health in the first place.

Health care consumers are suckered, led like lemmings, and sacrificed like pawns to feed health care industry interests instead of being guided toward better individual health through concerted societal and rescue industry caring health efforts. Fortunately, opportunity and recourse exist for health care consumers to achieve and maintain health without depending on commercial rescue industry assistance or involvement.

Achieving true health concerns what needs to be done right not what is being done wrong.

Health is an inherent life quality delivered at birth to most body vehicles to be defended purposefully and protected through the preventative elimination of existing and impending risks that threaten body vehicle health, function, and survival.

Without the appropriate behavioral and lifestyle choices to preserve health and prevent illness and health deterioration from occurring, rescue industry systems profit to do the deed and fill the need at consumer and societal expense, by delivering costly health care that offers body vehicle damage control and repair often for preventable human diseases.

Maintaining health with a transparently functioning body vehicle dramatically eliminates the need to seek health care delivered artificially through commercial rescue industry products and services.

Since the health care system thrives on intervening for illnesses and health deterioration, then striving to remain healthy averts falling into rescue industry traps that foster dependification for rescue industry products and services. Health care industry interventions also entangle worried consumers into running around scared busily completing time-consuming gauntlets of intimidating tests and treatments driving up personal expenses and suffering rather than increasing own health.

Ideally, the appropriate utilization of available health care services is as a **backup plan** to complete screening evaluations to detect silent health conditions hidden in susceptible and higher-risk individuals and to intervene sooner to limit progression and harm from developing or established health disorders and underlying illnesses.

Rescue health care is not the go-to, easy way out to compensate for behavioral indiscretions and unhealthy lifestyles that shirk personal health maintenance responsibilities and lead to health disrepair demanding corrective measures marketed by the commercial rescue industry. Healthy behaviors and lifestyles avoid many of the pitfalls of health care delivery systems that turn into money pits for consumers and society. Directing proper attention, time, and energy to maintaining rather than recovering body vehicle health reduces *lifetime* payments to the commercial rescue industry system for health care.

7 HEALTH MAINTENANCE

Two basic life principles make choosing healthy easier and minimize *lifetime expenditures*:

1. **Living** is simple.
2. **Trust** the basics.

Health maintenance is more about having the will to pursue life strategies that achieve the best possible health and longevity than about possessing the willpower to avoid behaviors, foods, and substances that are toxic to the body vehicle.

Health maintenance encompasses all human behaviors that ensure smooth, transparent, and uninterrupted body vehicle functioning at optimal DNA genetic program code specifications.

Body vehicle health maintenance inherently integrates with body vehicle fueling.

The human body is a biological, physical entity magnificently designed to synchronize oral nutrient intake with the appropriate digestive processing to transform ingested natural whole foods into usable energy to sustain body vehicle life. Commercial processing and refinement of natural crude, whole earth foods artificially modify whole food properties including the nutrient balance and composition to change the pace of delivery and biological effects of nutrients transiting down the gut to impact digestive functioning and body vehicle metabolic operations.

Disturbances of the tactical relationships of digestive organs and functional sequences of gastrointestinal operations to alter the natural synchrony of fuel delivery and digestive processing within the gut, as occurs following gastric bypass surgery that reroutes digestive anatomy, profoundly affect body vehicle metabolism to produce enormous health repercussions. Therefore, industrially manufactured, fake foods and surgical options should not be convenient defaults readily accepted as preferred methods to address failed body vehicle nutritional management and solve obesity and other excessive fueling disorders in humans.

7.1 HEALTH NUT

Health nut is a term likely contrived by commercial industry elements threatened by any real consumer health-directed efforts. Ridicule of individuals enlightened with a true sense of health consciousness directed away from commercial industry involvement is uncanny. Subversive elements twist industry break-away mind-sets as being unconventional and nonconforming with usual commercial food industry norms.

Branding individuals who seek genuine health as outcast health nuts safeguards health misperceptions that maintain commercial food industry status quos and, additionally, subverts grassroots efforts to break free from industry clutches and spread true health mindfulness to others.

Industry consistently works to distort human perceptions and understanding of "natural" and "organic." Orchestrated marketing campaigns stretch the definition of natural and organic to include artificially crafted, commercially manufactured, and mass-produced food industry products having unnaturally long shelf lives to survive large-scale commercial distribution and prolonged storage. Industry discredits simple, genuinely natural, inexpensive, and commercially unprofitable health conduct alternative to industry-supported options as being substandard, inferior, and unconventional compared to commercially endorsed health behaviors, which are promoted as being more convenient, fashionable, high-tech, "scientifically proven," mass accepted, and expert and celebrity endorsed.

Peer pressure from close friends and associates who are trapped by addictification and dependification and misguided by industry to endorse commercially sponsored health maintenance options may coercively derail health efforts to pursue naturally healthy behaviors independent of commercial industry involvement. Therefore, breaking away from industry subterfuge and pressures to untangle the real truths behind essential body vehicle health maintenance and basic human survival needs is challenging on many fronts.

7.2 NUTRITIONAL MORALITY

Morality applies to conformity with specific principles and appropriate code of conduct and avoidance of behaviors derailing, detracting from, and disabling that morality. Learning to distinguish between good and bad and right from wrong body vehicle fueling behaviors lays the foundation for a nutritional morality that extensively benefits the body vehicle system in many ways.

Nutritional morality is founded on a specific **code of nutritional conduct** providing ground rules that guide dietary behaviors to be commensurate with maintaining optimal body vehicle health and existence. Nutritional morality helps preserve the physical and biological sanctity of the body vehicle system to allow the inner body vehicle driving life force to accomplish the intended life purpose without unwelcomed interruption from preventable fueling disorders.

Nutritional morality develops by valuing the appropriate nutritional measures essential for healthy living and setting a precedent to correctly follow body vehicle fueling behaviors and lifestyles that defend and preserve health. Becoming nutritionally moral involves adopting and adhering to the set of ground rules that guide which body vehicle nutritional, behavioral programs are acceptable and allowable to run.

The basis of nutritional morality is recognizing and understanding the differences between correct and incorrect fueling to maintain optimally functioning body vehicle system operations. Nutritious fueling choices are made more deliberately without compromise or exception when nutritional morality guides personal fueling decisions.

Adherence to a nutritionally appropriate code of conduct is analogous to faithful observance of behavioral doctrines determined to produce a trouble-free personal and social existence for the long run, whereas voids in nutritional morality create nutritional vulnerabilities opening industry opportunities for commercial manipulation and exploitation, which result in costly body vehicle breakdown and deterioration.

Disgust is a primitive human emotion serving as a body vehicle survival mechanism that inherently protects individuals against high-risk experiences that are potentially harmful, toxic, or life-threatening. Unhealthy, extensively processed and refined commercial food products should disgust and be shunned like unacceptable and inappropriate behaviors and conduct. Consumers without a sense of nutritional morality are easier to misguide and manipulate like puppets on a string to dance to the tune of commercial industry deceptions that lead to unnecessary and avoidable adverse health consequences, which increase life expenses and suffering.

Foods detrimental to the body vehicle are like criminals that can break into and violate the body vehicle system to corrupt mind software and compromise body vehicle hardware upon gaining body vehicle access and entry. Criminal foods that destroy body vehicle nutritional integrity and undermine body vehicle function and health should never be brought home under any circumstances to be shared personally and with loved ones at the dinner table. Food establishments that heavily serve addictification food products are like dens of iniquity or houses of ill repute, which present irresistible temptations for vulnerable individuals to engage in "sinful" feeding behaviors that condemn healthful virtues.

Addictification food establishments should be avoided altogether if adequate nutritional self-control is sufficiently lacking to prevent making poor dietary choices at these facilities. Consequently, if visiting the home of a supposed friend or some commercial eating establishment derails healthy nutritional behaviors, then going there in the first place is best avoided. Just as individuals involved in failing relationships who are disrespected by partners understandably seek divorce to end being subjected to personal abuse and suffering, consumers who are entangled in relationships with food products that abuse and disrespect body vehicle health need to divorce those food products miserably failing to benefit their health.

A life philosophy that eliminates unhealthy behaviors and lifestyles achieves health more successfully.

Individuals who strongly possess a life philosophy that embraces genuinely healthy living more easily refrain from deleterious circumstances and behaviors and from purchasing and consuming toxic substances.

Ultimately, all capable adults are personally responsible for learning the appropriate nutritional morality and are obligated to maintain the health of their body vehicles properly.

Parents and guardians are responsible for teaching and promoting appropriate nutritional morality and proper body vehicle maintenance to children and dependents. Trusting self-serving commercial industries focused on profitability to virtuously promote nutritional morality and conscientiously meet true human dietary needs creates personal vulnerabilities ultimately costing individuals and society dearly. Industry intends to secure money or *lifetime* by "hook" or by "crook" and works first to gain consumer trust and then to establish perpetual consumer dependency on industry services and products, irrespective of any potential to cause adverse consumer health consequences.

8 FUNCTIONAL LONGEVITY

Functional longevity means to maintain maximally productive body vehicle operations and physical output of running body vehicle genetic program codes over the intended body vehicle life-span.

There is no immortality or fountain of youth (yet).

Aspire to achieve youthfulness to maximize personal life potential by maintaining biologically transparent body vehicle operations and keeping the natural aging process from accelerating.

Body vehicle genetic programs, encoded in DNA inherited from biological parents, govern all aspects of human physical existence. These genetic programs are amenable to modification and corruption through extraneous environmental influences and the natural aging process. Under extreme or repeated physical, chemical, and emotional body vehicle stresses genetic program codes become modified unpredictably, potentially creating detrimental mutational changes that undermine healthful body vehicle existence. Body vehicle DNA codes may not be modifiable to increase longevity, but repeated engagement in maladaptive behaviors risks shortening anticipated global and component body vehicle functional survival times.

Unhampered behavioral and physical wear and tear and a lack of appropriate personal maintenance care adversely challenge and provoke the operations of body vehicle survival programs. Make body vehicle behaviors obey a health-driven mind and intentionally select appropriate behavioral programs that preserve body vehicle health to maximize functional longevity.

Recognize and delete viral programs and malware corrupting the mind to carry out mindless behaviors such as excessive feeding, unnecessary alcohol consumption, and other expensive, addictification behaviors that reduce functional longevity and cause illness and suffering—and often emotionally produce feelings of guilt, shame, anger, sadness, apprehension, and loneliness. Reboot and reprogram body vehicle functional operations to original factory specifications, without the malware and unnecessary add-ons and popups that deleteriously disturb healthy body vehicle behaviors.

Take back personal control to live a life free from harmful external commercial manipulation.

9 PLANET EARTH AND THE STORY OF THE GARDEN OF EDEN

Living is simple; trust the basics.
Trust what Mother Nature made,
because everything else is made for profit.

9.1 FOOD

Food is a generic term that applies to both Mother Nature–made natural crude and unmodified whole earth foods and industrially manufactured processed and refined earth fuels that can power and energize body vehicle system operations.

The body vehicle converts food into energy to carry out physical actions and accomplish life goals. Food is composed of complex biological signaling molecules that communicate with body vehicle sensors to physiologically control and direct body vehicle behaviors, emotions, and biochemical operations.

The commercial food industry deliberately manipulates chemical and physical food properties and qualities through processing and refinement to create food products that surreptitiously drive body vehicle nutritional activities to generate industry profits.

Certain foods provide a distinct survival advantage by optimizing health and maximizing longevity when eaten, while other foods lead to a survival disadvantage by assessing a health and survival penalty to increase the risk for illness and shorten life-span when consumed.

Concept foods have made-up names and made-up ingredients.

Concept foods carry commercially made-up food names and refer to artificially created food products not existing naturally within the planet earth environment. Commercial foods having made-up names are often artificially formulated and industrially manufactured through extensive processing, which extracts and subtracts natural food ingredients while adding numerous other unnatural and artificially produced ingredients and contaminants.

The *nutritional subtraction and artificial addition routines* of commercial, industrial food manufacturing processes unbalance the natural qualities, composition, and wholesomeness of earth fuels, which, in their undisrupted state, best fulfill body vehicle nutritional needs.

Characteristic ingredients composing concept foods may be chemical, artificial, processed, refined, and even natural, which are variously combined to gratify consumer taste preferences, meet cultural and ethnic demands, and achieve commercial industry objectives.

Examples of concept foods having made-up names include pasta, brownie, hotdog, hamburger, French fries, ketchup, mayonnaise, sandwich, juice, cake, smoothie, pretzel, pizza, ice cream, and so on. All are invented food products not existing naturally on earth that are prepared and manufactured artificially for commercial purposes.

Similarly, **junk food** refers to the *junk in the foods* and represents some concocted hodgepodge of artificially crafted, formulated, and combined processed and refined food ingredients and chemical additives made available for human consumption.

Additionally, concept foods comprise broad biochemical nutrient categories such as protein, carbohydrate, sugar, and fat commonly used to refer directly to various commercially sold food products. Concept names conveniently cater to human food and nutritional misconceptions and are most amenable for creative portrayal using sophisticated marketing schemes devised to influence and drive up consumer purchase and consumption of artificially created food products. Creative concept food names more readily allow for industry **gotcha moments,** whereby industry commercially captures consumers who rely on food product labeling terms to help guide dietary selections when purchasing foods.

9.2 CRUDE FUELS

Crude fuels are whole, unadulterated, and unprocessed, genuinely organic, living organism, earth-produced foods in their natural state and composition. These can dynamically participate directly in the grand recycling of biological life elements such as carbon inherent to all earth life-forms.

Crude fuels include

1. *Plants and direct plant products,* such as fruits, vegetables, pure whole grains, nuts, seeds, maple tree syrup, and legumes such as beans, peas, and lentils.
2. *Fresh animal flesh and direct animal products,* such as meat, poultry, seafood, fish, eggs, and milk. (Many of these require decontamination through cooking maneuvers to reduce the risks of transmitting any harbored infectious organisms.)
3. *Insects and direct insect products,* such as honey.

The name is the ingredient,
meaning that the crude fuel name is entirely the natural whole food
ingredient.

Therefore, the designated name and appearance of crude fuels identify all contained ingredients. For example, apple is the ingredient of an apple, and the ingredient of a pear is pear, a carrot is carrot, chicken is chicken, cashew is cashew, and so on. The crude fuel name universally embodies all the whole food contained nutritive ingredients having beneficial sustentative qualities to promote and enhance body vehicle health and existence naturally.

Crude fuels are directly available for the body vehicle biological system to break down sequentially and systematically into basic nutrients that optimally nourish and sustain body vehicle cellular functions and viability. The entire body vehicle physical structure continuously undergoes refurbishment, repair, and replacement dependent on energy and the availability of the highest quality replacement parts or nutrients to maintain body vehicle components at original "factory-installed" specifications.

Crude fuels deliver "original factory parts" straight from the manufacturer "Mother Nature," directly in a *one-step* process without any intervening artificial, commercial modifications with nutritional subtractions or additions.

Unadulterated crude fuel whole foods naturally contain and deliver fuel and other nutrient biomolecules directly produced by the earth environment that best communicate with body vehicle system sensors to supply vital biological information, which optimally directs body vehicle nutritional behaviors, metabolic functions, and survival.

The best time to consume and deliver fresh crude fuel nutritional 'goods' into the body vehicle is easily determined and naturally gauged because crude fuels undergo recognizable ripening, decomposition, and spoilage easy to *see, smell, taste,* and *feel* and requiring no "best by" or "freshness expiration" dates.

Natural, unprocessed crude fuel, whole earth foods have built-in portion control that harmonizes with body vehicle nutrient and fuel gauges to biologically regulate food consumption precisely. Crude fuels are first sensed by the body vehicle visually and through smell, and then tasted in the mouth to signal and communicate with fueling and satiety centers in the brain, which regulate eating to synchronize body vehicle feeding with nutritional needs.

After initial interaction with body vehicle sight, smell, touch, and taste sensory portals, ingested whole earth crude fuels communicate internally through complex physiologic and biochemical means during the ensuing digestive breakdown into basic nutrients such as sugars, proteins, fats, vitamins, minerals, fiber, and water that ultimately nourish body vehicle cells.

Uncontrollable eating with repeated cravings for pears, strawberries, bananas, broccoli, peas, carrots, and many other natural crude fuel whole earth foods are unlikely to occur, as frequently happens with processed and refined food products that are artificially prepared and specially formulated deliberately to arouse food cravings and promote addictification. Therefore, crude fuels can be eaten freely with limited regard to restrict quantity and sacrifice quality nutritional fueling.

Crude fuels essentially satisfy the following properties:

1. require no labels
2. require no ingredient lists
3. require no nutrition facts
4. recognizable internationally
5. often naturally delivered in serving size quantities
6. consist of 100% Mother Nature–made genuinely organic earth foods
7. can be conveniently ingested at any time during waking hours
8. provide nutrient fuels that cleanly produce carbon dioxide (CO_2) and water (H_2O) when metabolically burned to power body vehicle cells
9. carry ideal compositions and proportions of vitamins and other nutrients to supply body vehicle energy–generating and detoxification processes appropriately
10. correctly deliver the energy and cellular building block components that best integrate with body vehicle nutrient requirements and processing capabilities to maintain the biological balance and repairs for body vehicle operations to run smoothly
11. globally ubiquitous
12. extensively diversified with innumerable variations to satisfy countless taste preferences

9.3 COLOR

Natural crude fuel whole earth food colors literally reflect vital compositions of internally contained life-sustaining nutrient biomolecules necessary for optimal body vehicle operations and existence. A varied diet that includes whole natural foods from all colors of the rainbow best supplies the basic nutrients needed to sustain body vehicle health.

Nutritional variety is the spice and key to a long and healthy life. Therefore, expanding the color spectrum of natural crude fuel nutritional experiences to eat assorted colored plants along with a variety of fresh animal flesh naturally maximizes health and promotes functional longevity.

9.4 INTACT WHOLE EARTH FOOD PRINCIPLE

Natural whole earth foods are not equal to the sum of their industrially disrupted, processed, and refined component parts.

Enterprising commercial food markets have opportunistically jumped on the consumer-driven whole food movement bandwagon and created food stores dedicated to selling overpriced, container packaged, and artificially manufactured and processed food products sold as whole earth foods to nutritionally misinformed consumers. Industrial processing and refinement of whole earth foods separate, extract, alter, unbalance, and transform natural whole earth food component qualities, composition, form, and balance to disturb essential food characteristics that naturally signal body vehicle fueling sensors. Food processing disrupts the biologically intended nutritional information that truly natural whole earth foods communicate to the body vehicle when eaten. All food processing and refinement steps *subtract* some essential quality, property, or component from Mother Nature–manufactured whole earth foods.

The changes imposed by processing whole natural foods would be analogous to the effects produced by altering the unique global qualities of individuals through freeze-drying, roasting, mechanically pulverizing, or chemically breaking down and separating whole persons into component molecules. Processed and refined humans would never embody the same identity, qualities, characteristics, and personality traits existing within whole persons.

Cellular DNA software, which encodes the system of communication happening between the body vehicle and available crude fuels provided on planet earth to power body vehicle cellular needs, has evolved over innumerable symbiotic life cycles shared between humans, animals, plants, and microorganisms present within earth's vast and integrated biologic ecosystems. Food processing separates and removes natural food ingredients to disturb natural food qualities and composition and reduce the diversification of nutrient components available for interacting with the body vehicle, losing the nuances of complex chemical and biological, nutritional communication that otherwise takes place when whole natural foods are consumed.

Body vehicle fueling programs governing how the body vehicle powers physiologic operations run on internal clocks, which time feeding behaviors and digestive activities precisely according to body vehicle nutrient and energy needs for survival.

Natural whole earth crude fuels best synchronize with feeding timers, with the digestive breakdown products of crude fuels signaling internal body vehicle sensors to direct and complete body vehicle nourishment activities as required to satisfy body vehicle nutrient and energy needs efficiently in a timely manner. Artificially processed food products "doctored" with additives confuse body vehicle sensors evolved over millennia to gauge natural food qualities and composition guiding body vehicle nutritional behaviors correctly.

Excessive ingestion of industrially altered body vehicle fuels that miscommunicate with body vehicle fueling sensors disrupts natural body vehicle fueling programs to compound the adverse effects of other environmental, physical, and emotional body vehicle life stresses.

Body vehicle nourishment and satiety baselines adaptively reset to compensate for increased life stresses and the continual ingestion of industrially altered fuels delivering excessive energy, resulting in impaired body vehicle regulation of feeding that predisposes to overeating and addictification. Eventually, sustained overfueling with processed foods recalibrates the properties of body vehicle fueling programs to new norms geared toward excessive ingestion of unbalanced nutrients to accommodate overfueling, which causes metabolic disturbances leading to obesity and other physical and emotional illnesses that deteriorate life quality and shorten body vehicle survival.

9.5 SATIETY

Satiety is that sense of having fulfilled the nutrient and fuel needs of the body vehicle sufficiently for the time being. The satiety balance point lies somewhere between having had too much and experiencing the need or urge to get more nutrients and fuel for the body vehicle system. Satiety regulation occurs through complex physiologic body vehicle mechanisms that shut off the body vehicle feeding drive and desire to continue eating or seeking food.

Control of satiety depends on a multitude of complex interacting body vehicle physiologic programs relying on information delivered from various body vehicle sensors that gauge the state of internal nutrient and fuel reserves and needs and, additionally, determine the properties and qualities of ingested nutrients and fuels attempting to satisfy those needs.

In addition to being regulated by body vehicle nutritional requirements and the physical properties and quantity of food consumed, satiety is also affected by the physical and emotional states of the body vehicle and the effects of extraneous medications and other chemical substances taken into the body vehicle. The brain, therefore, processes fueling and other information received from various inputs and then dispatches commands to body vehicle hardware to execute fueling responses with the appropriate behaviors to fulfill nutritional needs and achieve proper body vehicle nutritional balances. The body vehicle processes nutritionally related data and dispatches fueling responses by integrating numerous chemical, physical, hormonal, and neurological program loops run by DNA blueprint codes present within various specialized body vehicle cells.

Two highly integrated hormonal regulators of satiety are **ghrelin,** released by an empty stomach to stimulate hunger, and **leptin,** released by fat storage cells when full to inhibit hunger, with both hormones competing to trigger respective brain sensors to control fueling behaviors.

Physiologic perturbation of satiety signaling can lead to uncontrollable over-eating or dangerous underfeeding. Leptin released by fat cells adequately filled with fat energy stores should theoretically suppress further body vehicle fueling activities, thereby conveniently linking fat reserves to satiety. Unfortunately, persistent overfueling with continual ingestion of excessive calories and fat, despite possessing adequate or even abundant stores of fat energy, as occurs in obesity, desensitizes brain sensors to continuous leptin stop-fueling signals.

A balanced intake of unadulterated, unprocessed crude fuel whole earth foods, which signal uncorrupted fueling messages to body vehicle system sensors for accurate nutritional data interpretation, best informs and satiates body vehicle fueling and feeding survival drives. Satiety recognition requires learning to identify the body vehicle signaling that correctly informs when adequate body vehicle fueling and nutritional completeness are reached to allow eating to stop.

Processed and refined addictification food products deliver adulterated nutrient compositions to disturb satiety signaling so that internal body vehicle nutritional assessments fail, skewing satiety to occur only when the body vehicle reaches some toxicity point of excessive and unbalanced food ingestion.

Commercial food industries surreptitiously target satiety signaling by chemically manipulating food property qualities to corrupt food nutritional data input to the body vehicle to keep the body vehicle feeding voraciously with hunger turned up full throttle for commercial industry food products. Continued eating after body vehicle nutritional needs are sufficiently and appropriately satisfied with a nutritionally balanced meal indicates that further eating is occurring for alternative reasons, such as to drive pleasure, escape pain or suffering, or feed an addictification crave.

10 COMMERCIAL FOOD INDUSTRY

The **commercial food industry** is that mass conglomerate of commercial business enterprises that manufactures and supplies conveniently available and readily prepared processed and refined food products having unnaturally extended shelf lives, which are produced artificially by mechanically and chemically manipulating, formulating, and adulterating natural crude fuel whole earth foods.

10.1 THE UNNATURAL INCONSISTENCY OF COMMERCIAL FOOD PRODUCT CONSISTENCY

Commercial food products are artificially engineered to deliver the same appearance, taste qualities, and nutrient characteristics across all time and space. For example, strict industrial formulation and quality control measures applied under exacting standards identically reproduce the commercial food products sold in the previous year in the State of Washington to meet the same consumer taste expectations and food product experiences the following year in the State of Florida.

Nature and evolution are about consistent variability and change.
Industry rides a fixed food product formulation that consistently
reaps financial rewards across time and space.

Through crafty marketing expertise, winning commercial food product formulas that are embodied reproducibly in signature foods become staged perfectly for display with the most appealing and seductive appearance and qualities, which entice humans to purchase and consume food products that biologically ensnare consumer behaviors to turn industry profits.

Consider how highly successful, iconic fast-food chains consistently offer and serve exactly those *same* food products across time and space that *billions* come to desire and expect everywhere anytime. The commercial food industry employs highly specialized food engineers and flavor chemists to skillfully utilize various chemical industry products and methods to create winning, secret processed food product formulas for consumers to ingest and desire continually.

Food processing that serves to generate revenues for commercial industries disrupts natural whole earth foods to drastically alter the composition, proportion, and delivery of original natural whole food nutrients. During food processing, certain whole earth food nutrients are deliberately removed or disproportionately concentrated to retard food spoilage or more potently trigger and captivate smell, taste, and touch sensors that govern human food palatability and consumption. Various food elements, chemicals, and vitamins are then added artificially in unnatural quantities and composition to enhance flavor, replace nutrients lost or removed through processing, and further stabilize mixed food product ingredients to slow natural product spoilage and increase food product shelf life and sales opportunities.

Tearing apart the natural "wholesomeness" of whole earth foods to separate out industry-defined "good stuff" from "undesirable" food components instead produces artificially designed industrial strength food substances that are nutritionally foreign to the body vehicle. Chemical, physical, and compositional alterations made to natural crude fuel whole earth foods to artificially increase the likelihood of consumption disrupt natural body vehicle feeding satiety signaling, predisposing to overeating that promotes obesity and leads to other fueling-related health disorders.

Many artificial food ingredients deliberately added to extend food shelf life and to achieve characteristic flavor, texture, smell, and appearance qualities and enhance the palatability of signature processed foods, provide no nutritional value and must be actively detoxified and eliminated by the body vehicle following ingestion to protect the body vehicle from toxic chemical harm. However, commercial food industries sell food processing as allegedly being accomplished to enhance the taste experience and nutritional value of natural foods, while creating designer taste experiences that commercially drive food sales and consumption at the expense of natural nutritional experiences and sustenance.

10.2 COMMERCIAL FOOD ADDITIVES

Chemical food additives are industrially manufactured substances concocted in laboratory settings that are commercially added to processed foods to alter the flavor, retard spoilage, allow immiscible ingredients to mix, or artificially replace some natural whole food property lost through commercial food processing. Since chemical food additives other than vitamins are not found naturally in crude fuel whole earth foods and serve no specific body vehicle biologic purpose, the body vehicle does not recognize these substances as nutritionally vital or usable. Most chemical food additives play no biological role in cellular metabolic operations that harness energy to produce simple carbon dioxide and water and are not structurally or functionally utilized, conservatively recycled, or strategically stored by the body vehicle for future use. Instead, the body vehicle recognizes chemical food additives as *foreign toxins,* termed **xenobiotics,** that require detoxification and clearance through the liver and kidneys for elimination from the body vehicle into the stool, urine, exhaled breath, or sweat.

Thousands of artificially derived chemical food additives have been added to processed and refined food products over the past several decades. Many of these food additives are not strictly scrutinized or controlled by the **Food and Drug Administration (FDA),** which has entrusted oversight and surveillance responsibilities to industries manufacturing and selling these chemicals to vouch for their safety, essentially leaving the fox to guard the henhouse.

A very limited partial listing of industrially manufactured chemical food additives commonly found in processed food items includes the following: glycerin, soy lecithin, tocopherols, fructooligosaccharides, azodicarbonamide, ammonium sulfate, sodium citrate, sodium phosphate, sodium acid pyrophosphate, sodium benzoate, sodium stearoyl lactylate, carrageenan, calcium propionate, sodium propionate, propionic acid, sodium hydroxide, methylparaben, propylparaben, dextrose, various FD&C Red, Blue, and Yellow food dyes, monocalcium phosphate, potassium sorbate, Polysorbate 80, maltodextrin, monosodium glutamate, beta-carotene, BHT, BHA, TBHQ, magnesium oxide, aspartame, acesulfame, dipotassium phosphate, gellan gum, "artificial flavors," malic acid, ethyl vanillin, caramel color, citric acid, xanthan gum, monoglycerides, ammonium bicarbonate, guar gum, monocalcium phosphate, calcium sulfate, calcium disodium EDTA, calcium peroxide, microcrystalline cellulose, cellulose gum, carboxymethylcellulose, lactic acid, polydextrose, propyl gallate, titanium dioxide, PGPR, etc., etc., etc.

A reference collection that conveniently lists and numbers a multitude of chemical food additives approved for human consumption is the **European Union E Number (100–1500s) Food Additive Listing.**

Grocery store shelves are unlikely to stock listed chemical food additives for consumers to buy and incorporate into favorite home food recipes for individual or family consumption. Calorically "light" versions of artificially prepared commercial food products commonly incorporate a greater abundance of artificial additives that serve as fillers to substitute for removed crude fuel natural whole earth food ingredients.

10.3 FDA GRAS FOOD POLICY

Chemical substance manufacturers create and produce thousands of chemical products yearly to fill the needs and demands of modern human existence. For many of these manufactured chemicals, the biological safety and the scale and details of biologic effects in humans and other living organisms are undefined or unknown. Modern societies create agencies such as the FDA to determine the safety of manufactured chemical products for human use and consumption.

The FDA has devised a food policy known as **GRAS** (generally recognized as safe) that designates which chemical food additives "experts" consider "safe" for human use, which then exempts these identified additives from requiring rigorous scientific safety testing before approval for human consumption. The federal government exempts food additives from safety testing when a *general recognition and agreement or consensus* exists without severe conflict among qualified, trained experts that a specific additive is considered safe based on available published or unpublished studies, any experience gained through common usage of these additives, and any other available data.

GRAS and other food additive safety designations by "experts" raise many questions:

1.   Are the time frames and capacity of expert panels to review and consider available scientific studies and safety data in detail sufficient before food additive approval for release to society?

2.   Are "experts" deciding the safety of chemical food additives the best available, most qualified, and unbiased without financial interests to affect safety determinations?

3.   Are the scientific studies unbiased and data selected for consideration in safety designations comprehensive and of the highest quality to definitively address the potential short and long-term risks to consumers using additives?

4.   Were the direct and indirect funding sources for available studies that generated safety data to determine the human safety of food additives fully known and disclosed?

5.   Did the safety parameters applied in making determinations accurately reflect the potential health and survival risks posed to consumers using products over more extended time periods than allotted within additive safety studies?

6.   How sensitive were the studies to detect human risk, and were safety data measurements detailed and complete?

7.   Did safety determinations consider behavioral and economic, as well as physical, developmental, and reproductive effects on short- and long-term human users, or were safety determinations primarily based on lab animal data and short-term human use of additive chemicals?

8.   Which commercial entities are likely to profit following safety designations from select panels of experts providing a governmental seal of approval, which comprehensively authorizes commercial use of chemical food additives by millions or billions of users?

These questions illustrate only some of the many shortcomings and uncertainties that impact safety considerations preceding formal approval of chemical food additives for human consumption.

Limitations affecting scientific experimentation and available technical instruments used in research studies compromise the ability to detect the human harm entirely that industry manufactured products cause, and consequently, to fully determine product safety for human use. Available scientific studies and experience often unsatisfactorily settle many of the lingering concerns surrounding the safety of chemical food additives before governmental agencies formally approve additives for general commercial use. Consequently, a better definition of GRAS would stress that manufactured chemical substances are scientifically designated to be safe for human consumption based on the absence of detecting human toxicity by searching for potential toxic effects under numerous scientific limitations. Consumers would be more informed to decide whether to risk ingesting GRAS approved chemical additives if provided with easy to understand summaries outlining measured toxicities; naming entities funding and carrying out safety studies; describing general procedures used in studies to obtain safety data and listing significant limitations of safety determinations; providing essential omissions and untested facets in generating safety data; and recording the time frames required for approval decisions and time-span devoted by studies to complete scientific observations and measurements.

Despite existing quandaries surrounding the human safety of ingesting various chemical food additives, expert FDA panels routinely vote to grant formal government approval to allow the use of chemical additives in the manufacture of processed food products consumed by humans. Additionally, food additive safety designations are also prone to gaming for individual and system gain and to surreptitious influences from paid lobbyists and self-serving special interest groups that stand to prosper obtaining requested governmental approval for additives.

Furthermore, many science professionals working for the FDA and other government agencies that generate GRAS decisions, legislate policies, and enact regulations to protect society against industry, have also previously been employed or had personal research work funded by the same industries being regulated and monitored to create an underlying potential for bias and conflicts of interest in making safety determinations.

Human allegiances run deep, and personal bonds developed through close working relationships are difficult to violate solely to create general policies and regulations that would subsequently introduce professional hardships for personal allies.

10.4 GMO (GENETICALLY MODIFIED ORGANISM) MUTANTS

GMOs are mutated plant, animal, insect, and microbial organisms that possess biochemically or technologically altered genetic codes controlling their development, growth, function, or structure. Specific "wild-type" biologic traits naturally found in living organisms can be increased, reduced, replaced, or eliminated for scientific and commercial purposes by using genetic modification. Biochemical technologies modify DNA or other organism genetic controls to change natural organism properties and create *genetically engineered mutants*.

Commercial industries rely on genetic technology to transform the biology of living organisms predictably to obtain economic advantages and meet industry standards or consumer demands more quickly. Economically profitable uses of genetic engineering include exaggerating or diminishing natural wild-type organism features and adding previously absent or removing present qualities or characteristics to increase organism commercial appeal, or possibly, manipulating organism properties to accelerate growth or confer resistance to natural predators and herbicides or weed killers.

Genetic technology eliminates unpredictable, slower, and less economic or unprofitable evolutionary drift, natural selection, and breeding from determining organism attributes. Targets for genetic modification include organism color, size, smell, shape, taste, growth, behavior, biochemical properties, and survival under certain adverse circumstances, and the proportionate balance and composition of organism components.

GMO constructs behave, appear, or function differently compared to unaltered natural wild-type biological organisms. For example, corn may be genetically modified to grow faster and taller, be more yellow, taste sweeter, or resist weed killers and insects.

One concern about GMO foods engineered to resist insects is that if simple insect life-forms, whose cellular metabolic operations share some similarities with those of humans, avoid or die by consuming a genetically modified food made for human consumption, can that food indeed be safe for humans to consume? Agricultural **GMO** alterations that increase crop yields by introducing pesticide qualities into plants cultivated for humans to consume may have profound ecological effects on the food chain to deleteriously affect human survival on earth. Major disturbances in the earth ecosystem occur when the toxic effects of foods mutated to resist insects unintentionally wipe out vital insect populations, such as bees, which are crucial to cross-pollinate plants that maintain the existence of humankind.

Scientific studies have detected that the insect biomass serving as the initial foodstuff for small animals in the food chain, and bee populations crucial to cross-pollinate plants that ultimately feed biological life, have gradually dwindled over the past decades, possibly as a result of deliberate human alterations of natural food properties as well as toxic effects on earth ecosystems through modernization and pollution of the earth environment.

GMO distortions result in organism changes, such as those developing in various disease states, including tumors, whereby mutations affect strategic cellular characteristics, causing cells to behave aberrantly from the usual checks and balances controlling normal cellular biological activities. Mutations introduced into biological organisms may then pass down genetically to future progeny or descendants of mutated cells to further disturb natural earth ecosystems.

Mutation of natural earth foods using genetic technology to modify selective food properties or nutrient compositions is inexact and may unintentionally disrupt other beneficial food traits linked genetically to cellular components targeted for modification. Genetic modification of organisms may inadvertently delete or detrimentally alter beneficial off-target food qualities genetically linked to genes targeted deliberately for deletion or alteration. Consuming GMO food products may then provide a false sense of security with body vehicle nutritional requirements not actually being met as expected or required for proper body vehicle function.

Furthermore, toxic GMO plant qualities passed down through the food chain eventually to be consumed by humans may well end up concentrating within the body vehicle to produce even greater untoward health consequences. Artificially induced mutations in foods consumed by humans and animals may unintentionally produce toxic or immune sensitizing food elements, which then harmfully react within the body vehicle to cause metabolic disturbances or abnormal immune activity to precipitate body vehicle toxicity, autoimmune disorders, or cancer.

Ultimately, foods are genetically modified to drive up food product sales and increase commercial industry profitability and not to benefit human health. **Cash crops,** such as corn, wheat, soy, and sugarcane, which can be mass planted and harvested efficiently using automated technologies and supply secondary world markets profitably, are most likely to be genetically modified to maximize crop yields for market availability.

Adoption of genetically engineered crops in the United States has progressed steadily between 1996 and 2018.

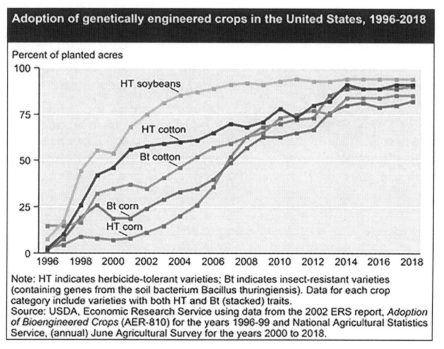

Note: HT indicates herbicide-tolerant varieties; Bt indicates insect-resistant varieties (containing genes from the soil bacterium Bacillus thuringiensis). Data for each crop category include varieties with both HT and Bt (stacked) traits.
Source: USDA, Economic Research Service using data from the 2002 ERS report, *Adoption of Bioengineered Crops* (AER-810) for the years 1996-99 and National Agricultural Statistics Service, (annual) June Agricultural Survey for the years 2000 to 2018.

Most genetically engineered (GE) corn and cotton seeds now have both herbicide tolerance (HT) and insect resistance (Bt).

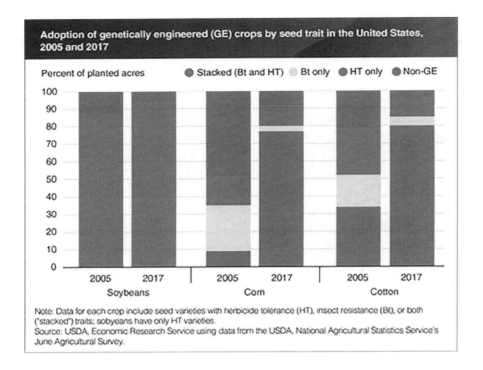

Adoption of genetically engineered (GE) crops by seed trait in the United States, 2005 and 2017

Note: Data for each crop include seed varieties with herbicide tolerance (HT), insect resistance (Bt), or both ('stacked') traits; sobyeans have only HT varieties.
Source: USDA, Economic Research Service using data from the USDA, National Agricultural Statistics Service's June Agricultural Survey.

Within earth's vastly integrated ecosystems, delicate symbiotic evolutionary balances exist among all living organisms. These delicate evolutionary balances may suffer deleteriously when unnaturally rapid and unprecedented commercially designed biological changes are deliberately imposed onto natural earth foods to selectively introduce qualities or characteristics exclusively to satisfy commercial industry interests.

Given the complexities and uncertainties surrounding GMO products, immediate and delayed body vehicle and societal health consequences resulting from GMO consumption are undefined and unknown, and claims to the safety of GMO food products should be approached with the utmost wariness and skepticism.

11 SENSORY STIMULATION

Sensory stimulation enables the body vehicle to experience the environments within and outside of the body vehicle that define physical existence and shape the emotional and intellectual understanding of the world. Body vehicle sensory portals essentially plug human lives directly into the externally surrounding and internally contained physical worlds.

Sensory stimulation activates body vehicle awareness to produce feelings of pleasure, leading to personal happiness and gratification, or pain, producing disappointment and suffering that give meaning to daily living and drive human behaviors, which are factors that industry seeks to manipulate and command at any cost. Feeder and breeder sensory portals carry higher precedence for the commercial industry to target and control due to their prime roles in human survival.

11.1 TASTE PERVERSION

The addictification food industry creates powerful taste illusions that provide life distractions and control human choices and actions. Life is difficult enough, so why not "interrupt" humdrum and difficult life routines to indulge in special moments of taste pleasure, now!

The distraction of sensory signaling and human attention occurs when informational data fed through specific sensory portals are prioritized to take precedence over competing informational data streaming through other sensory portals, whose information delivery is selectively suppressed and deferred to allow more immediate attention and responses to prioritized signaling.

Consequently, sensory portal signaling from less insistent body vehicle sources become muted or extinguished entirely to redirect body vehicle attention to sensory portals that are delivering critical survival information or are being stimulated more intensely.

11.2 TASTE PORNOGRAPHY

Humans experience deep pleasure, satisfaction, and relief from suffering performing activities that gratify feeding and breeding drives, which commercial industries heavily target to reprogram and exploit consumer behaviors. Industries sell cosmetic, fashion, and hygiene merchandise and services to appeal to human breeding drives indirectly by offering commercial options that purportedly enhance personal appearance, youthfulness, vibrancy, desirability, and virility to augment breeding opportunities and reproductive advantages, while pornography industries target breeding drives directly through services and products that pleasure human reproductive "breeder" organs.

Since society forbids self-pleasuring of reproductive "breeder" organs publicly, then a globally accepted, promoted, and unrestricted public self-pleasuring alternative involves hyperstimulation of highly sensitive oral "feeder" taste organs ad libitum with potent taste indulgences. **Taste pornography** invokes obscenely decadent and intensely pleasurable oral sensory taste experiences that strongly arouse primal feeding impulses and craves.

Addictification food industries create sinfully "tasty" food goodies to hook consumers into indulgently pleasuring oral taste sensors through uncontrollable eating that labors to achieve perfectly legal gustatory orgasms without restraint. Oral taste sensors and brain pleasure-reward centers adaptively desensitize with continual pleasurable stimulation and, consequently, require progressively higher levels of stimulation to reach expected levels of pleasure and satisfaction, which conveniently multiplies commercial food industry profits as the consumption of food industry products escalates progressively to meet personal pleasure expectations. Taste pornography pleasures become that oral pacifier that directly soothes painfully harried and stressed-out human lives.

The addictification food industry works hard to capture all available commercial opportunities to satisfy consumer oral taste pornography demands under any circumstances. Unfortunately, taste pornography indulgences also lead to **gigolo moment regrets,** when only temporary appeasement of taste pleasure craves leaves a heavy sense of regret in the wake of unhealthy behaviors that produce excessive caloric baggage.

11.3 CONSUMER TASTE TESTS ARE ADDICTIFICATION TRIALS

Commercial food industries formulate secret recipes for maximal human addictification, which are then gratuitously confirmed and refined using humans to taste test artificially manufactured food products. Unknowingly, humans freely consent to reveal addictification triggers by enthusiastically participating in industry taste testing trials. Conveniently, no consent is required for participants in taste trials to divulge what commercial food manipulations best control and enslave human behaviors orally through the sense of taste. Willpower and self-control are no match to resist enticing flavor ingredients, which food engineers and flavor chemists ingeniously concoct to produce powerful taste sensations that captivate primal urges and impulses to capture human existences commercially.

The food industry intentionally disturbs the sense of taste and food palatability to steer taste recognition away from experiencing natural crude fuel whole earth food qualities and toward accepting patented industrially created flavor formulas that provide novel flavor sensations that arouse the utmost taste pleasures artificially. Food engineers and flavor chemists work diligently to formulate consumable food products that biologically titillate, excite, fool, and ultimately exhilarate the senses of taste, "mouth feel" texture, and smell to generate powerful brain craves that drive individuals to seek to recreate these pleasurable oral taste experiences repeatedly. Taste testing trials then reliably confirm which flavor and taste combinations deeply engage and drive human eating and feeding behaviors.

By subverting, usurping, and enslaving taste bud experiences wired directly into brain stem circuits that govern primal urges and impulses, human feeding craves become owned and controlled to generate industry profits.

11.4 CLUES TO INDUSTRIAL FOOD MANIPULATION

Select words included in the ingredient lists on food package labels divulge that food substances contained inside the packaging are chemically and mechanically **processed** and **refined**.

For example, *high, partially, light, syrup, oil, juice, concentrate, puree, extract, flour, paste, crisps, malt, starch, cream, invert, oligo, instant, isolate, dried, hydrogenated, modified, fractionated, partially defatted, fortified, cultured, flavored,* and *artificial* are all terms that commonly precede or follow natural crude fuel whole earth food ingredient names on food product labels and reveal that some form of chemical or mechanical industrial food processing or refinement occurred prior to delivery of final food products to consumers. Two natural food names combined into one phrase, such as *almond milk,* also indicates the presence of food processing.

11.5 ENTERTAINMENT AND INDULGENCE FOODS

Entertainment and indulgence food products are processed and refined *treat foods* made to potently arouse the taste senses to provide immediate pleasure and moments of personal runaway escape, emotional excitement, or stress release. Frequent consumption of various indulgence food products acts as a gateway to enhance the likelihood of addictification for numerous related commercial food industry products formulated to deliver similar taste experiences. Potentiated consumption of treat foods with "I can't get enough" and "I want more" feelings commonly occurs at parties and celebrations, which plentifully supply indulgence goodies to be consumed freely to enhance the pleasurable enjoyment of festivities at hand.

The addictification food industry promotes mindless munching of conveniently prepackaged indulgence treat foods, which often masquerade under healthy-sounding names to suggest these processed food options are healthier to consume. Routine reliance on entertainment, indulgence, and convenience commercial industry food products to make difficult life experiences more tolerable or "palatable" eventually costs consumers dearly on many different levels. Body vehicle health depends on learning to properly separate out basic maintenance fueling, which optimizes body vehicle function and survival, from indulgence and entertainment activities, to be enjoyed selectively with self-control and appropriate discretion on limited occasions.

Candy and gum are typical examples of chemically engineered oral indulgence food substances that potently deliver on-demand taste pornography. The wizardry of concocting taste pornography flavor experiences to provide multitudes of invented indulgence and entertainment oral sensory taste illusions is exemplified best by the brilliant efforts of flavored jelly bean manufacturers, which masterfully create chemical flavor fantasies that trick taste experiences to keep consumers desiring and coming back for more.

Industry formulated **on-demand indulgence taste products** disrupt natural body vehicle feeding experiences by misinforming fueling sensors of the mouth, digestive tract, and brain, which evolved to understand and gauge fueling information supplied through natural crude fuel whole earth foods. Processed and refined food products are nutritional *imposters* that portray commercially contrived versions of idealized food product qualities, which artificially stimulate taste sensors to drive incessant feeding and promote food product consumption on large scales to profit industry while providing consumers hollow nutritional experiences.

12 INGREDIENT LISTS AND NUTRITION FACTS: FINE PRINT DISCLOSURES AND DISCLAIMERS

Mother Nature delivers foods naturally free from fabricated packaging, containers, attached labels, or informational writing.

Mother Nature provides natural crude fuel whole earth foods directly on trees, bushes, or shrubs; in water or dirt; and flying, swimming, running, slithering, or crawling through the earth, entirely without commercial packaging or labeling.

Labels on containers and wrappers packaging industrially prepared foods include legally obligatory nutritional language known as **ingredient lists and nutrition facts.** Ingredient lists and nutrition facts amount to food product **disclosures and disclaimers** that itemize food product alterations, artificially added ingredients, and the content, deficiency, and potency of select nutrients scientifically known to nutritionally impact body vehicle health.

Food package ingredient lists and nutrition facts disclose how industrial food processing and refinement artificially altered the composition and nutritional components of natural crude fuel whole earth foods. Ingredient and nutritional disclosures on food packaging labels are **legal notifications** that disclaim possible immediate or future body vehicle nutritional imbalances or adverse health consequences that may occur by consuming the artificially modified and manufactured food products.

The print listing ingredients and nutrition facts on food package labeling has noticeably progressively shrunken in size, deliberately creating *fine print* difficult for many older adults to discern and read comfortably without the use of corrective eye lenses. Consumers shopping for food items and trying to make nutritionally healthy food purchases should not have to bring magnifying glasses to read food product labels.

In addition to tiny difficult-to-read print, other misleading food labeling practices deceiving consumers and hiding the toxic realities of processed and refined food products include widely separating food ingredient lists from the nutrition facts labelling on packaging and using noncontrasting colors to blend label writing into background colors, making it harder to read food product information (e.g., small black print writing on a dark blue background).

Ingredient lists summarize the full complement of processed and refined food substances and known additives formulated and combined to produce enticingly tasty designer food product creations. Listed food ingredients serve as a roll call to credit the multitudes of individual artificial food and chemical industry contributions incorporated into final processed food products.

Substituting ingredient lists and nutrition facts with a large *skull and crossbones,* displayed prominently on processed and refined food product packaging, would better alert unwary consumers concerning the actual qualities and benefits of the processed food products concealed within the packaging. If industry highly regarded the nutritional value, health benefits, and human safety of ingredients composing artificially produced foods, text size of listed ingredients would dominantly occupy package wrappings since the ingredients denote the actual food constituents that consumers ingest.

Given that many processed and refined food product packages list many contained ingredients, labels prominently displaying ingredient lists and nutrition facts with large, easy-to-read print would likely cover entire packaging surfaces to obscure visibility windows revealing artificially created designer food products stealthily hidden within the packaging.

12.1 EXPIRATION DATES

Product expiration dates, termed **freshness dates** or **best before dates,** are alerts stamped onto food packaging to provide time limits for "safe" human consumption of industrially manufactured food products, and indirectly estimate when substantial chemical and biological decomposition and deterioration exists to warrant discarding of processed food items. Expiration dates insinuate that to consume food products before expiration dates is safe with limited potential for causing adverse health effects and human toxicity. Manufactured chemicals, including those routinely used as commercial food additives, also have product expiration dates. Although food packages display an overall expiration date for the manufactured food products, the expiration dates applying to the individually mixed-in additives are omitted from food package labels, despite the possibility that some of the additives will chemically expire well before the labeled expiration date for the composite manufactured food products.

Survival among earth life-forms is a constant struggle that involves a continuous competition for scarce natural food resources that provide energy and essential nutrients similarly required by all living organisms to sustain their biological existence. Natural whole earth foods are best for humans to eat when ripe and fresh before significant decay occurs after animals are sacrificed, and plants are harvested for consumption. The flavor of unprocessed natural whole earth foods changes with ripeness to disappear rapidly and become unpalatable as foods go bad on store shelves and during storage.

Chemical and biological decomposition of foods, termed **spoilage,** commences immediately following the harvesting of plants and the sacrifice of animals to be eaten by humans. Spoilage is a natural biological process essential for regenerating biological life, which works to release seeds from plants for germination and decompose dead organic matter into basic life molecules that are recycled in the earth environment to keep other living biological organisms alive. Spoilage occurs substantially through the chemical breakdown of earth foods reacting with oxygen in air or through bacterial and mold microbial decomposition of food products, as microbes compete with humans to feast on available food nutrients to sustain their own growth and viability. Refrigeration slows down the rate of oxidative and chemical breakdown of foods and the growth and biological activity of microorganisms attempting to consume food nutrients.

The overall taste experience of processed foods is an industrially crafted orchestration of artificial and chemical flavors, textures, consistencies, and aromas teaming up to pleasurably stimulate oral taste sensors to promote food product consumption and addictification. Food processing and refinement markedly alter the taste, flavor potencies, and biologic qualities of natural earth foods to change food palatability and shelf life for commercial purposes.

Food spoilage proceeds continuously to progressively decrease the freshness and fraction of remaining food nutrients and steadily increase the percentage of spoilage-generated chemical and biological decomposition by-products and growing microorganisms, all which humans eventually consume in various proportions when eating foods.

Human system sensors are built to recognize natural earth food spoilage and rot, which are conspicuously putrid and aversive to the senses to prevent consumption of spoiled or rotten foods. Artificial food manipulations and additives fool and confuse body vehicle smell and taste sensors to impair their natural abilities to discern subtle food spoilage. The human senses do not readily detect accumulating chemical breakdown by-products progressively generated within artificially manufactured and preserved food products that are spoiling. As processed foods decompose, residual food flavors reflect the concentrated effects on taste sensors of remaining sugars, fats, salt, artificial flavoring agents, and added chemicals until advanced staleness and the rancid taste of spoilage-generated by-products become obvious to the human senses.

Consequently, artificially preserved processed and refined commercial food products require expiration date labeling, which estimates when substantial chemical decay or microbial contamination of food ingredients may be present to pose possible health hazards upon ingestion.

Molds and bacteria are living microorganisms that feed and grow on decaying biologic matter to decompose and recycle basic earth elements contained within life matter back into the earth for reutilization. Conspicuous food rot and visible mold growth on decaying foods suitably serve as natural indicators of food spoilage. Industrially processed foods are specially formulated and contain artificial additives to kill and inhibit the growth of molds and bacteria on treated foods to interfere with microorganism decomposition of food products. Stalling or completely preventing microbial consumption of devitalized biological food products extends opportunities for humans to consume artificially treated foods.

Unfortunately, foods artificially formulated to delay and prevent visible mold growth and food rot that conveniently signal and gauge food spoilage continue to generate and accumulate unseen and difficult to identify chemical and other biological decomposition by-products, while stored or situated on shelves awaiting purchase and consumption.

Human cells evolved to share many biological features with primitive bacterial and mold microorganisms, which are targeted indiscriminately and killed or prevented from consuming and growing on chemically treated and artificially preserved food products. Consequently, scientific claims indicating that artificially preserved food products with their potent chemical additives and progressively accumulating decomposition by-products are entirely safe for humans to consume are extremely suspect.

Therefore, the "freshness date" stamped on processed food packaging is analogous to the "expiration date" that labels various other household chemicals, such as cleaners, paints, pharmaceuticals, and beauty and hygiene products, which alerts that decomposition has affected manufactured product integrity to decrease product potency and pose possible hazards to humans using expired products.

12.2 PRESERVATIVES

The preservation of crude fuel natural whole earth foods involves manufacturing steps that strategically extract and concentrate specific natural whole food constituents, and then artificially formulate and treat extracts or concentrates with certain additives and chemical substances called **preservatives.** Preservatives artificially slow down food constituent decomposition to prolong the commercial availability of food and beverage products for human consumption. Therefore, preservatives artificially pervert and prevent natural biological spoilage of foods.

Food preservatives are often chemically formulated substances potently active in very minute quantities to retard natural food spoilage and unnaturally extend food product shelf life sometimes for years. Preservatives can act as **antibiotics** to sanitize foods by killing or inhibiting the growth or function of microorganisms that normally consume and grow on foods to cause spoilage. Preservatives can also function as chemical **antioxidants** or **stabilizers** that slow and interfere with food spoilage resulting from chemical reactions occurring spontaneously among contained food product ingredients, and through chemical interactions taking place between food product ingredients and oxygen in the air.

Frequent ingestion of potently reactive preservative-type chemicals over a lifetime, particularly through regular consumption of processed and refined food products, can saturate body vehicle tissues and cells with potent chemicals that can disrupt native body vehicle biochemical, metabolic reactions. The body vehicle purposefully generates and uses oxidant molecules to work strategically within many body vehicle life–sustaining metabolic operations. Antioxidant effects of preservatives can interfere with the actions of naturally generated cellular oxidants carrying out important metabolic and immune system roles. The body vehicle possesses complex metabolic, biochemical capabilities to detoxify poisonous chemicals and an elaborate immune system to resist invading rogue microorganisms from gaining unwelcome access into the body vehicle system, which combine to protect body vehicle health and survival continuously. Protective body vehicle metabolic and immune functions clear away externally introduced or internally produced toxins and neutralize attacking microorganisms to defend against inadvertent body vehicle breakdown and demise.

The liver and kidneys are the primary metabolic domains biochemically safeguarding body vehicle existence. The immune system of defense cells circulate protectively within the blood and anchor within various organs such as the liver, spleen, skin, and gut lining barrier membranes.

The body vehicle additionally contains trillions of indwelling microorganisms estimated to outnumber body vehicle cells by a factor of more than 10 to 1, which symbiotically coexist with the body vehicle to preserve health and produce vital biologic substances necessary for the body vehicle to function and survive.

Chemical preservatives having antibiotic properties that are ingested into the body vehicle can indiscriminately kill susceptible indwelling microorganisms to adversely alter strategic symbiotic relationships between resident microorganisms and body vehicle cells, potentially to trigger protective immune responses that may become abnormally sustained and lead to autoimmune health disorders.

Cellular detoxification and immune system activities intimately rely on forming and utilizing specific oxidants to accomplish protective biological actions. Furthermore, protective metabolic and immune functions that collectively destroy incipient cancer cells developing spontaneously within the body vehicle under the stresses of daily living also generate oxidants to carry out their work.

Chemically reactive antioxidant food preservatives disperse throughout the body vehicle to indiscriminately bind up body vehicle generated oxidants and compromise detoxification and immune system operations, impairing protective cellular and tissue responses against toxins and invading microorganisms to predispose the body vehicle to toxicities and infections. Disturbed immune function with aberrant immune activity may also lead to the development of autoimmune disorders and cancer.

Additionally, metabolically reactive chemical food additives may damage delicate digestive system barrier linings upon ingestion to produce leaky gut membranes, through which toxins and unfriendly bacteria normally confined to the gut can penetrate to access the blood and enter protected body vehicle areas, to increase body vehicle toxicity and infection risks to compromise health and survival further.

Lastly, preservatives acting as antibiotics may eliminate the strategic balances and composition of gut microorganisms necessary to protect against invasion and attack by unfriendly pathologic microbes, thus rendering the body vehicle more vulnerable to opportunistic infections that undermine body vehicle health.

Chemical preservation of food is akin to the process of embalming a corpse since during food preservation, devitalized or sacrificed crude fuel whole earth foods are sanitized, treated to prevent spoilage well beyond natural decomposition times, and cosmetically enhanced to create a presentable appearance for a long wake on the shelf.

In defense of commercial food processing industries, food preservation is not intended to poison consumers with preservatives and other additive chemical ingredients. Food preservation considerately extends consumers a courtesy to save money by allowing foods to last indefinitely on store shelves or in storage until foods are purchased or consumed, thereby minimizing wastage occurring when foods "prematurely" spoil and must be discarded. Undoubtedly, food preservation provides consumers much more than they bargained to receive.

12.3 COMMERCIAL FOOD ADDITIVES

Chemical food preservatives, taste stabilizers, texturizing agents, emulsifiers allowing immiscible food ingredients to mix, and various other food additives, such as artificial sweeteners, colors, and flavors, are all artificially manufactured substances concocted through large-scale industrial, chemical processes.

Not only do the various individual food additives have the potential to cause body vehicle toxicity but the aggregate effects of mixtures of these additives may induce even greater overall toxicities against body vehicle health and survival.

The manufacture of commercial food additives employs complex formulations between multitudes of potentially toxic chemical ingredients that are combined to produce final form chemical additives. Many of these chemical formulations unpredictably generate minute quantities of toxic chemical reaction by-products that unavoidably contaminate the manufacturing processes synthesizing the additives.

Impurities generated during the chemical manufacture of food additives, which are chemically inseparable from the additives, are additional sources of toxins that become inadvertently introduced into the body vehicle upon ingestion of additive-containing foods. These undesirable impurities generated chemically through the industrial manufacture of foods and food additives are incorporated collectively into final processed food products usually below amounts detectable by usual food purity testing or, alternatively, may even acceptably fall within levels deemed to be "safe" for human consumption per industry standards to be unwittingly ingested in processed foods.

99.99% product purity translates to 1/10,000 potentially toxic particles introduced as contaminants within a given quantity of substance consumed, potentially to accumulate significantly within the body vehicle during a lifetime of consuming contaminated products. For instance, 6 ounces of food product providing 10,000,000,000,000,000,000 total molecules of food substance having 99.99% product purity would undesirably deliver 0.01% (1/10,000) or 1,000,000,000,000,000 total molecules of impurities that contaminate the body vehicle.

Many processed foods contain higher than 1% (1/100) concentration levels of preservatives, and other potential toxins incorporated per food serving size, and therefore introduce substantial amounts of these toxic substances into the body vehicle upon food product consumption.

Some of the unique chemical properties of food additives that are employed to formulate processed food product ingredients may be the exact source of toxic body vehicle effects. Oil and water do not mix and separate after standing for a while even after vigorous mixing. Similarly, food ingredients that dissolve into oil will separate from food ingredients that dissolve with water. Chemical agents called **emulsifiers** act as detergents that split up and disperse individual oil and water molecules to disrupt their natural tendency to separate from each other, thereby permitting smooth blending of oil- and water-based ingredients into a more uniform mixture.

Some of the more commonly used food emulsifiers are polysorbate 80, carrageenan, and carboxymethyl cellulose, which are added to foods in small, 1% quantities to disperse and allow mixing of ordinarily immiscible food product ingredients that otherwise separate out within processed foods in the absence of emulsifying agents.

Body vehicle membranes possess oil and water characteristics that allow directionality of function and containment of critical cellular and tissue contents. A protective mucus slime layer having oil and water properties and known as **biofilm** also coats the lining membranes of the gut. The detergent properties of emulsifier agents chemically dissolve and strip away this mucus slime layer protectively coating intestinal lining cells and disrupt the oil and water matrix of cellular and tissue membranes.

Stripping away the gut mucus slime layer and disrupting gut cell membranes renders intestinal lining cells defenseless and compromises gut barriers, predisposing harmful bacteria and toxins ordinarily confined to the gut to readily cross into the blood. Scientific studies on the biological safety of food additives screen for apparent illness, biologic or metabolic disruption, or death occurring in test animals or human subjects receiving additives at relatively higher doses over shorter time periods and may not assess for subtle biological, cellular, or behavioral effects developing after additives are consumed repeatedly at lower doses over prolonged durations.

Subtle and undetected adverse health effects accumulate to cause serious harm following repeated and prolonged substance usage, especially in genetically susceptible individuals and developing children, and may even compound the harmful effects of other chemical substances, such as medications being taken for specific reasons.

Commercial producers of industrially manufactured food products and chemical food additives can conveniently defend food contamination with tiny amounts of potentially toxic substances determined to have negligible adverse health effects, when substances receive GRAS approvals following scientific inquiries by "experts" in the field.

12.4 FOOD CONTAMINANTS

Large-scale manufacture and preparation of food products in industrial facilities additionally risks unintentional food product contamination during the manufacturing process through numerous other avenues, including

1. incorporation of environmental impurities and other contaminants such as pesticides and herbicides harbored by original raw food ingredients that are introduced during processing into final food products
2. utilization of spoiled food ingredients
3. unrecognized bacterial and mold contamination of food ingredients and food products
4. accidental inclusion of insects and small animals or animal components, such as hair, which may fall into and mix within food products being produced on large scales in factory facilities.
5. inadvertent or excessive addition of chemical ingredients introduced unnoticeably or through mechanized processing errors during routine food production
6. contamination of food products while being transported on conveyor belts during the manufacturing process, as has been surmised for dangerous **phthalate** (plastic softener) contamination of macaroni and cheese food products

Governmental food inspection agencies such as the FDA set levels and limits for contaminants that industrial food producers can "safely" deliver to consumers in industrially mass-produced processed food and beverage products.

Unrecognized and unregulated contamination of foods with pesticides, herbicides and weed killers, antibiotics and various other antimicrobials, hormones, and potent fertilizers introduced into the environment and the food chain are also increasing in modern, industrialized societies, which incorporate large-scale food production and manufacturing practices catering to growing world population food demands.

Residues of chemical cleansers used to scrub and sanitize industrial vats utilized for large-scale production of food products and chemical food additives are additional sources of impurities that contaminate industrially prepared food products.

Complete food product purity is inconceivable when the industrial manufacture of processed and refined food and beverage products is mechanized and involves numerous automated steps and the timeline between harvest or sacrifice of individual natural whole earth food ingredients and product preparation, store delivery, and human consumption can be several months or longer.

The difficulties in maintaining complete product purity during commercial manufacturing are highlighted during the industrial production of commercial-grade apple sauce, whereby hundreds of thousands of apples are processed daily using automated technologies that stream apples rapidly on conveyor belts under limited worker oversight, making the thorough scrubbing of all pesticide residues and herbicides and the meticulous physical removal of insects and rotten parts from all passing apples virtually impossible.

It is unsurprising that multitudes of industrially prepared commercial food items are recalled regularly after causing epidemic human illnesses and creating potential population health risks because of food product contamination with microbes, toxic chemicals, and other foreign substances. Ingesting industrially prepared foods with all intentionally added or inadvertently included contaminants and impurities introduced during production challenges body vehicle health and survival.

The immediate and future body vehicle toxicities resulting from excessive ingestion of food additives, environmental and production contaminants, and a myriad of other unknown chemical by-products generated during progressive spoilage of packaged foods laced with preservatives are *unknown.*

It is reassuring that fresh, natural, crude fuel, whole earth foods can be more easily inspected to confirm freshness and remove obvious contaminants, and then thoroughly scrubbed to reduce contamination with undesirable impurities before ingestion or use in recipes.

12.5 CONTAINERS AND WRAPPERS

Containers and wrappers encase and store commercially prepared foods and beverages awaiting purchase and consumption. Storage containers are industrially manufactured products made from various substances, which are molded and constructed into assorted shapes and sizes and often additionally treated with protective coatings applied to inside storage vessel surfaces in contact with contained foods or beverages.

Synthetic petroleum-based hydrocarbons, such as plastics; real, "organic" substances, including natural rubber, wood, and other plant-based materials; glass, porcelain, and ceramic; or metals, particularly aluminum and tin, are some of the elements commonly utilized to make food and beverage storage containers and wrappers. Storage containers and inner container surfaces not made of nonreactive or more chemically inert ingredients, such as glass and porcelain, are often impregnated with preservative substances to slow the natural chemical degradation and disintegration of container materials.

Decomposition of storage vessels and any substances coating inside vessel surfaces releases numerous chemical substances, which leach into and contaminate food products or goods being contained or wrapped, especially when foods are heated within storage vessels to accelerate release of container chemicals, and during prolonged storage of foods and beverages that remain in contact with chemically decomposing vessels.

Container vessel chemicals entering the body vehicle through ingestion of contained consumable products can exert toxic health effects to cause various health conditions including cancer, immune compromise, and glandular or hormonal dysfunction, and can perturb the natural composition, balance, and activity of indwelling symbiotic microbial organisms to compromise body vehicle health even further.

The potential for the toxic mineral lead to leach from storage vessels into contained food and beverage products and cause severe neurotoxicity especially in developing children is one reason why lead use in dishware and beverage containers is banned. The growth and prosperity of container recycling industries reflect the increasing human reliance on storing foods, beverages, and other physical items in disposable, artificially manufactured, and frequently nonbiodegradable containers that pose numerous health and survival risks to humanity.

The world would be less polluted chemically if humans substantially prepared and ate freshly grown, natural, crude fuel, whole earth foods at home to reduce the need for using toxic containers. The body vehicle cleanly combusts natural, crude fuel, whole earth foods such as fruits, vegetables, nuts, seeds, and animal flesh essentially entirely into carbon dioxide and water, with remaining waste products eliminated as biodegradable feces and urine that recycle safely back into the earth environment.

12.6 BPA OR BISPHENOL A

BPA (bisphenol A) is a chemical compound commonly used in the manufacture of plastics, particularly of containers made to encase consumable foods and liquids, and additionally constitutes the thin plastic film that coats the internal surfaces of metal and aluminum cans in contact with container-stored food and beverage products.

BPA has been detected progressively in human blood and tissue samples since being introduced and utilized industrially in the manufacture of food storage containers. Scientific studies have associated rising blood and tissue levels of BPA in humans with infertility, increased cancer risk, and childhood obesity and behavioral health problems.

BPA is one such example of many other unlisted, unrecognized, or undefined toxic chemical substances composing storage containers which can migrate into and indirectly contaminate stored food and beverage products to poison the body vehicle when consumed along with container-stored products, potentially leading to numerous immediate and delayed adverse health consequences.

12.7 PFCs (PERFLUORINATED CHEMICALS) AND PFASS (POLYFLUOROALKYL SUBSTANCES)

PFCs (perfluorinated chemicals) and **PFASs** (polyfluoroalkyl substances) are used in manufactured products to resist grease and stains and in cookware to prevent sticking.

Fast-food packaging wrappers, cartons, and boxes are commonly treated with PFCs and PFASs to keep food products from bleeding through and sticking to packaging. PFCs and PFASs leach from packaging materials into contained foods and then are ingested along with food products to accumulate and linger within body vehicle tissues. PFCs and PFASs have been scientifically linked to cancer, thyroid disorders, and compromised immunity in humans.

12.8 TROJAN HORSE

The **Trojan horse** tale embodies the concept of unsuspected compromise and destruction occurring from within and fittingly applies to body vehicle fueling choices when special, well-deserved "feel good" food rewards enticingly wrapped in seductive packaging are introduced into the body vehicle as an indulgence or gesture of goodwill consequently to wreck body vehicle health.

The original mythical tale about the Trojan horse describes a lengthy stand-off in ancient Greece between two warring armies. One army, secured inside an impenetrable self-sustaining fortress, successfully repelled all attacks from an army gathered outside the stronghold. The army outside the fortress deceived the army inside to let down its guard and open its doors to accept into its protected compound an inviting Trojan horse gift secretly concealing the enemy, which then invaded, captured, and destroyed the fortress from within.

Therefore, a Trojan horse surreptitiously lowers resistance to pierce the veil of defense to conquer, subjugate, and destroy.

Once introduced through the mouth, a Trojan horse invader
unmercifully unleashes concealed contents that attack and break
down the body vehicle system from within.

Consequently, avoid introducing that Trojan horse into the mouth, because it will attack the body vehicle system from the inside to wreak havoc and destruction in its path.

Among the major accomplishments of advanced and modern civilizations, sanitation with societal waste and sewage disposal has been a crowning achievement. Reducing environmental pollution, providing a clean water supply, and furnishing sanitation services to remove and dispose of societal wastes and contamination dramatically improve human health and survival.

Paradoxically, while modern society increasingly focuses efforts on reducing and cleaning up the contamination of external living environments, humans progressively contaminate and pollute their internal body vehicle environments. Chemical pollution of the body vehicle occurs obviously through toxic environmental exposures and less noticeably through consumption of processed food product additives, ingestion of pharmaceutical agents and health supplements, inhalation of recreational substances of abuse, and absorption of beauty and hygiene products through the skin and oral cavity membranes. Analyses of hair and nail samples in human populations disclose the widespread degree of toxic human exposures to chemical substances over time.

The body vehicle demands the very best fuel and maintenance care to function at the highest levels, which infinitely surpass any levels achievable by the most intricately engineered and manufactured machines, such as the finest race cars or modern fighter jets. If owner's manuals for outlandishly expensive, commercially manufactured machine products provided specific fuel and maintenance care guidelines to ensure optimal product durability and performance, few owners would foolishly ignore manufacturer recommendations and needlessly face the prospect of paying exorbitant costs to repair an expensive machine breakdown brought on by neglecting recommended product care.

Unfortunately, many ignore providing their body vehicles with appropriate fueling and maintenance care, despite risking the potential consequences of losing health and having to pay astronomical costs to repair body vehicle damages to restore health, with the caveat that no comparable commercially available replacement parts exist for irreparably damaged body vehicle components.

Fortunately, Mother Nature conveniently supplies the most premium fuels and nutrients in naturally appropriate compositions and packaging and at the lowest costs necessary to maintain optimum body vehicle health and performance over intended body vehicle lifetimes, ultimately to greatly reduce health care costs and personal suffering.

12.9 BUYER BEWARE

Think naturally outside the box and independently of containers.

Be on guard for foods packaged with ingredient list and nutritional facts labels divulging industrial alteration of foods from their natural forms. Read all food product labels carefully and thoroughly. Ignorance is no excuse for suffering adverse health consequences by eating packaged and processed industrial food products laced with chemical ingredients and other contaminants, which are deliberately added or inadvertently taint food products during manufacture or through migration from packaging and wrappers.

Unnaturally long food product expiration times plainly broadcast dangers to body vehicle health and survival lurking inside the packaging.

13 GLOBALISM GROWTH

In modern industrial societies, automated and mechanized industrial production, expanding communication technologies, and growing transportation modalities facilitate the growth and international globalism of businesses to enhance the opportunities, penetration, and profitability of addictification industries in new markets having burgeoning consumer demands.

The commercial food industry aims to profit by servicing new markets or by growing people bigger, and preferably by doing both.

As addicitifcation industries increasingly globalize, the human size grows progressively more massive worldwide.

13.1 BODY MASS INDEX OR BMI

The body vehicle has a structural framework that functions as a scaffold to hold body vehicle flesh. The body vehicle structural framework consists of the bones, ligaments, muscles, and other fibrous elements designed to optimally support and move around the entire body vehicle.

Body vehicle flesh can be divided simplistically into two basic categories: **working flesh,** such as the brain, muscles, and various body vehicle organs, including the heart, lungs, liver, kidneys, intestines, and blood, and **cargo flesh,** such as the fat cells that store fat energy and also comprise the tissues that pack body vehicle cavities to keep the organs in place. Body vehicle health and longevity deteriorate faster when the structural framework supports and carries too much flesh or has insufficient flesh to mobilize the body vehicle.

A crude analogy to illustrate the importance of having an appropriate balance between the body vehicle supporting and working elements and the cargo components considers optimal size relationships among structural and working elements and carried cargo for a pickup truck.

Pickup truck structural components include vehicle frame and chassis, suspension system, and wheels and axles; working parts consist of the engine and transmission, and cargo is what loads into the cargo bed for transport and does not contribute to vehicle work.

Consequently, if a particular pickup truck has a maximal cargo load carrying capacity of 2,500 lbs., then trucking around loads weighing more than 2,500 lbs.

for extended periods of time would accelerate the wear and tear of various truck components, such as the engine, transmission, suspension system, brakes, and tires, to shorten the expected life-span of working parts and also of the truck itself.

A small and underpowered engine, flimsier suspension, and weaker transmission also lead to imbalances that lessen the performance and life-span of truck components and the truck itself, especially under increased work demands imposed on the vehicle.

Likewise, medical science defines an optimal range of sizes for the body vehicle associated with lower risks for illness and premature death and higher odds for maximizing body vehicle health, function, and survival. Ideal proportions exist between the total mass of the entire body vehicle and the size of the structural framework having to support that total mass.

The **Body Mass Index (BMI)** is defined as the total body vehicle mass (structural framework + working and cargo flesh) in kilograms divided by the body vehicle height in meters squared:

$$BMI = MASS \text{ (kilograms)} \div HEIGHT^2 \text{ (meters}^2) = kg/m^2$$

whereby 1 kilogram (kg) ≈ 2.2 pounds (lbs.), and 1 meter (m) ≈ 39.4 inches (in). A sample BMI calculation for a 5 foot 6-inch-tall adult weighing 155 lbs. is as follows:

155 lbs. ÷ 2.2 lbs./kg ≈ 70.5 kg, and 5 ft 6 in = 66 in ÷ 39.4 in/m ≈ 1.68 m
$BMI = 70.5 \text{ kg} \div (1.68 \text{ m})^2 ≈ 25 \text{ kg/m}^2$

The **optimal body vehicle BMI range = 18.5–24.9 kg/m²** and is statistically associated with the lowest illness and mortality risks and best odds of health and survival. BMI levels **above 24.9** are considered **overweight** and **below 18.5 underweight**.[4]

Therefore, the BMI is a mathematically derived relationship between the entire amount of body vehicle (mass) and the frame size (height) that completely supports or carries around the whole body vehicle. The height in meters squared essentially designates the area (height²) of a square platform that supports the body vehicle mass. As mass increases, a constant platform area calculated by squaring the height becomes less capable of safely holding up an enlarging body vehicle. Simply, *BMI calculates a **health ratio** between weight (mass in kilograms) and height* (in meters squared).

BMI calculations for various height and weight relationships relate to body vehicle *health and survival odds* and the risks of experiencing certain disease states and premature death. The risks of developing health problems and shortening the life-span to die prematurely increase progressively beyond the extremes of the optimum BMI range.

---

4. Online BMI applications readily calculate BMI values for various individual height and weight measurements.

A BMI above 30 may reduce life expectancy by a few years, while a BMI above 40 or substantially below 18.5 may lower life expectancy by decades, as evidenced by the reality that very few 5-foot-tall individuals weighing 300 pounds or 6-foot-tall individuals weighing 100 pounds reach 80 or 90 years of age.

When the BMI is too low, the body vehicle has insufficient working flesh to motor around all the structural and flesh components, whereas at a high BMI too much flesh is overloading the body vehicle structural framework, which sounds various alarms that include elevations in blood pressure, sugar, and cholesterol levels; back, hip, and lower extremity pains; breathing difficulties; excessive tiredness and fatigue; and numerous other symptoms.

Therefore, BMI extremes are associated with higher odds for the body vehicle to break down and die for various reasons.

When gambling to maximize health and survival in the game of life, body vehicle physical sizes matter, and the BMI serves as a useful parameter corresponding to the odds for body vehicle health and survival within a broad range of nutritionally influenced body vehicle dimensions.

13.2 IDEAL BODY WEIGHT OR IBW

The **ideal body weight (IBW)** is an alternative scientific computation that approximates a biologically appropriate balance between body vehicle height and weight, which is useful for calculating pharmacologic medication dosing in humans. The IBW also serves as a guide specifying the desirable weights for various heights that lower health and mortality risks but has limits estimating the appropriate weight for tall men and short women.

> *Male IBW estimate*: 106 lbs. of weight for the first 5 feet of height plus 6 lbs. of weight for each additional inch of height above 5 feet (add 10% extra weight for a large body vehicle frame size and subtract 10% weight for a small frame size).

> *Female IBW estimate*: 100 lbs. of weight for the first 5 feet of height plus 5 lbs. of weight for each additional inch of height above 5 feet (add 10% extra weight for a large body vehicle frame size and subtract 10% weight for a small frame size).

Thus, the ideal body weight (IBW) target range falls within 10% of the calculated IBW for height (IBW ± 10%).

13.3 OBESITY

Obesity is the body vehicle state of being overfueled and carrying greatly excessive nonworking cargo flesh as fat fuel reserves that increase risks for developing detrimental health consequences and a shorter body vehicle life-span.

By definition, obesity = BMI $\geq$ 30 kg/m^2, according to the Centers for Disease Control and Prevention (CDC).

Obesity develops gradually as body vehicle fuel consumption continually outpaces body vehicle fuel energy demands and utilization capacities.

Fat is the most concentrated storage form of body vehicle fuel energy. A body vehicle that repetitively fuels excessively will over time progressively accumulate surplus fuels in **fat cells** distributed strategically throughout the body vehicle that are ready to release stored fat energy on-demand for metabolic utilization.

Fatness reflects possession of overly abundant body vehicle fuel surpluses consisting of more fuel than a body vehicle can metabolically burn to meet routine fuel energy requirements for daily existence. Continual deposits of fuel into fat energy storage banks progressively increase body vehicle cargo flesh to compromise health and survival.

People do not choose to be obese.
Consumers are not at fault for overfueling and becoming obese and
unhealthy.

Individuals become obese because they are earmarked and cultivated by commercial industries, which employ target demographics and sophisticated marketing techniques to identify and manipulate the fueling, survival behaviors of vulnerable consumers. Commercial food industries search for the best bait and hook to capture the segments of humanity most vulnerable to fuel excessively and massively profit industry.

Addictification industry food engineering and mind control marketing techniques create human food energy sponges that insatiably absorb empty processed food calories to stoke primal feeding craves. Addictified consumers exchange their money to gorge uncontrollably on commercial food products to experience fleeting, artificially induced taste pleasures and feed industry profits.

Ultimately, consumers are manipulated, herded, and sacrificed to fuel industry prosperity with their *lifetimes,* analogously to how human lives were used to power machines in the movie *The Matrix.*

The societal obesity pandemic that is escalating to epidemic proportions exposes the diligent combined work accomplishments of addictification and rescue industries to increase their growth, penetration, and profitability within human societies. The increasing obesity epidemic, 32% of U.S. adults in 2012 estimated to climb to 40% by 2030 (according to the CDC), reveals the societal failures to control rampant obesity and the "sickening" successes of food industry tactics to keep human addictification growing. Consequently, the quest to fight obesity must begin from a deeply held conviction to strive for true health and longevity, adopted as the only appropriate means for the body vehicle to exist.

Reliance on outside institutions, such as the government and governmental agencies, processed food industries, pharmaceutical and health supplement rescue industries, or health care societies, to fight obesity is doomed to failure since these sectors profit immensely from societal food addictification and the consequent development of fueling disorders that require expensive rescue industry bail-outs leading to dependification.

Only the most gullible hens trust the fox to guard the henhouse.

Human expenses are corporate industry earnings.

Humanity funds the growing profits of corporate and commercial industries at its own expense and often to its own detriment. Corporate economic returns are immensely greater by investing advertising dollars to promote and finance addictification and dependification systems of human control and exploitation than by spending money to help humanity live healthier naturally. Human addictification and dependification are markedly profitable for commercial and corporate interests, while empowering humankind by promoting self-sufficiency free of commercial and corporate interests is unprofitable.

Obesity and attendant fueling disorders create lucrative business opportunities for commercial industries. Obesity is a pipeline supplying society with jobs and leading to commercial industry growth and prosperity at the expense of individuals and societal finances. Considerable business revenues, tax dollars, and livelihoods would vanish from society if human addictification and fueling disorders, which substantially drive the profitability of rescue industries and the economies of burgeoning world economies, ceased to exist and generate their enormous industry profit opportunities.

Numerous economic indicators plainly demonstrate how human lives fund addictification and rescue industry profits to cost society dearly at the expense of societal health and finances. A conspicuous ∫-shaped curve ubiquitously evident in various socioeconomic time plot graphs peculiarly reveals how human existence economically translates into commercial industry profitability.

The S-shaped **Humanity Economic Subjugation Curve ∫ (HESC)** reflects the inherent economic relationship between the growth of adverse human conditions, the increase in commercial activities imposing a costly toll on humanity, and the progressive rise in corporate and commercial industry prosperity.

For example, the following several pages chart various societal health and economic measures against time for economically relevant human circumstances, depicting strikingly similar HESC ∫-shaped curves.

Obesity rates have gradually increased over the past 40 years for both men and women from approximately 15% in the late 1970s to greater than 35% approaching the year 2020.

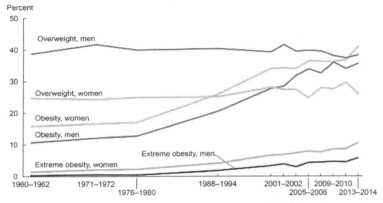

Trends in adult overweight, obesity, and extreme obesity among men and women aged 20–74: United States, 1960–1962 through 2013–2014

NOTES: Age-adjusted by the direct method to the year 2000 U.S. Census Bureau estimates using age groups 20–39, 40–59, and 60–74. Overweight is body mass index (BMI) of 25 kg/m² or greater but less than 30 kg/m²; obesity is BMI greater than or equal to 30; and extreme obesity is BMI greater than or equal to 40. Pregnant females were excluded from the analysis.
SOURCES: NCHS, National Health Examination Survey and National Health and Nutrition Examination Surveys.

https://www.niddk.nih.gov/health-information/health-statistics/overweight-obesity

Over the past four decades, children have also become progressively more obese with obesity starting younger in life with approximately 10% of 2- to 5-year-old children and 15% of teenagers considered obese by 2010 compared to a 5% obesity rate among all children in the mid-1970s.

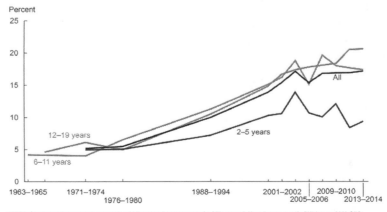

Trends in obesity among children and adolescents aged 2–19 years, by age: United States, 1963–1965 through 2013–2014

NOTES: Obesity is defined as body mass index (BMI) greater than or equal to the 95th percentile from the sex-specific BMI-for-age 2000 CDC Growth Charts.
SOURCES: NCHS, National Health Examination Surveys II (ages 6–11) and III (ages 12–17); and National Health and Nutrition Examination Surveys (NHANES) I–III, and NHANES 1999–2000, 2001–2002, 2003–2004, 2005–2006, 2007–2008, 2009–2010, 2011–2012, and 2013–2014.

https://www.niddk.nih.gov/health-information/health-statistics/overweight-obesity

The 1980s saw diabetes rates rise to parallel the progressive increase in obesity rates.

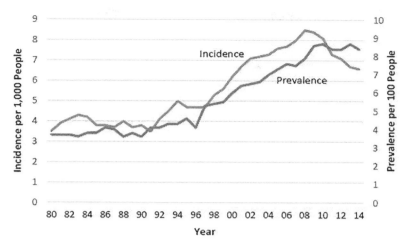

https://www.cdc.gov/chronicdisease/resources/publications/aag/diabetes.htm
https://gis.cdc.gov/grasp/diabetes/DiabetesAtlas.html
https://www.cdc.gov/diabetes/pdfs/data/statistics/national-diabetes-statistics-report.pdf
https://www.cdc.gov/diabetes/statistics/slides/maps_diabetes_trends.pdf

Coincidentally, outpatient visit and hospitalization rates for all digestive disorders also started to increase progressively from 1990 through 2004.

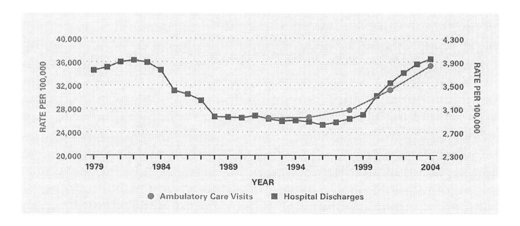

All Digestive Diseases: Age-Adjusted Rates of Ambulatory Care Visits and Hospital Discharges With All–Listed Diagnoses in the United States, 1979–2004. Source: National Ambulatory Medical Care Survey (NAMCS) and National Hospital Ambulatory Medical Care Survey (NHAMCS) (averages 1992–1993, 1994–1996, 1997–1999, 2000–2002, 2003–2005), and National Hospital Discharge Survey (NHDS). Niddk.nih.gov / Strategic Plans Reports / Burden of Digestive Diseases in the United States Report https://www.niddk.nih.gov/about-niddk/strategic-plans-reports/burden-of-digestive-diseases-in-united-states/burden-of-digestive-diseases-in-the-united-states-report#CHAPTER1

Likewise, rates for hospitalizations and outpatient medical attention for inflammatory bowel diseases similarly increased progressively between 1990 to 2004, with more recent data published in the journal *Gastroenterology* in January 2017 showing a continuation of this trend in modern, westernized societies.

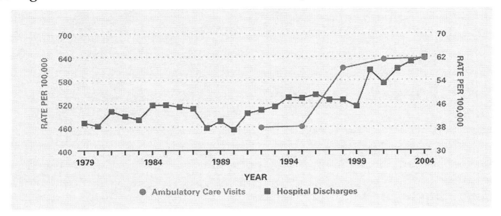

All Inflammatory Bowel Disease: Age-Adjusted Rates of Ambulatory Care Visits and Hospital Discharges With All-Listed Diagnoses in the United States, 1979–2004. Source: National Ambulatory Medical Care Survey (NAMCS) and National Hospital Ambulatory Medical Care Survey (NHAMCS) (averages 1992–1993, 1994–1996, 1997–1999, 2000–2002, 2003–2005), and National Hospital Discharge Survey (NHDS). Niddk.nih.gov/ Strategic Plans Reports / Burden of Digestive Diseases in the United States Report https://www.niddk.nih.gov/about-niddk/strategic-plans-reports/burden-of-digestive-diseases-in-united-states/burden-of-digestive-diseases-in-the-united-states-report#CHAPTER1

A 25% increase in the total daily U.S. per capita caloric intake of food calories between the late 1970s and 2010 coincides temporally with the rise in obesity, diabetes, and digestive health disorder rates.

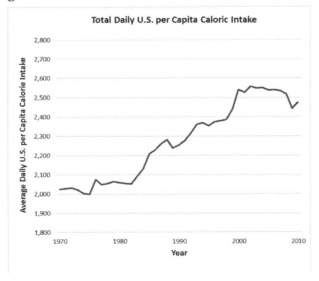

Source: Graph generated using Excel spread sheet data sets available from USDA Economic Research Service Food Availability (Per Capita) Data

The total daily U.S. per capita consumption of calorically dense processed and refined food products also increased from the late 1970s to 2010 with the intake of flour and cereal products increasing 45%, added fats and oils and dairy fats increasing 65%, and added sugars and sweeteners increasing 15%.

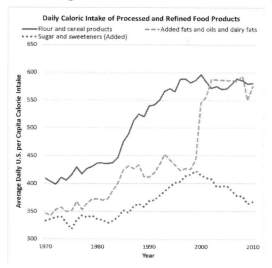

Source: Graph generated using Excel spread sheet data sets available from USDA Economic Research Service Food Availability (Per Capita) Data

The wheat industry has profited between the 1970s and 2014 from the increase in wheat consumption among U.S. consumers eating more calories in the form of flour and cereal products.

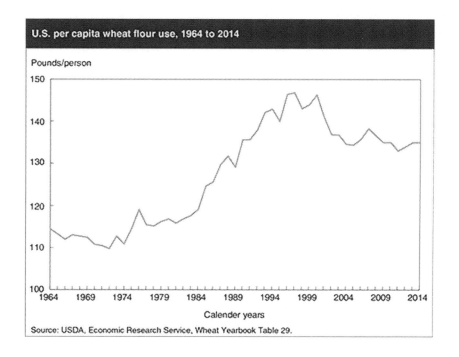

The corn industry has also thrived from the late 1970s as U.S. society has increasingly consumed corn sweeteners that contribute to the excessive caloric intake.

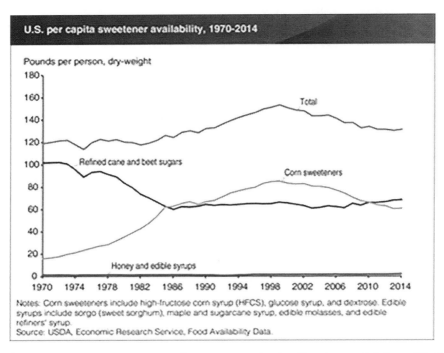

U.S. domestic consumption of various calorically dense high milk-fat dairy products additionally contributing to excessive caloric intake has also risen since the 1990s to parallel the increasing obesity rates.

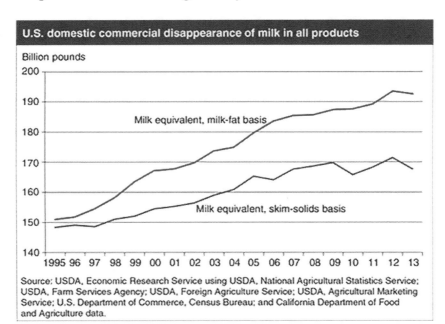

Increasing cheese consumption has been a significant part of the rising U.S. per capita domestic consumption of dairy products.

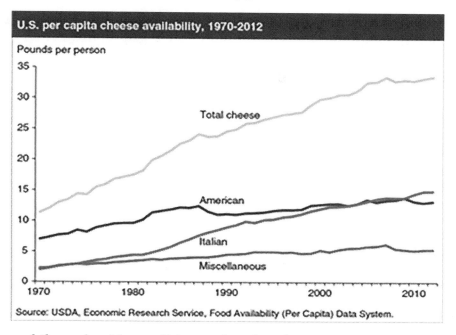

Meanwhile, as health conditions related to the inappropriate fueling of the body vehicle have escalated since the 1980s, the need for pharmacologic rescue interventions for various fueling associated health disorders has continued to grow unimpeded to progressively increase drug company revenues.

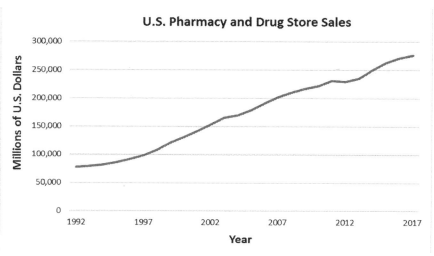

Data source: Graph generated using Excel spread sheet data sets available from https://www.census.gov/retail/index.html; census.gov / Business and Industry / Time Series / Trend Charts / Retail Trade and Food Services 1992–2018 / U.S Pharmacy and Drug Store Sales-Not Seasonally Adjusted; https://www.census.gov/econ/currentdata/dbsearch?program=MRTS&startYear=1992&endYear=2018&categories=44611&data-Type=SM&geoLevel=US&notAdjusted=1&submit=GET+DATA&releaseScheduleId=

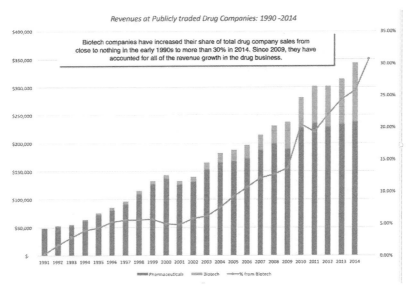

Source: http://aswathdamodaran.blogspot.com / Musings on Markets / Divergence in the Drug Businesses: Pharmaceuticals and Biotechnology. Aswath Damodaran, November 10, 2015; http://aswathdamodaran.blogspot.com/2015/11/divergence-in-drug-businesses.html. Reprinted with permission from the author, Dr. Aswath Damodaran.

U.S. society pays dearly for its progressive health decline as evidenced by a steady growth of U.S. national health expenditures as a share of Gross Domestic Product (GDP), which increased from 5% of GDP in 1960 to approximately 18% of GDP in 2015, despite worsening in the health status of U.S. society. Notably, national health expenditures increased over 12,000 % while the GDP grew less than 3500% between 1960 and 2015, creating ever greater economic demands on U.S. society to fund its health care needs.

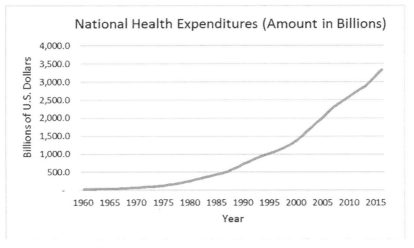

Graph 1. National health expenditures increased by 12,000% between 1960 and 2015. Source: cms.gov / Centers for Medicare and Medicaid Services Data

Graphs 1–4 illustrate the rising costs of U.S. health care with national health expenditures soaring since the late 1970s to parallel the increasing consumption of calories and processed and refined food products and rising obesity rates.[5]

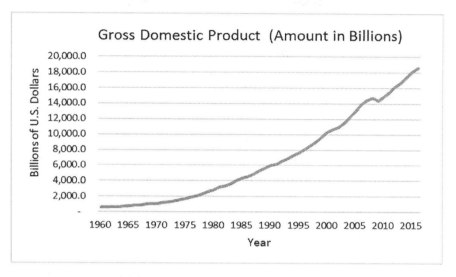

Graph 2. U.S. Gross domestic product increased by 3500% between 1960 and 2015. Source: cms.gov / Centers for Medicare and Medicaid Services Data

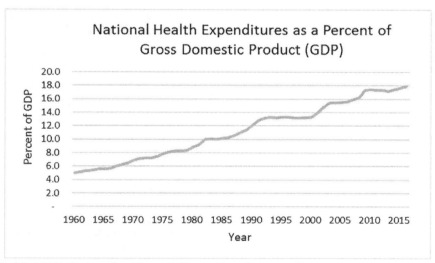

Graph 3. U.S. National health expenditures grew from 5% of GDP in 1960 to 18% of GDP in 2015. Source: cms.gov / Centers for Medicare and Medicaid Services Data

---

5 Graphs 1–4 were generated using Excel spread sheet data sets available at cms.gov / Centers for Medicare and Medicaid Services / Historical / NHE Summary including share of GDP, CY 1960–2016, https://www.cms.gov/Research-Statistics-Data-and-Systems/Statistics-Trends-and-Reports/NationalHealthExpendData/NationalHealthAccountsHistorical.html

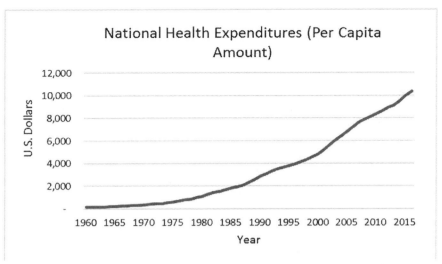

Graph 4. U.S. Per capita national health expenditures grew 7088% from 1960 to 2015
Source: cms.gov / Centers for Medicare and Medicaid Services Data

Based on average hourly earnings data from the current employment statistics survey (national), the average hourly earnings of production and nonsupervisory employees grew only approximately 1000% between 1960 and 2015.

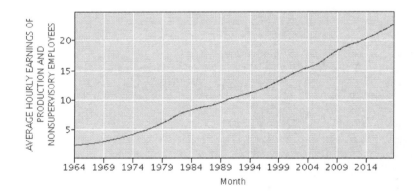

Graph data shows approximately a 900% increase in average hourly earnings between 1964 and 2015 of production and nonsupervisory employees with hourly wages increasing from $2.50/hr. in January 1964 to $22.81/hr. in September 2015, averaging roughly a 4% yearly wage increase. Extrapolating the 4% average yearly wage increase between the years 1964 to 2015 back to January 1960 provides an estimated hourly wage of $2.13/hr. for Jan 1960 that translates into an approximate wage increase of 1000% from 1960 to 2015, which falls markedly short to fund the 12,000% growth of national health expenditures during this period. Source: U.S. Department of Labor Bureau of Labor and Statistics / Data Tools / Databases, Tables & Calculators by Subject / Employment, Hours, and Earnings from the Current Employment Statistics survey (National), https://data.bls.gov/pdq/SurveyOutputServlet

Based on data available for the 10-year period from March 2006 to March 2016, average hourly earnings of all U.S. private employees increased only approximately

27% while the total and per capita national health expenditures skyrocketed 154% and 143% respectively during the same period.

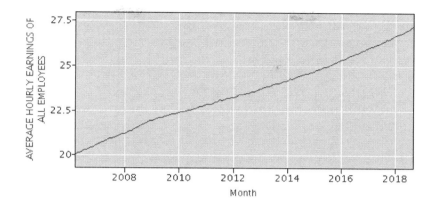

Average hourly earnings of all employees, total private, seasonally adjusted. Source: U.S. Department of Labor Bureau of Labor and Statistics / Data Tools / Databases, Tables & Calculators by Subject / Employment, Hours, and Earnings from the Current Employment Statistics survey (National), https://data.bls.gov/pdq/SurveyOutput-Servlet

Graphs 5–7 illustrate the rising U.S. federal and public debts between 1960 and 2015, which also increased sharply upwards starting in the late 1970s when obesity rates began to rise.[6]

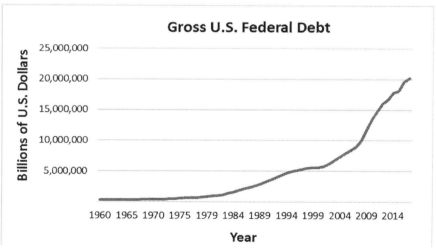

Graph 5. Gross federal debt. Source: whitehouse.gov / Historical Tables / Spreadsheets Table 7.1 Data

---

6 Graphs 5–7 were generated using Excel spread sheet data sets available at https://www.whitehouse.gov/omb/historical-tables/ Table 7.1 Federal Debt at the End of the Year: 1940–2023

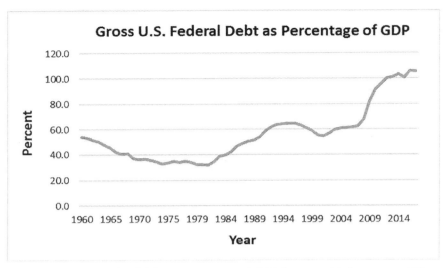

Graph 6. Gross U.S. federal debt as percentage of GDP. Source: whitehouse.gov / Historical Tables / Spreadsheets Table 7.1 Data

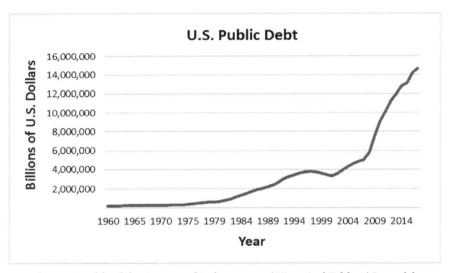

Graph 7. U.S. Public debt. Source: whitehouse.gov / Historical Tables / Spreadsheets Table 7.1 Data

Consequently, the bottom line is that declining U.S. health contributes greatly to societal costs and rising federal and public debt.

Meanwhile, as U.S. consumers spend more money to buy processed and refined food products and pay for the health consequences of poor behavioral and lifestyle choices, the financial costs paid by society fund the progressive rise in industry profitability.

The **Standard & Poor's 500 Index (S&P 500)**, which measures the stock value of the 500 largest corporations traded on the market in a moving average, has increased 2000% in value between the late 1970s and 2016 to mirror in a HESC curve the increases in obesity, consumption of calories and processed and refined food products, health expenditures, and federal and public debts perfectly.

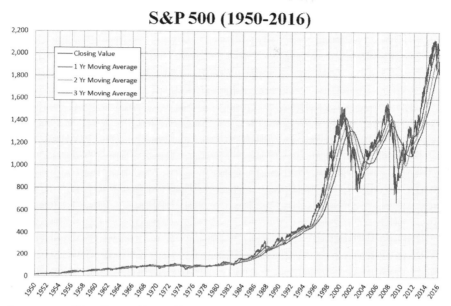

S&P 500 (1950-2016)

Source: en.wikipedia.org / https://en.wikipedia.org/wiki/S%26P_500_Index; https://commons.wikimedia.org/wiki/File:S_and_P_500_chart_1950_to_2016_with_averages.png#file

Humans need to stop being feed fueling commercial industry growth and profitability. A personal health contract eliminating the use of addictification industry-created products, which behaviorally exploit and chemically manipulate human existences surreptitiously to profit industry, successfully optimizes personal health to maximize longevity.

Healthy daily routines founded on the understanding that fueling is basic body vehicle maintenance help maintain optimal body vehicle health and functioning to reduce the need for rescue industry bail-outs.

Living is simple; trust the basics.
Trust what Mother Nature made, because everything else is made for profit.

Body vehicle metabolic functions and chemistry integrate best with natural crude fuel, whole earth foods. The body vehicle comes fully equipped at birth with all necessary physiologic sensors, gauges, and effectors to guide and perform all the appropriate operations to procure and biologically transform natural crude fuel whole earth foods to power the body vehicle system.

Body vehicle equipment conveniently present at birth for processing and delivery of fuel and nutrients for cellular utilization includes

1. intricate food processing and refinery system consisting of mouth tools, intestines, and other digestive organs
2. fuel and nutrient distribution and delivery systems composed of the cardiovascular system, blood, and lymph vessels
3. storage system located within fat, muscle, and liver cells for excess unutilized fuels
4. elimination system comprising the liver, kidney, lung, bowel, skin, and urinary bladder organs that rids the body vehicle of generated metabolic wastes from fuel burning
5. an elaborate system of alarms that alert to body vehicle system overload, deficiencies, or malfunction involving fueling and energy production and utilization, which include measurable vital sign indicators such as blood pressure and energy biomarkers such as blood sugar and cholesterol levels

14 TIME AND BIOLOGICAL FUNCTIONS

14.1 BIOLOGICAL TIME AND ENERGY

Time and energy parameters limit body vehicle activities and existence.

All naturally recurring body vehicle biological actions working on body vehicle clocks and timers use energy and demand minimum energy and time allotments to run programmed cycles of operation properly. Specific time allowances permit functioning body vehicle components to complete biological activities correctly. For example, heartbeat, breathing, intestinal contractions, reflexes emptying the bowel or urinary bladder, chewing and digesting food, sleep, menstruation, pregnancy, and pregnancy labor and infant delivery all require measurable amounts of time and energy to complete designated cycles of activity.

Biological body vehicle clocks and timers do not necessarily conform to artificially imposed social, occupational, economic, or recreational time schedules. Impatience with and failure to satisfy natural body vehicle time and energy requirements as necessary for existence create rescue industry patients.

The body vehicle physical entity globally encompasses a discrete and limited amount of actively available physical energy that must be intelligently budgeted and distributed accordingly to allow proper body vehicle functioning while avoiding squandering or misappropriation of precious body vehicle energies.

Every physical and metabolic body vehicle action expends time and consumes some fraction of the aggregate available energy contained within the entire body vehicle system.

Body vehicle lifetime and energy are continuously utilized eating, breathing, circulating blood, physically mobilizing, eliminating waste, worrying, staying warm, digesting food, repairing body vehicle wear and tear, recovering from illness, fighting infection, thinking, and so on.

When one body vehicle system component is more active and demands more energy to run, the body vehicle shifts energy balances and taps into stored energy reserves as necessary to meet those energy demands. Redistributing body vehicle component energies may create vulnerabilities or cause a malfunction in energy underfunded body vehicle systems.

Vital body vehicle life programs or physiologic "applications" (apps) that control heartbeat, breathing, digestive function, and maintenance of appropriate body vehicle temperature and blood pressure run continuously and have minimum energy requirements that must be met, or the body vehicle system may shut down and cease to work entirely.

When the body vehicle is insufficiently fueled, inadequately rested, or excessively challenged by greater physical and mental demands or during illness, the body vehicle reallocates energy distributions to maintain survival, possibly causing malfunction, disrepair, or shutdown of less vital life programs to create body vehicle health and survival vulnerabilities.

14.2 BODY VEHICLE MAINTENANCE SIGNALS

The body vehicle regularly signals basic maintenance and survival needs requiring attention. Routine body vehicle maintenance and survival signaling include

1. hunger to eat and fuel the body vehicle
2. thirst to drink water to rehydrate and replace lost body vehicle water
3. tiredness to sleep or rest to restore depleted body vehicle energy
4. coldness to warm up or hotness to cool down to maintain proper body vehicle working temperatures
5. urge to urinate or defecate to eliminate accumulated, stored toxic body vehicle wastes
6. loneliness to seek the company of others

14.3 STRESS

Stress is challenge to survival.

The primal inherently programmed body vehicle biological stress response is **fight or flight.** Stress stimulates the body vehicle to release the physiological stress hormones **adrenaline** and **cortisol.** Adrenaline and cortisol are produced by the adrenal glands, located above the kidneys toward the middle backside of the torso.

The body vehicle biologically has a neurochemical chain of command system called the **HPA (hypothalamic pituitary adrenal) axis** that directs fight or flight stress responses based on brain processing of information fed through internal and external body vehicle sensory portals.

When brain filters interpret delivered information as stressful or threatening to health or survival, dedicated brain executive function areas trigger the release of nervous and chemical impulses terminating their effects on the adrenal glands to stimulate the release of adrenaline and cortisol, which activate numerous downstream body vehicle survival responses.

Adrenaline and cortisol potently elicit multiple coordinated cascades of body vehicle physiologic actions that impact energy processing, utilization, balance, and storage; influence eating behaviors; affect blood sugar and cholesterol levels; alter fat reserves and distribution; and perturb blood pressure, pulse, and respirations. Adrenaline raises blood pressure, increases heart rate, quickens breathing, tenses muscles, and causes behaviors to be more aggressive, allowing the body vehicle to mobilize and respond quicker to threats.

Cortisol releases sugar from body vehicle stores to supply ready fuel for muscles to burn on-demand, shifts fats stored in peripheral sites centrally into the abdomen to be readily available for rapid conversion into energy by the liver, and promotes overeating to stockpile energy for potential scarcity or immediate utilization. Cortisol drives body vehicle energy processing to *store for war* by increasing fat fuel energy reserves particularly within the abdomen, leading to accumulation of belly fat and predisposing to obesity.

Stress modifies body vehicle cellular, tissue, and organ functions chemically and biologically on various levels to redirect metabolic activities and energy delivery to confront existing, potential, or perceived threats to health and survival. Adrenaline and cortisol potently affect body vehicle immune function to raise susceptibility for developing infections, autoimmune disorders, and cancer. Stress promotes cancer development, growth, and spread.

Exposure to excessively stressful conditions weakens and disrupts protective body vehicle intestinal barriers, rendering gut membranes less capable of containing toxic gut contents and microorganisms from leaking into the blood to access protected tissues and increase body vehicle risks to develop toxicities and infection that compound other harmful stress effects.

Stress not only provokes silent behind-the-scenes metabolic biological responses but also incites emotional reactions to arouse feelings of urgency, tension, anxiety, or a sense of impending doom and insufficient time available to accomplish basic biological body vehicle functions and personal activities.

Fear and worry surrounding the illusion, perception, or reality of an impending threat to personal health or survival trigger stress reactions. Sophisticated technologies that image and study the effects of stress on the brain demonstrate measurable changes in brain anatomy and functional activity induced by stress, which may impact complex human behaviors, social interactions, and life choices. Continual experience of excessive stress precipitates chronic irritability, anger, and energy deficiency with feelings of tiredness and fatigue, and predisposes to substance abuse, addictions, and other risk behaviors.

The risks of developing obesity rise with persistent stress as individuals seek runaway escapes from stress-induced emotional pain and suffering. Stress creates emotional pain and suffering demanding relief, conveniently provided through addictification products that temporarily pleasure oral sensors and through rescue industry pharmaceuticals that chemically reduce unpleasant stress experiences, which behaviorally condition individuals to develop commercial addictification or rescue bail-out dependification when resorted to with regularity.

Stress also reduces mental focus and increases distractibility to raise vulnerability to behavioral manipulation by commercial industries, which use subliminal cues to surreptitiously activate conditioned stress-escape behaviors that profit industry commercially. More extreme behavioral consequences of experiencing excessive life stresses may include being accident prone or going on wild shopping sprees with unrestrained spending that depletes personal finances to incur serious debt.

Continual stress may alter the natural body vehicle physical experiences of the world by changing baseline sensitivities of body vehicle sensory portals and physiologic responses of effectors, which adapt to compensate for repetitive or sustained adverse survival pressures exerted onto the body vehicle system.

Excessive body vehicle stresses may transform reversibly reactive and self-limited physiologic stress responses to become permanently sustained, resetting normal body vehicle physiologic activity set points to stress-induced response levels that compromise body vehicle health and survival. Therefore, repeated body vehicle exposures to stressful circumstances that engage **FIGHT** or **FLIGHT** physiologic responses eventually recalibrate normal body vehicle functioning to remain at stress-heightened alert levels to cause numerous adverse health consequences, including

1. high blood pressure or hypertension
2. elevated blood sugar levels or diabetes
3. altered appetite predisposing to overeating leading to obesity
4. belly fat accumulation producing torso obesity with a fatty liver, increased body vehicle inflammatory activity, and other adverse metabolic effects to worsen diabetes, cholesterol levels, and blood pressure
5. salt and water retention leading to edema or swelling of tissues to raise blood pressure and stress the heart muscle, which must pump around more body vehicle water against higher blood pressures
6. altered immune responses that impair resistance to infection and increase the risks of developing cancer and autoimmune disorders
7. impaired tissue and wound healing
8. heightened vigilance and anxiety that interfere with vegetative body vehicle functions including rest, sleep, sexual performance, menstruation, and bowel and urinary bladder activity

9. increased susceptibility for developing behavioral health and substance abuse conditions
10. reduced capacity of intestinal barrier membranes to restrict gut toxins, bacterial products, and microorganisms normally confined to the gut from leaking through to protected blood circulation

14.4 DELAY OF GRATIFICATION

Delaying gratification of basic body vehicle maintenance needs creates stress and suffering, priming behavioral impulses to seek immediate relief to increase vulnerability for commercial exploitation.

Addictification and rescue industry products coincidentally provide convenient commercial, quick-fix escape solutions that offer immediate relief from pain and suffering but only temporarily delay the inevitability of having to satisfy repressed biological maintenance needs (e.g., consuming an energy drink instead of resting when tired does not cancel the pent-up need to rest).

In modern societies, familial, social, occupational, and economic demands compete for time and energy necessary for fulfilling personal biological needs, pressuring individuals to stall, forgo, sacrifice, and neglect their need to eat food, drink water, rest and sleep, move and exercise, eliminate waste, enjoy intimacy, think uninterrupted, and seek personal meaning to life just to fulfill extraneous societal demands.

Existing contrary to satisfying basic needs promptly compromises body vehicle system integrity and depletes body vehicle energy reserves that become redirected to repress, suppress, and postpone timely responses to body vehicle biological needs.

Some common time and energy thieves hindering body vehicle biological maintenance include

1. oppressive personal and occupational requirements to increase economic productivity and earnings
2. heavily scheduled agendas brimming with numerous obligations that eliminate all vestiges of available free time and energy
3. constant availability and accessibility for all through perpetual electronic device connectivity
4. continuous attention directed toward operating electronic gadgets and communication devices
5. endless watching of television and engagement with other media device programming

Inappropriate suppression, postponement, interruption, or disregard for body vehicle urges signaling the need for body vehicle biological maintenance produces tension and suffering inciting survival responses to seek immediate relief from pain.

Stress develops from neglecting body vehicle physical and emotional mainte-nance needs and failing to respond to body vehicle biological clocks and rhythms promptly, which then facilitates addictification and dependification for available commercial industry conveniences that only temporarily appease unfulfilled body vehicle biological demands to prolong stress suffering.

Industry readily cashes in on the human willingness to default on self-maintenance obligations by selling convenient commercial runaway escape options that further deprive the personal need to maintain the body vehicle suitably.

Excessive cravings for and use of commercial industry products and services that temporarily pleasure the senses or provide momentary runaway escapes from suffering indicating insidious addictification for those products or services are clues suggesting the presence of excessive underlying personal stresses. Anticipation and prompt fulfillment of body vehicle maintenance needs prevent behavioral derailment into primal fight or flight survival programming that disrupts emotional balance and self-control to increase vulnerability for addictification and rescue bail-out dependification.

14.5 CONSUMERISM AND INDUSTRIAL PRODUCTIVITY

Whereas most individuals work to earn a living, commercial industries work to turn a profit. Working individuals who earn a living to survive function as acces-sories to carry out industry profit directives. In commerce, time is of the essence that creates opportune economic moments for commercial industries to profit.

Making more money in less time summarizes the usual objectives of commer-cial business enterprises. **Productivity** measures human work output as the rate of production of goods and services having economic value divided by the costs of production. Productivity revenues determine cash flow of commercial industry systems. Simply, positive productivity means cash is flowing into and profitably funding the commercial industry systems, while negative productivity means that system cash is flowing out and being lost from the business systems.

Primary objectives for productivity-driven business entities are to maximize cash inflow and earnings while limiting cash outflow. Productivity work efforts achieving positive cash flow into the system indicate the profitable use of worker lifetimes to capture consumer *lifetimes.*

In competitive commercial markets, industry work demands continually increase as commercial industries progressively squeeze every bit of profit from work efforts and monetary investments. Goods need to be produced faster and more cheaply, and services supplied more efficiently at lower costs, for businesses to prosper locally and on the stage of growing world markets. Revenue-driven time compression eliminates workflow activities losing or failing to earn income for industry systems.

Commercial industries hire **efficiency experts** to streamline worker actions and work-related activities to lower business expenses and maximize productivity.

When market demands decline or industry competition stiffens to challenge business survival, workers are often paid less and expected to work harder and accomplish more to compensate for declining business industry revenues. Business entities target worker efforts and demand worker sacrifices to achieve commercial industry profitability. As commercial entities push productivity to ensure industry profitability, workers labor harder and sacrifice more while earning relatively less to permit the commercial systems and the fortunate few to thrive economically.

Extensive data analyses of various economic indicators by the **Economic Policy Institute (EPI)** to study the relationships between worker productivity and commercial industry profitability reveal that over the past few decades as corporate profits are soaring most are toiling, receiving limited compensation for their increasing work efforts.

EPI data analyses of worker productivity and compensation for the decades stretching between the years 1973 and 2013 have shown a progressive divergence between worker productivity rates and compensation. During these years, worker productivity rates increased faster than the average and median worker compensations, and family income rose for work efforts. Total economy productivity surged approximately 145% while real hourly compensation of production and nonsupervisory workers climbed 18% and real median family income grew only 27%. Additionally, hourly worker productivity rose approximately 80% while the average hourly compensation for salaried, self-employed, and wage workers went up 39%, and the median hourly compensation advanced only 10%.[7]

Furthermore, between 1979 and 2013, the wages of the top 1% of earners grew 138% while wages for the bottom 90% increased only 15%. Additionally, during this period, very high wage earners saw a 41% increase in their hourly wages, while the hourly wages of middle-wage earners remained stagnant rising only 6%, and the hourly wages of low-wage earners decreased by 5%. Particularly between the 1990s and 2013, corporate profits out-paced GDP and labor income growth by approximately 2 to 1 as worker productivity increased, markets globalized to provide cheap global labor, and worker wages grew very slowly if at all.[8]

Consequently, corporations and very select individuals thrive from higher worker productivity and increased consumer spending. As workers toil producing more at work for less compensation and then spend their hard-earned wages existing unhealthily and paying premiums to correct mounting adverse health consequences from poor behavioral and lifestyle choices, corporate profits soar across the board.

7. http://stateofworkingamerica.org/chart/swa-wages-figure-4u-change-total-economy/; http://stateof-workingamerica.org/charts/productivity-and-real-median-family-income-growth-1947-2009/; http://stateofworkingamerica.org/chart/swa-wages-figure-4v-change-hourly-productivity/.

8. https://www.epi.org/publication/raising-americas-pay/; https://www.epi.org/publica-tion/why-americas-workers-need-faster-wage-growth/; https://www.epi.org/publication/charting-wage-stagnation/; https://www.theatlantic.com/business/archive/2013/03/corporate-profit s-are-eating-the-economy/273687/.

Industrial productivity dehumanizes worker behaviors into commercially defined mechanical actions or **labor units** that are systematized and measured, as exemplified by assembly-line processes initiated in the early 1900s by the automotive industry under the auspices of Henry Ford.

Productivity automates human biological time and energy to create **human machines,** expected to deliver services or produce products perpetually robotically while **on-the-clock,** without inconvenient and unprofitable interruption of workflow activities to address personal body vehicle biological needs for necessary maintenance or breakdowns.

Industrially quantitated human work actions or labor units are assigned discrete **monetary and time values**.

Human labor units are then maneuvered and manipulated strategically to extract the greatest work output at the lowest business costs and times allotted to maximize commercial industry profits from human labors. Therefore, commercial productivity converts human life forces into becoming revenue-generating industry machines.

Human limitations and the difficulties in forecasting human productivities and work outputs accurately and hence in predicting the potential industry profitability from on-the-clock human machines are leading to the gradual replacement of humans in the workforce by robotic machines and computers, which can carry out industrial worker tasks perpetually with minimal interruption to meet business revenue expectations dependably.

During the modern era of continuous universal electronic connectivity through portable laptop computers and cellular smartphones, worker productivity and working for industry take on new meanings. Electronic connectivity melts work into play to bleed play of regenerative human biological time and energy. Humans continually plugging into electronic media devices work round-the-clock for commercial industries, which drain personal play time and energy for work or employ sophisticated marketing schemes to manipulate online media device users simply for commercial purposes.

As previously noted, productivity measures human work output as the rate of production of goods and services having economic value divided by the costs of production.

Simple formulas express industry profits and worker productivity.

$$\text{PROFITS} = \text{PRICE} - \text{COSTS}$$

$$\text{PRODUCTIVITY} = \frac{\text{WORKER OUTPUT}}{\text{LABOR COSTS}}$$

Industry profits increase by selling more products and services and lowering overhead costs of materials, supplies, and labor to produce and deliver goods. Quicker supply of consumer demands by producing more products and services in less time and at lower production costs also increases industry profits.

Productivity and consumer demands drive industry profitability.

In busy modern societies, increasing worker efforts and efficiency and limiting worker schedule interruptions for attending to nonproductive activities, such as bathroom and meal breaks, vacations, and sick time, are routinely used to lift worker output at fixed costs to maintain productivity and industry profitability. Likewise, using fewer workers paid lower wages to accomplish the same job also reduces work costs to raise productivity and industry profits.

Productivity can also be expressed in **work units** that have a determinable commercial market economic **cost-value** derived by subtracting away the costs of creating from the market price obtained selling work units. Industry productivity goals are to optimize the cost-value ratio of work units by shrinking the costs of materials, supplies, and labor to nothing while maximally driving up the value of delivered work units by raising the unit price and increasing unit reimbursements as much as markets will bear. Consequently, under productivity demands, industries aim to reduce work unit costs by using the least and cheapest materials and supplies and employing the fewest workers paid the lowest wages over the shortest times for production, while charging as much as possible for delivered work units.

Productivity-driven industry operations exploit workers and consumers more easily when industries own a monopoly or the exclusive rights to deliver and produce particular work units, especially when legislation fails to oversee and regulate or even supports industry activities.

Productivity demands generate economic time pressures.

Economic time pressures create monetary stresses forcing workers to work more efficiently. Monetary time stresses drive workers to compress body vehicle software codes and streamline body vehicle program operations to run the least number of lines of commands to execute only the actions that maximize revenues and reduce expenditures for industry.

Industry demands for profitability and monetary efficiency redirect workers' energies to earn industry more money and squeeze out any worker times available for focusing on personal body vehicle maintenance. In commercially competitive societies, human value and the worth of human activities are being progressively misperceived as equaling the potential for generating revenue or increasing economic productivity. Economic time pressures distort the value of human lifetime activities to be appraised according to the estimated economic worth or propensity of the activities to generate or lose revenue rather than to be appreciated solely based on any intrinsic worth or inherent human value of the activities. Therefore, economic time pressures would value expressing or being in love or engaging in humanistic activities according to revenues generated or lost while loving, caring, or being humanistic.

Under economic time pressures, productivity-driven work processes take precedence over individual human maintenance needs and the demands of unique personal life circumstances, and occupational constraints force workers to defer or suppress fulfilling personal needs and biological requirements. Consequently, in industrially competitive market economies, workers regularly accept *lifetime* trade-offs and sacrifices frequently amounting to surrender of personal lifetime to acquire economic returns or prevent economic losses for themselves or industry.

Biologic time requisites to accomplish basic body vehicle maintenance or to recover from illness are then routinely managed to suit economic time constraints and occupational or financial expectations. When time is money, seconds translate into economic profit or cost, and every working moment is accounted for economically to relegate time requirements for completing body vehicle biological functions as inconvenient and costly. Consequently, humans forfeit biologic times in busy modern, industrialized, technological societies to achieve higher earnings and raise industry profit margins.

Economic time pressures that force individuals to exchange dwindling lifetime to acquire some financial reward create dilemmas that increase life stresses, especially when personal returns are marginal or negative on precious lifetime sacrificed to pursue economic goals.

Stress challenging body vehicle survival especially develops when occupational productivity demands infringe on and siphon away personal biological time and energy obligatorily needed to run vital body vehicle survival programming. Body vehicle biological clocks do not behave on-demand consistently or with precision. Industry requisites routinely compel humans to voluntarily alter natural body vehicle clocks and biologic functions to conform to economic time and to suppress or postpone biological functions that inconveniently interfere with economic productivity and industry profitability. Coincidentally, industry also produces and sells commercial products of convenience that artificially alter biologic functions on-demand, when inescapable surrender to repressive economic pressures demands artificial manipulation and suppression of inconveniently intrusive body vehicle biologic functions and urges.

Commercial rescue and addictification industry products available for individuals to endure industry-inflicted pressures include laxatives, antidiarrheal agents, sleep aids, sedatives, birth control pills, energy boosters, and numerous other rescue industry remedies, as well as industry-prepared convenience and fast-food products, all of which conveniently help individuals cope and resist natural body vehicle biologic demands and urges.

The stresses and pressures created by the productivity demands of industry successfully serve to perpetuate industry profitability in many ways. Human work productivity stresses that produce delay of gratification stresses lead to increased consumption of addictification and rescue industry products and services to cope with stress fallout.

Forcing children to shorten or eliminate meal times, creative play, bathroom activities, or other human biological times to fulfill oppressively tight agendas and heavily scheduled daily routines, conveniently indoctrinates and conditions the children for future commercial industry system exploitation and control.

Industry productivity benchmarks increasingly gauge the delivery and allocation of health care resources to consumers to stress health care workers and reduce rightfully deserved consumer health care benefits. High rescue industry productivity translates to efficient high-volume delivery of expensive health care services to maximize revenues financially feeding rescue industry systems. Productivity in delivering health care to consumers requires paring down and streamlining services to only those generating collectible revenues that ensure system profitability.

Health care services and products have to be delivered progressively faster at the lowest expense, employing the fewest number of paid health care workers, and using the shortest facility times and least amount of equipment costing industry revenue, while providers are pressured to comply by simplifying health care routines to satisfy minimum standards of care passing payer scrutiny and peer review.

Profit-driven health care mills seize on productivity principles to implement aggressive business strategies to maximize health care billings and limit available health care services and products to those predictably turning a profit. Accumulating scientific knowledge complicates the understanding of the immensely intricate human body vehicle system to demand more thoughtful consideration and greater caution from health care providers, when advising or performing diagnostic and therapeutic maneuvers to manage human health disorders. The sophistication of technological developments and the scientific breakthroughs to test for and treat human diseases and disease predispositions are growing exponentially. The increasing complexity of health care options also leads to the generation of ever more elaborate health care guidelines for health care providers to follow in executing their health care work. Mounting rescue industry productivity demands and escalating health care options further stress health care workers already concerned with the inherent liabilities of caring for complex human health care needs within increasingly litigious societal environments.

Health care providers experience physical and mental exhaustion, leading to provider **burnout** from the oppressive health care pressures to meet growing societal health care needs profitably despite shrinking revenues, which are increasingly redirected to profit corporate and commercial industry systems, ultimately at the expense of health care consumers. Provider burnout then unsurprisingly leads to health care provider professional work dissatisfaction and attrition from servicing health care consumers and opportunely serves commercial industry systems as leverage to manipulate and control the behaviors of professionally weakened health care workers.

The **health care productivity contradiction** expresses that as ever more sophisticated diagnostic and therapeutic health care options become rampantly available within the health care domain and the complexity of human health matters grows exponentially, less health care workers are expected to deliver progressively more health care services in shorter times and at lower costs to an increasing number of ever more complicated and demanding health care recipients. Consequently, the productivity mill mentality of commercial health care delivery applies poorly toward meeting the health care needs of individuals presenting with increasingly challenging personal and medical issues in an intricate world progressively driven by economic demands.

Individuals who seek health care rarely present with health needs neatly fitting into discrete disease categories easily serviced using business-focused health care delivery templates, which incorporate productivity efficiency formulas that marginally satisfy the simplest of health care delivery guidelines. Adequate interactive time spent between health care providers and recipients to address health problems and patient concerns carefully, and formulate realistic, efficient, and economic health care delivery solutions individualized to patient needs, undoubtedly lowers health care delivery costs and improves societal health to benefit all much better than can productivity-driven health care delivery behaviors.

Unfortunately, spending adequate interactive time and delivering humanism during health care encounters are not profitable or even adequately reimbursable strategies for health care delivery systems, which predominantly focus on servicing time demands deliberately to maximize system profitability. Humanism especially threatens to subtract time away from more monetarily profitable commercial health care delivery activities and may instead be used as a conduit to promote more profitable health care delivery. Ostensibly, humanistic encounters occurring within institutional health care settings between providers and recipients may even be scripted to identify intervention opportunities that allow deployment of profitable services, such as administration of pain-relieving medications, which incidentally are blamed as contributing toward societal narcotic addiction problems leading to lethal drug overdoses.

Hospital environments progressively enslave nursing staff to push around intrusive **computers on wheels (COWs)** like a ball and chain during direct patient contact to document in the EHR all reimbursable health care activities and interactions and to pad the medical record with information that may be used to protect against future legal liabilities and lawsuits.

Quick procedural turnaround times for health care services delivered repetitively in assembly-line fashion conveniently minimize opportunities for any human interactions that may slow and detract from profitable, productivity-driven workflow. Profit-hungry commercial health care industry systems undervalue and rarely adequately compensate necessary interactive face-time deservedly spent between health care providers and recipients. Third-party payers customarily pay substantially less for administered health care services failing to involve technological or laboratory testing, surgical procedures, or programmed ancillary specialty interventions, such as physical or occupational therapy. Alternatively, expensive health care ticket items comprising convenient pharmaceutical treatments, invasive surgical interventions, and technological assessments employing laboratory and radiologic studies that profitably pad productivity bottom lines are handsomely reimbursed to rescue industry providers and institutions.

With health care delivery productivity and profit margins on the line, health care consumers are more likely to be routinely subjected to costlier health care delivery options and practices to address personal health care needs. Health care delivery systems carefully track system profitability and consumer throughput, which increase by incorporating easy-out prescribing of pharmaceuticals, using expensive technologies to perform diagnostic testing, or resorting to high-tech procedures and surgical options to address consumer health complaints.

Conservative health care management strategies that incorporate intensive, interactive face-time to individualize health care and provide appropriate preventative health counseling, which are likely to produce better health outcomes and health care savings for consumers and society, are undesirable, revenue-reducing, conservative strategies that threaten commercial health care industry earnings.

Productivity incentivizes system games producing system financial gains.

Rescue industry prescriptions for medical products and services are **tickets-to-ride** for rescue industry system players to keep industry system monetary games going, revenues flowing, and rescue system players in the game playing. Providers writing the most orders executed by the system and consumers maximally utilizing system products and services become **all-star members** within health care delivery systems focusing on financial productivity goals. Rescue industry **get-the-money** productivity goals to achieve higher industry earnings on made investments reward for doing or may penalize for not doing expected health care delivery maneuvers under specific circumstances, as defined by directives generated by rescue industry professional organizations and policymakers and employers of health care providers.

Health care providers failing to practice according to devised rescue industry standards may experience significantly reduced practice revenues or suffer punitive measures including fines or professional liabilities for transgressing expected industry practices.

When the focus on productivity ceases to yield humanistic returns in delivering health care, then productivity demands short-change health care recipients and generate negative sentiments in providers entrusted and privileged to serve the health needs of humanity. Additionally, when the primary force that drives health care delivery is productivity based and bent on wringing out maximal economic profitability from health care system operations, then the morale and gratification of health care staff pressured to care for human needs under business productivity models devised to sell inanimate commercial industry wares plummets and disappears.

14.6 BOREDOM

Boredom is a universal human experience that increases vulnerability to addictification runaway escapes and rescue bail-out dependification. **Boredom** is suffering developing with the weariness that follows tedium and monotony in daily routines leaving little room for creativity and self-discovery.

Boredom occurs in the absence of adequately stimulating life experiences, especially when expectations for excitement are unmet and the resourcefulness to plan interesting or exciting activities or enjoy solitude is limited. Humdrum daily routines carried out aimlessly with minimal reflection or imagination induce personal boredom that produces restlessness and feelings of captivity causing suffering, whereas life journeys having personal goals that provide direction and destination points to allow purposeful life navigation with ample opportunities for self-discovery generate excitement.

Daily routines satisfying personal goals that are meaningful, instill a sense of human belonging, and lead to personal accomplishment with humanistic enrichment enhance the life experience to prevent boredom. Taking time to reflect on day-to-day existence increases the enjoyment of life experiences and allows appreciation of passing life moments to keep life interesting and boredom away.

Commercial industry goods and media programming create distractions that diffuse boredom through numerous modalities, mainly by providing sensory stimulation to captivate attention and usurp valuable lifetime from distracted spectators, who unsuspectingly surrender precious lifetime moments otherwise available for learning, creativity, solitude, introspection, self-discovery, and healthy physical activities. Electronic media devices, which become the focal point for bored, wandering thoughts producing personal feelings of uneasiness or anxiety, take over and commercially drive minds that relinquish opportunities to think independently and free of commercial industry influences or propaganda.

When personal imagination fails to fill precious moments of passing free time creatively, industry capitalizes by offering addictification options to relieve the stress of boredom with products that tactically fuel primal human urges. Stress and boredom prime and condition individuals for exploitation with addictification industry runaway escapes and rescue bail-out interventions that quickly alleviate pain and suffering on-demand. For example, industry may advertise some pick-me-up to make the day better and imply that purchasing and using their product is an answer to a bad day that should be relied upon indefinitely.

Repetitive relief of stress and boredom suffering by pleasuring oral taste sensors with commercial food products that potently arouse primal feeding impulses and craves facilitates the loss of behavioral control to enable unrestrained eating predisposing to obesity. Addictification food industries opportunely groom vulnerable consumer victims into becoming eating machines, which insatiably consume excessive industry calories to derive short-lived oral pleasures to temporarily relieve stress, boredom, or pain in exchange for giving up *lifetime* to sustain addictification and rescue industry profits.

14.7 XS AND NOW

Addictification and rescue industries thrive when consumers expect immediate gratification of demands and fulfillment of desires with excess.

> ***Instant gratification and surplus govern modern societal behaviors.***

The **wow of excess and now** seduces consumer greed.

Fast-paced lives impatient with human biological limitations and societal constraints and governed by on-demand expectations for satisfaction from daily routines and interactions with others, society, and industry have launched human existence into **now-time**! *Bigger, larger, faster, more, better, extra, two or more for one, today, now, immediate, no waiting, on time,* and *have it your way* are common terms catering to and feeding societal consumer demands and expectations.

Now-time living is counterregulatory to thoughtful impulse control. Through continual visual, auditory, and taste sensory portal overstimulation of excitatory brain centers, and habitual immediate gratification of individual biological urges, desires, wants, and craves, the body vehicle threshold for impulse control becomes reset to make patience truly a virtue.

Within the incessant orgasm of crazed human existences, quiet, restorative moments of peace, comfort, and uninterrupted solitude, which provide an opportunity for creative and reflective thought, are often eliminated from jam-packed schedules and overburdened personal agendas.

Industry panders to and financially thrives on frenzied lives lacking rest, who become wearied and resigned to welcome any conveniently available commercial industry products or services, which offer an artificial escape or some purported edge in the tired fight against imagined or industry-created personal antagonists, competitors, or foes. Every waking moment in modern daily existence can easily be overwhelmed using commercial products or services fulfilling any human whim, want, or crave and depleting every available personal moment of solitude and quiet at consumer expense. Excessive personal, societal, and occupational demands in technologically modern, industrial societies have unsurprisingly fostered the creation, penetration, and robust growth of the *FAST*-food industry.

FAST foods feed rushed, frenzied, impulsive, demanding, and immediate excitement-seeking personal existences driven by industry-shaped expectations, technology, and personal economic ambitions. Fast-food restaurants are low-cost body vehicle fueling stations selling relatively cheap-quality and artificial flavor–enhanced food products to rapidly power up stressed-out, overworked, and tired lives rushing through crazed daily existences.

FAST foods conveniently provide instant gratification by immediately dispensing potent designer taste pleasures that provide runaway escapes and temporarily appease primal hunger craves inexpensively, which are ideal features that combine to generate and perpetuate dependence on the fast-food industry to fuel the body vehicle. Fast-food drive-thrus become **drive-by** consumer killings, pumping passing drivers full of cheap, toxic food products while robbing drivers of *lifetime* and destroying driver opportunities to prepare and eat healthy meals at home.

The constant rush of modern daily living begs the question that seeks to understand the ultimate purpose and destination of the mad frenzy of human activities which continually sacrifice meeting basic biologic human needs simply and naturally.

15 HOW BODY VEHICLE FUELING COMPONENTS WORK

15.1 SENSE OF SMELL

The **sense of smell** embodied within the nose allows recognition of distinctly identifiable earth substances and biological entities, which exist simply as a gas or that emit gas molecules into the air to create characteristic odors, aromas, fragrances, and scents.

The sense of smell provides flavor subtleties to the sense of taste. Smell helps humans distinguish and identify freshness and spoilage of living or devitalized and decaying natural earth foods. Sensory portal receptors in the nose chemically detect different "smell" molecules, and then send signals through nerves directly from the nose receptors into the primitive brain, which governs reflex survival instincts, urges, and behaviors.

Various animal species and primitive life-forms, such as insects, emit biologically potent gas molecules, termed **pheromones,** that spread through the air in a cloud to motivate or induce stereotypically characteristic behavior patterns in receptively programmed organisms of the same species. Pheromones are chemical communication signals that intimately govern biologic impulses involving mating, sexual reproduction, and community behaviors when sensed or smelled by same species members.

Natural earth foods in their native biological states are typically not potently fragrant, except for their associated flowers, which attract bees and other insects to help plants cross-pollinate. Commercial products frequently utilize fragrances and scents to deceive and exploit the sense of smell to arouse emotions and excite primal behavioral impulses and urges. For example, consider the pleasant emotional experiences that commercial fragrances and scents such as "baby fresh," coconut, "fresh air," "pine fresh," and "lemon scent" elicit, with their strong smells frequently lingering in the air to be detectable from far away.

Few natural biological smells are detectable by humans over any significant distances, except possibly for skunk, smoke, and the putrid stench of decaying organic matter, which warn of danger and compel one to flee or seek immediate refuge.

15.2 MOUTH OR OS, THE SACRED "O"-HOLE FOR FUELING

The **mouth "O"-hole,** also known as the **OS,** is the main fueling portal for the body vehicle and functions as the "kitchen," where ingested crude fuel natural whole earth foods are prepared for subsequent digestive transformation into usable nutrient and energy forms in the gut. Complex oral sensory portal receptors act as **oral feelers** to identify and gauge the chemical and physical properties of substances placed into the mouth. After oral sensing, the mouth mechanically and chemically readies ingested foods for subsequent intestinal digestion, which completes fuel and nutrient breakdown for blood absorption and cellular delivery.

The mouth is intimately linked through dense nerve and chemical inputs to primitive and higher-order functioning areas of the brain and to the gut, which communicate critical information concerning oral digestive activities. Therefore, during eating, the mouth talks to the brain and digestive system to give a nutritional "head's up" to "tell" what is being delivered down the food pipe to nourish and power the body vehicle system.

Notably, the mouth is a strategic control point that dramatically impacts body vehicle health, survival, and life quality and uniquely affects human body vehicle existence both by what goes into it as well as what comes out of it. Nutritionally unbalanced or chemically doctored foods fed into the mouth misinform the body vehicle system to disrupt the natural biological signaling necessary to drive feeding behaviors correctly.

Mastering control of the mouth provides the best opportunity for a long, healthy, and happy life. Coincidentally, some commercially successful OS stimulator artificial food products that potently stimulate oral feelers to commandeer feeding behaviors and impulses curiously also have names ending in -*os*.

The main working components of the mouth include

1. *teeth* that cut, tear, rip, disrupt, and grind solid food fibers into tiny pieces, pulp, or a liquid
2. *salivary glands* that moisten, dissolve, liquefy, and chemically dismantle orally introduced solid foods and complex liquids into smaller molecules
3. *the tongue* that mechanically compresses, mixes, and senses the chemical taste properties of ingested foods and liquids
4. *cheek and throat muscles* that retain, push, and direct consumed liquids and chewed foods down the food pipe for delivery into the gut for further digestion
5. *chemical and neurological sensors* that densely line the mouth cavity, tongue, and throat to detect and measure various properties of ingested foods and beverages such as chemical composition, shape, taste, texture, consistency, and temperature, and

then signal acquired information to the brain and digestive tract for further processing

6. *microbial organisms,* which inhabit the oral cavity and contribute to oral and body vehicle health and disease predispositions and are nourished or disrupted by the effects of orally introduced substances including foods, beverages, medications, recreational drugs, alcohol, tobacco, and oral hygiene products

Processed and refined food products containing chemical additives, particularly preservatives, exert immediate effects on oral tissues and microbial organisms upon contact that become amplified during chewing. These effects may adversely impact oral health and hygiene to increase risks for developing foul breath, dental caries with loss of teeth, oral tumors, and loss of salivary gland function with the loss of saliva production leading to a dry mouth that causes additional health problems.

15.3 TASTE BUDS (ORAL SENSORS)

Taste buds are complex neurochemical sensors that line the mouth cavity roof, cheeks, tongue, and throat and the beginning portions of the esophagus swallowing tube, and that biochemically recognize distinct chemical qualities of orally introduced substances. Nerves and biochemical signals from taste bud sensory receptors transmit oral information concerning the chemical attributes of substances placed into the mouth to appropriate brain centers for processing. Taste sensors connect to the primitive brain similarly to smell sensors, so that stimulating specific combinations of oral taste buds may induce pheromone like effects to activate stereotypical behaviors in susceptible receptive individuals.

The body vehicle assessment of food freshness and palatability, the experience of pleasure, and the determination of body vehicle fueling satiety are intimately linked to taste bud stimulation. Taste bud sensory experiences can be trained to cultivate acquired tastes and distort judgments for the palatability of foods and beverages. The extensive and integrated network of sensors and gauges of the mouth, digestive tract, blood vessels, and other body vehicle organs, which measure chemical and physical properties of ingested nutrients and fuels, work in concert to furnish nutritional information to the brain that directs feeding behaviors to meet body vehicle nutritional needs.

Oral sensory portal receptors require sufficient biological exposure time to detect and characterize ingested food properties accurately and then send collected information to register onto appropriate brain centers for further dispatch.

A comprehensive **oral inventory** of substances placed into the mouth requires adequate chewing time to thoroughly break down and orally identify the molecular properties of ingested food components responsible for biochemically guiding eating behaviors and digestive activities. Bypassing or shortcutting that strategic oral phase of digestion cheats front-line body vehicle sensors from correctly assessing ingested fuels and nutrients to perturb subsequent body vehicle system nutritional actions. Therefore, the critical first step oral phase of digestion that senses and gauges ingested nutrient and fuel properties is short-circuited by eating fast and swallowing foods without chewing thoroughly, or similarly by gulping down instead of slowly sipping complex liquids such as juices or blender-made beverages.

Incomplete sensory recognition and digestive preparation of ingested foods by the mouth diminishes the overall quality of oral digestive efforts to reduce the level of nutritional information delivered from the mouth to the brain, which negatively impacts feeding behaviors to compromise body vehicle nutrition and predisposes to overeating. Furthermore, the artificial stimulation of oral taste bud sensors with commercially manufactured food products to orally upload taste sensory misinformation to the brain may disturb eating behaviors and predispose to addictification for commercial food products.

15.4 TASTE

Taste is an oral sensory experience that recognizes some distinct combination of complex chemical qualities and physical characteristics of solid or liquid foods. Specific oral taste bud sensors are grouped based on their ability to biologically discriminate between basic familiar taste categories of sweet, sour, salty, savory (*umami*), and bitter with possibly more categories to be discovered in the future.

Food substances placed into the mouth physically and chemically stimulate different groups of oral taste sensors at various intensities. The combinations of stimulated taste buds and their levels of stimulation integrate with the experience of any scents or smells that foods emit to provide the identifiable characteristic taste qualities of foods called **flavor.** Flavor is a unique gustatory food experience that evokes recognition of earth plant, animal, or mineral substances and occurs through a complex interplay between the oral chemical effects of food attributes, the smell stimulating properties of foods, and subsequent brain processing of delivered taste and smell information.

A natural crude fuel whole earth food diet maintains high sensitivity, recognition, and discriminatory accuracy of oral taste sensor functions for natural whole earth food flavors.

> *The 4 S tastes—Sweet, Salty, Sour, and Savory—stimulate salivation,*
> *not satiation.*

Food engineers and flavor chemists biochemically manipulate the **4 S tastes** to interfere with natural satiety and feeding impulses and promote uncontrollable eating as evidenced through consumer taste testing trials.

Commonly, substances toxic to the body vehicle are bitter tasting. **Bitter** has powerful satiety or *stop eating* effects when bitter taste sensors located in the mouth and incidentally substantially along the entire length of the digestive tract are engaged and, consequently, is rarely used commercially as a taste enhancer. (Think 100% chocolate cocoa and green bananas slamming the brakes on the urge for continued eating.) Conversely, sugar and fat, especially in combination, potently stimulate sweet and savory taste sensors of the mouth and pleasure-reward centers of the brain to drive feeding to continue unabated.

Dietary choices condition body vehicle fueling programs to expect and seek a certain amount daily of sweetness or fat from foods. Obesity develops when body vehicle fueling required to satiate the desired levels of sweetness or fat to reach pleasure-reward expectations regularly exceeds body vehicle fuel energy needs and utilization capacities. Surplus fuels exceeding body vehicle energy burn are stored for future use to accumulate progressively as body vehicle fatness.

15.5 FACILITATORS AND ACCOMPLICES

Specific combinations and intensities of basic sweet, salty, sour, and savory tastes, as well as taste-enhancing properties of laboratory-synthesized chemicals, potently stimulate body vehicle taste and smell sensors to activate feeding program loops to run automatically without filtering or interference from higher-order brain controls. **Artificial sweeteners** and **flavor enhancers** (e.g., aspartame, sucralose, sorbitol, saccharin, monosodium glutamate) powerfully stimulate oral taste sensors that engage brain feeding responses to blind natural taste experiences and impair the brain nutritional gauging that controls satiety and, eventually, distort the discriminant capacity of oral taste sensors toward natural flavors and sweetness. Artificial flavors and sweeteners disturb the natural sense of fueling satiety to provide a false sense of appetite, as experienced when various "snacks," "appetizers," and "desserts" are consumed voraciously.

Synthetically designed chemicals that potently couple to body vehicle taste and smell sensors reprogram brain circuits and rewire feeding behaviors to compel eating beyond body vehicle nutritional needs. Industrially manufactured food and beverage products that are strategically formulated to target taste experiences and influence eating behaviors also undermine the nutritionally affiliated functioning of sensitive brain circuits, gut sensors, cellular metabolic processes, and gut microorganisms to compromise body vehicle fueling activities and energy processing more globally.

Eating taste-enhanced, artificially manufactured foods and beverages, vaping nicotine, smoking tobacco products, and chewing potently flavored gum on a regular basis alter the sensitivities and discriminatory capacities of oral taste sensors to disturb natural taste experiences and perturb the normal palatability for subtle taste qualities present within healthy natural whole foods.

15.6 FUELING, FEEDING, TEETH, AND EATING

Body vehicle fueling supplies the body vehicle with the energy substrates necessary to power metabolic operations and sustain body vehicle existence. Feeding introduces foods through the body vehicle mouth, digestive tract, or a vein to supply the body vehicle with nutrients and fuels. During routine oral feeding, known as **eating,** food is placed into the mouth, chewed, and swallowed to fill the stomach and gut, which then complete nutrient breakdown for blood absorption and delivery for cellular utilization.

Eating activities trigger a series of biologically programmed physiologic and biochemical digestive events eventually leading to intestinal absorption of essential nutrients and energy substrates. *Teeth are oral tools* that function under *voluntary* control to cut, shred, crush, and grind solid foods placed into the mouth in preparation for *involuntary* food processing by the gut and other digestive organs. Teeth mechanically assist the release of nutrients from ingested foods, ensuring a more thorough nutrient release downstream in the digestive tract to optimize nutrient absorption for cellular utilization. Regular flossing and brushing of teeth preserve the mechanical capabilities of a crucial component of food digestion that reduces larger ingested food portions into smaller size particles to facilitate further chemical food digestion with saliva in the mouth, and enzymes, acid, and bile in the gut.

Flossing and brushing teeth keep food residues and bacteria from caking and hardening on teeth to form plaque and tartar buildup, which can lead to gum disease and dental decay and loss, which impairs chewing capabilities to reduce dietary options and hamper nutrient release from foods to compromise body vehicle health.

The mouth, therefore, functions as a kitchen to prepare foods to be "cooked" further downstream within the gut for eventual body vehicle utilization. Eating requires the correct oral technique to initialize the transformation of crude fuel whole earth foods into usable nutrient and energy constituents that supply body vehicle needs. The proper eating technique is to place food into the mouth; chew the food thoroughly into a paste, pulp, or liquid by working tongue, cheek, and jaw muscles to mix, moisten, and chemically digest the food using saliva; and finally, swallow to clear the orally prepared food bolus down into the stomach for further digestive processing.

Tips for proper eating include the following:

1. Load smaller portions and bites of food into the mouth at any one time to allow comfortable and thorough chewing with mouth closed to moisten and digest mouth contents entirely down to a pulp or liquid before swallowing.

2. Practice *chewing a mouthful of food with eyes closed* a few times to focus undistracted on food qualities and to train oral sensors

to appreciate food flavors and textures and to recognize better when food reaches the correct consistency for swallowing.

Chewing with eyes closed allows for more **mindful eating** that directs attention toward food qualities and the eating process. Human senses exhibit survival **primacy** and prioritize visual and auditory sensory receptor inputs delivered to the brain from the eyes and ears ahead of taste and chewing sensations originating from the mouth. The primacy of human senses is highlighted under circumstances when direct orders are given to soldiers on guard duty to keep their eyes and ears open and their mouths shut. Consequently, engaging while eating in activities that distract attention away from eating, such as reading, watching television, or interacting with other media devices, interferes with the delivery of oral sensations to the brain to reduce the oral signaling and brain recognition of food information coming from the mouth. Therefore, closing the eyes while chewing allows the brain to focus better on sensations originating from the mouth to enhance oral food awareness and promote more thorough chewing. When feeling rushed and eating too fast during meals, eating speed can be slowed by chewing mouthful contents with eyes closed.

Two additional tips follow:

1. Sip liquids sparingly while chewing only to moisten foods to promote better mixing with saliva and allow easier swallowing with a more thorough clearance of mouth contents down into the stomach.
2. Swallow mouthful contents entirely before reloading the mouth with more food to repeat the eating process.

Chew, chew, chew!
The stomach doesn't have any teeth.
Chew your food and take your time; mealtime is a sacred time.

15.7 LIFE CONNECTIONS

The **digestive tract** or **gut** attaches directly in line to the mouth to receive swallowed mouth contents for further mechanical and chemical processing and refinement. The adult human gut consists of approximately 30 to 35 feet of tubing or expanded pouchlike compartments that connect serially to work in digestive sequence beginning from the mouth and ending at the rectal anus opening.

The gut functions as a lengthy natural whole earth *food processor* and nutrient *refinery* to prepare ingested foods to nourish body vehicle life functions and, consequently, makes the ingestion of already processed and refined commercial food products superfluous. The digestive tract is a *temporary holding tank* that safely contains, propels, and disassembles ingested crude fuel whole earth foods into basic nutrients and fuels for timely delivery into the blood for distribution to supply cellular metabolic demands. The gut operates like a long conveyor belt loaded up with passing nutrients and fuels that the body vehicle gradually pulls out according to body vehicle nutritional needs. The body vehicle continuously transports the gut around to feed as necessary to sustain body vehicle life. Consequently, the brain and gut have evolved an intricate communicative relationship that collectively ensures body vehicle function and survival.

Ingested life-sustaining nutrients and fuels communicate vital chemical, physical, and biological information to body vehicle oral, gut, and brain cells during digestion. Gut sensory portals recognize sweetness (natural and artificial), fat, bitter, and *umami* (savory) taste qualities of ingested foods, which in turn modulate feeding activities. Many brain neurochemicals involving human thoughts, emotions, and behaviors are also present within gut tissues. The intimate neurological and chemical connection between the brain and gut help explain why medicines used to treat behavioral health conditions, such as anxiety and depression, can unintentionally disturb gut function or even are sometimes intentionally prescribed to treat gut disorders.

The digestive tract additionally houses innumerable indwelling symbiotic microorganisms, which regulate gut function and the working relationships between the gut and brain to impact body vehicle eating behaviors, health, and survival. Finally, the digestive tract also works as an excretory and waste management system that disposes of nutritionally spent ingested crude fuel earth foods and other body vehicle refuse generated in the context of daily existence. Successive digestive tract compartments are separated by check valves that prevent system back-flow to promote forward movement of digesting nutrients and fuels progressively propelling down the gut, and containment of accumulating wastes for eventual expulsion from the body vehicle.

Each digestive compartment is a functional department with a job to do and accomplishes specific operations that combine with the actions of other gut compartments to reduce crude fuel, whole earth foods into smaller molecules absorbable into the blood. Consecutively arranged digestive chambers are specialized to sense, gauge, and process specific nutrient compositions or food qualities most suitable for digestion. During the sequential delivery of crude fuel, whole earth foods down the digestive tract, the successive fulfillment of digestive responsibilities by individual gut compartments depends on the completion of digestive work within preceding gut compartments.

Optimal digestive preparation of nutrients and fuels for absorption into blood and delivery to body vehicle cells for metabolic utilization ultimately depends on the combined totality of gut activities completed within individual digestive tract compartments. Undoubtedly, an excellent evolutionary rationale exists for the development of such a long and complicated system of tubes to process and refine natural whole earth foods, enclose innumerable symbiotic microorganisms, and manage generated digestive waste products.

Digestion and cellular nutrient delivery proceed in a *safe mode* of body vehicle metabolic operations when the body vehicle fuels appropriately with crude fuel whole earth foods that utilize the entire length of the gut for digestive processing and nutrient absorption into the blood.

15.8 DIGESTION

Digestion is a chemical, mechanical process that transforms ingested crude fuel, whole earth foods into forms suitable for blood absorption and ultimate metabolic utilization to power body vehicle life–sustaining cellular operations. Digestive activities within the intestines commence even before food is delivered down into the gut.

The anticipation and thought of food and the act of eating are potent stimulants of gut motility and secretion of various hormones and digestive juices such as acid, bile, and enzymes by the stomach, intestines, liver, and pancreas, which work collectively to break down and prepare ingested foods to energize the body vehicle.

The initial brain or **cephalic phase** of digestion works like *autostart* on a car to rev up and ready the gut engine in preparation for food to drive down the gut for digestive processing and accounts for up to a quarter of intestinal digestive activity associated with eating. The oral and subsequent intestinal processes that sequentially dismantle larger ingested food nutrients into tiny molecular particles absorbable into blood require adequate biological time to accomplish correctly. Digestive work is analogous to breaking down large, solid concrete slabs into the individual sand, stone, and cement powder ingredients to be reutilized and reconfigured in alternative construction projects.

Processing chambers of the digestive system are lined with complex working barrier surfaces composed of integrated structural, neurologic, vascular, hormonal, and immune system of defense cells that intimately communicate with each other and the rest of the body vehicle while accomplishing vital nutritional operations. The intestinal barrier cells protectively interface between ingested foods and gut-dwelling microorganisms and all other internal body vehicle cells. Intestinal barrier linings possess intricate fuel and nutrient sensors, and super selective pores and biological transporters that selectively extract and absorb readied and available nutrients and fuels from passing foods undergoing digestion.

Stimulated gut sensors continuously regulate intestinal pores to open and close biologically and transporters to carry fuels and nutrients across gut membranes into the blood based on the metabolic needs of the body vehicle, as well as on the chemical properties and concentrations of passing nutrient and fuel molecules. The barrier lining surfaces of the digestive system are where the internal body vehicle domain and external environment meet and clash to enhance, maintain, or compromise the quality of body vehicle life and health.

Digestion involves a complex interplay between a multitude of body vehicle components and the ingested foods being digested, with the constituents of digestion elaborately signaling the rest of the body vehicle. Intestinal barrier cells, digestive organ secretions, ingested foods, products of food digestion, and residing gut microorganisms all interact to direct digestive operations and inform the brain and rest of the body vehicle with neurobiochemical "feedback" concerning ongoing digestive activities.

Maintaining the correct balance of digestive signaling ensures body vehicle health and well-being. Disturbances in the balance of digestive signaling lead to gut and body vehicle malfunctions and illnesses and possibly to the death of the body vehicle system. Consequently, numerous factors modify digestive signaling, including

1. properties of ingested foods and their products of digestion
2. food additives
3. use of medications, vitamins, and health supplements
4. body vehicle age and physical and emotional state of health
5. surgical alterations to native gut anatomy and other digestive organs, such as the gallbladder and pancreas
6. balance, composition, and activity of resident gut microorganisms

15.9 ESOPHAGUS

The **esophagus** is an approximately 10-inch-long transporting tube that connects to the oral cavity at the throat to transfer by squeezing and pushing, swallowed liquid and chewed food boluses down past the heart and lung organs of the chest cavity into the abdominal cavity stomach pouch for further digestive processing.

Esophageal health disorders are increasing in prevalence in societies experiencing rising obesity rates and a growing reliance on processed food and beverage products to supply nutritional needs and on pharmaceutical agents to maintain personal health.

Corrosive and allergic-like inflammatory injuries of the esophagus, resulting from toxic chemical and immunologic effects of irritating foods and pharmaceutical substances and caustic backsplash injuries from refluxing stomach acid and bile, are rapidly becoming common scourges in obese modern societies excessively consuming processed food products.

15.10 STOMACH

The **stomach** is a large, expandable, muscular pouch connected in line to the esophagus, which continues crude fuel earth food digestion after receiving swallowed liquids and chewed saliva digested food boluses passing down from the esophagus. The stomach kneads, churns, and mixes swallowed food boluses with stomach acid, mucus, and digestive enzymes to squeeze out and release nutrients further and convert the food boluses into a thin liquid, which becomes squirted through a small funnel-like opening into the beginning portion of the small intestine for additional digestive processing or rapid absorption into the blood.

Proper food digestion in the stomach reduces ingested food contents to tiny particles or a liquid absorbable directly or eventually into the blood through pores or transporters lining the small intestine. After the stomach adequately completes digestive activities, any remaining solid food residues are forcefully expelled into the small intestine for additional processing and nutrient extraction, or for delivery down the gut into the colon to feed residing microorganisms.

In response to contained stomach contents, sensor cells lining the stomach release specific chemical hormone substances and neurologically signal the brain and other gut components to coordinate stomach and intestinal digestive processing according to body vehicle feeding activities and nutritional needs. Ingestion of copious fluids during meals is best avoided to prevent excessive dilution and premature washout of digesting stomach contents before the stomach adequately completes its digestive operations.

15.11 STOMACH ACID

Stomach acid, included as standard body vehicle equipment at birth, is a corrosive substance produced by specialized acid-producing cells lining the stomach wall that helps digest food and assists in the performance of many other essential digestive and physiologic body vehicle gut functions.

Stomach acid creates the correct acidity and chemical environment for proper digestion of ingested foods by helping to dissolve remaining solid food particles entering the stomach from the esophagus, activating important digestive enzymes required to complete breakdown of nutrients for eventual absorption into blood from the intestines, and chemically converting certain minerals such as iron into forms suitable for gut absorption. Therefore, some of the many known stomach acid functions include

1. breaking down and dissolving swallowed foods for further digestive processing and absorption by the intestines
2. providing the appropriate stomach acidity (pH) to activate enzymes secreted by the stomach to enhance food digestion and absorption

3. promoting gut absorption of minerals and vitamins such as iron, calcium, and vitamin B_{12}
4. sterilizing ingested foods by killing swallowed microorganisms to prevent body vehicle infections particularly involving the gut and lungs
5. complementing the intestinal, pancreatic, and liver digestive functioning to help ingested foods complete digestion

Consequently, blocking stomach acid production and secretion medically with pharmaceuticals to relieve symptoms caused through overeating and consuming unhealthy foods, interferes with proper gut digestive operations and absorption of essential food nutrients and, additionally, predisposes to gastrointestinal and lung infections developing from swallowed microorganisms not killed by stomach acid that pass down the gut or reflux back up the esophagus to spill into the lungs.

15.12 SMALL INTESTINE

The **small intestine** is a long, slender, muscular tube measuring approximately 20 feet in length that contains a massive inner surface area lined by barrier cells arranged in deep piles like that of a thick shag rug. The small intestine mechanically mixes and chemically digests food residues and liquids delivered from the stomach to complete digestion of ingested foods and beverages, and then employs complex biological mechanisms to absorb water, simple fuel molecules, and basic salt, mineral, and vitamin micronutrients necessary for sustaining body vehicle operations and existence.

Barrier cells lining the small intestine that contact digesting food contents are equipped extensively with nutrient and fuel digesting enzymes, transporters, and pores that work selectively to break down and absorb passing nutrients and fuels. The small intestine also secretes specialized chemical hormones to integrate and coordinate intestinal digestive activities with the functioning of other digestive organs such as the liver, gallbladder, and pancreas. Small intestinal digestive operations combine with the effects of digestive secretions from the liver and pancreas organs to prepare contained gut nutrients and fuels for absorption into the blood to feed the body vehicle system.

Three inner fitting sleeves composed of tightly wound muscle fibers arranged in different orientations wrap around an innermost layer of small intestinal barrier membrane lining cells in contact with chemically digesting food, and mechanically massage the intestinal food contents to help release nutrient and fuel molecules for absorption through gut barrier membrane transporters and pores.

The small intestine extracts most of the ingested food nutrients and fuels that supply body vehicle nutritional requirements necessary to sustain body vehicle survival. The small intestine is also the largest immune organ of the body vehicle system, containing an enormous network of the immune system of defense cells that continuously monitor and protect body vehicle intestinal barriers against breaches and attack from ingested toxins and harmful microorganisms.

Immune defense system cells are primed to attention in the small intestine, learning to recognize any threatening intestinal contents passing through. Small intestine immune cells ready for action then migrate and distribute throughout the remaining body vehicle system to be on alert waiting to be reminded of their small intestinal encounters with objectionable elements. Subsequent recognition of any undesirable body vehicle invaders then leads primed immune system cells to react and ardently protect body vehicle health.

Many body vehicle immunological disorders and allergies may originate from sensitized gut immune cells that have become overly activated or inappropriately turned on within the gut by traversing intestinal contents. Gut sensors, immune cells, and barrier linings interact intimately with ingested foods, products of digestion, residing gut microorganisms, and digestive secretions, and then signal and communicate with the brain and other body vehicle organs to couple digestive activities with overall body vehicle operations.

A multitude of factors may modify small intestinal digestive activities, including the age, emotional state, nutritional needs, and physical condition of the body vehicle; underlying body vehicle illnesses; food types and chemical food additives consumed; medications and health supplements ingested; and the abundance, variety, and activity of residing gut microbial organisms.

Eating the wrong foods and ingesting chemicals irritating to body vehicle immune cells may pose numerous body vehicle liabilities compromising to health, well-being, longevity, and survival. Celiac Sprue with gluten intolerance is one example of a digestive health disorder becoming more prevalent in modern industrial societies. Celiac Sprue involves a major reactive inflammatory injury involving small intestinal membranes in genetically susceptible individuals repeatedly exposed to high levels of gluten, which is extracted from wheat, barley, and rye grains and then ubiquitously added in high concentrations to various industrially formulated and processed commercial food and beverage products consumed by humans.

15.13 LARGE INTESTINE, COLON, OR LARGE BOWEL

The **colon** is an approximately 5-foot-long, relatively voluminous and larger-caliber tube lined with partial dividers that occupies the abdominal and pelvic cavities in an inverted "U" shape and connects serially through a check valve directly to the preceding thinner caliber small intestine to form the terminal portion of the gut. The colon operates as a water conservation organ, nutritional waste recycling center, and waste holding tank and houses trillions of resident microorganisms estimated to minimally equal and possibly outnumber body vehicle cells by at least 10- to 100-fold.

The small intestine dumps undigested food matter; food residue wastes produced during intestinal digestion; any toxins ingested orally or cleared from the blood through the liver into the gut; liver bile components; and water into the colon that all mix with residing colonic microorganisms. The colon absorbs water from stool to concentrate and solidify fecal wastes for convenient expulsion from the body vehicle, while colonic microorganisms extract any vestiges of nutrients and fuels delivered into the colon for nourishment and to feed colon lining cells. The colon, therefore, is a home for vast numbers of microorganisms that work symbiotically with the body vehicle.

15.14 FECAL FLORA AND GUT MICROBIOME

The body vehicle literally contains, transports, and symbiotically coexists with an immense population of living microorganisms known as the **microbiota.** The microbiota occupies all body vehicle surfaces, crevices, cavities, and tubes that contact the external environment, such as the gut, skin, skin structures, mouth, upper respiratory tract, and external genital urinary structures including the vaginal cavity in females.

The **gut microbiota** or **fecal flora** is predominantly composed of an enormous population of bacteria and a small percentage of yeast and other more primitive microbes that live substantially confined to the colon, and functions as another body vehicle organ system that works intimately with and for the body vehicle to promote body vehicle health and survival. Essentially, microbial floras are intricately complex living biological machines employed by, working with, dwelling within, and dependent on their human hosts.

The **microbiome** comprises the totality of all the residing predominantly **bacterial** body vehicle microorganisms and their generated biological products, which interact symbiotically with the body vehicle to modulate the cellular operations and functions of the body vehicle to ensure body vehicle and microbiota existences. Additional microorganisms that inhabit the body vehicle structure include **viruses** grouped into the **virome** and **yeast** and **fungi** categorized within the **mycobiome,** which constitute two -*ome* classifications that are less well characterized or understood scientifically.

Everyone carries a unique microbiome signature identified by a distinct population, composition, balance, and function of microbial organisms. At birth, the human microbiome is limited in diversity and composition and substantially resembles the microbiome of the mother. During the first few years of human life, the microbiota dynamically changes to become richer in composition and diversity as the body vehicle acquires and cultivates microorganisms based on the living environment, diet, lifestyle behaviors, intimate human associations, and exposures to chemical agents including medications, health products, and food additives. After the first few years of life, the makeup of the microbiome begins to stabilize and becomes more permanent by adolescence to reflect the consistency of an individual daily human existence.

Drastic changes to any factors that affect daily human existences, such as the diet, lifestyle, state of health, living environment, use of pharmaceutical and chemical products, and human associations, can significantly affect and alter the composition, diversity, richness, balance, or function of the microbiome within as little as a few days. The statement "you are what you eat" rings true in many ways because the body vehicle begins to acquire gut microorganisms through the mouth immediately during birth and maybe earlier while still in the womb. Ingesting foods and liquids, placing objects into the mouth such as thumbs, pacifiers, and eating utensils, swapping spit during kissing, and swallowing nasal mucus draining inhaled microorganisms down into the throat are some of the ways microbes gain access into the human gut.

The gut microbiota is chiefly composed of several thousand different kinds of bacterial species with total microorganism numbers minimally equaling the estimated 4 trillion cells of the body vehicle and possibly amounting upwards of 10–100 trillion, with various yeasts and other primitive nonbacterial microbial life-forms comprising roughly a smaller 5% fraction of aggregate gut microorganisms. Additionally, vast numbers of viruses that are yet to be quantified inhabit body vehicle cells as well as the indwelling bacterial microorganisms. Therefore, the digestive tract minimally houses approximately 10–100 times more microorganisms than the number of all native body vehicle cells combined.

Consequently, more than 90% of the DNA containing living cells embodied within the entire human body vehicle structure are foreign microorganisms that reside on body vehicle surfaces or within body vehicle cavities or tubes, with most of these microorganisms localizing predominantly in the colon and other parts of the long gut tube. Conversely, of all living cells comprising the whole body vehicle structure, less than 10% originate from human DNA, while the remaining 90% arise from symbiotic microbial inhabitants possessing foreign DNA.

All living biological organisms require fuel energy and other vital nutrients to exist and function. A complex biological interplay between the body vehicle and the indwelling microbiota governs the existence of both entities living together symbiotically. Gut microbial organisms exist within functionally structured communities to carry out specific interdependent biological activities that maintain body vehicle system health and survival.

Since the human microbiota depends entirely on the human host to ensure its survival, the microbiota has a vested interest to modulate the fuel energy balance, extraction, and utilization and impact the nutritional behaviors of its host to exist and thrive. The residing gut microbiota feeds on the undigested food residues and digestive food wastes delivered down the gut, and on any nutrients contained in digestive and intestinal secretions and debris shed from gut barrier lining cells.

Colon lining cells are, in turn, fed directly by metabolic products produced by the gut microbiota, which additionally fosters intestinal immune cell development and competence to safeguard body vehicle health against invasion from unfriendly microbial intruders.

Human resistance to illness and disease is a shared undertaking between the body vehicle immune system and microbiome activity and is contingent on maintaining the proper nutritional health of the body vehicle that supports a healthy indwelling microflora. The body vehicle is, therefore, a living biological entity composed of a stable structural framework that houses and transports a vast, dynamically active, and functionally responsive population of bacteria, yeast, and other microorganisms that dwell within as vested working passengers.

The body vehicle system is like a giant spaceship traveling through the world universe, with the human body vehicle cells and tissues composing the shell structure that holds and transports a diverse multitude of dependent indwelling life-forms, with all elements working interdependently to journey symbiotically through earth time and space.

The human body vehicle with all contained microbial inhabitants is a cohesive biological system that navigates the complex earth ecosystem attempting to maximize own survival under a variety of earth challenges. Therefore, the body vehicle system is not alone and carries enormous responsibilities to properly maintain and protect both the external earth and internal body vehicle environments to ensure own health and existence.

Some scientifically described and hypothesized functions of the vast fecal microbial flora include

1. production of certain micronutrients essential for body vehicle survival needs (e.g., vitamin K and certain B vitamins)
2. regulation of body vehicle energy balances and utilization to protect against or predispose to the development of obesity
3. harvesting of residual energies from incompletely digested foods delivered down the gut to supply body vehicle energy needs
4. decomposition of fecal wastes into usable nutrients that directly nourish cells lining the colon (e.g., glutamine, butyrate)
5. interaction with the body vehicle immune system to promote and direct intestinal immune system development and functional competency to protect against infections and intestinal overgrowth of unfriendly opportunistic microorganisms
6. modulation of body vehicle immune balance and activity to regulate genetic propensities toward the development of various autoimmune disorders such as Crohn's disease, ulcerative colitis, multiple sclerosis, psoriasis, and rheumatoid arthritis
7. control of the transit of nutrients, fuels, and waste contents through the gut to impact bowel activity and nutrient absorption
8. connection with the body vehicle experiences of the surrounding world through biological effects on mood, emotional balance,

and sense of well-being to affect behavioral expression and predispose to health conditions such as anxiety and depression

9. affecting the susceptibility for cancer to develop within the colon and other body vehicle tissues

10. impacting body vehicle vascular health by promoting the metabolic breakdown of ingested animal flesh components into substances that increase risks for atherosclerosis or hardening of the arteries to develop. (Phospholipid breakdown into TMAO)

11. biochemical transformation and metabolism of various pharmaceutical drugs and other chemical agents passing down the gut to affect the blood delivery and biologic availability and activity of orally ingested medicinal and other pharmaceutical products

Healthier microbiomes promoting healthy human existences can be designed and cultivated through appropriate nutritional and lifestyle choices.

Body vehicle factors that affect the composition, diversity, balance, and richness of the intestinal flora include individual genetics, age, health, living environment, diet, physical activity, and sleep. Extraneous influences on the intestinal flora include ingested medicines; health supplements; food additives, preservatives, and contaminants; alcohol; and inadvertently swallowed hygiene products, such as toothpaste and mouthwash, that possess sanitizing, antiseptic, or disinfectant, antimicrobial properties. Effects on the microbiome, in turn, affect body vehicle physical and mental functioning. Richer and more diversified fecal microbial compositions are associated with longevity, a greater sense of well-being, better physical and mental health, and reduced likelihood of obesity.

Human frailty, illness, obesity, autoimmune disorders, and disease states such as cancer tend to have more restricted and less diversified fecal floras. Diets based on heavily consuming various plants increase diversification and richness of fecal microbial populations. Mother Nature does the best job of directly providing the appropriate feed for the body vehicle system through natural crude fuel whole earth foods, which optimally deliver the form, composition, and content of nutrients to sustain healthier and more diversified body vehicle microbiotas.

Extraneous factors that compromise the integrity and constitution of the microbiome include poor nutritional sustenance that creates body vehicle nutrient imbalances; regular ingestion of "sanitizing" products such as alcohol beverages; consumption of chemical food additives having antimicrobial properties such as preservatives; usage of recreational drugs, antibiotics, and other pharmaceutical agents including health supplements.

Substances affecting the intestinal microbiota gain direct gut access after oral ingestion or are indirectly eliminated into the gut through liver bile after blood filters through the liver carrying substances injected into a vein or absorbed through the skin, lungs, or nasal, vaginal, rectal, or eye mucous membranes after contact.

Processed food products manufactured using few nutrient ingredients often limited to refined flours, sugars, fats, and salt laced with artificial chemicals provide minimal nutritional value and increased toxicity to the microbiota. Food products that require minimal intestinal work to digest and absorb quickly into the blood immediately from initial gut segments deprive lower-gut microbes of receiving adequate nutritional sustenance.

When vital nutrients are rapidly siphoned off into the blood in earlier gut segments where microbial populations are sparse and in relatively low numbers, the bulk of the gut microbiota residing in lower parts of the small intestine and the colon that dependently await gut nutrient delivery become starved to disturb the microbiome activity and balance. Keeping protective gut microbial organisms in appropriate balance and working symbiotically with and for the body vehicle requires feeding the body vehicle with healthy diversified natural crude fuel whole earth foods, which digest utilizing the entire 30–35 feet of the gut to feed intestinal barrier cells and residing gut microbes more thoroughly.

Maintaining a healthy composition, diversity, balance, richness, and activity of the microbiome also depends on avoiding toxins such as antibiotics, food preservatives, chemical food additives, nonessential pharmaceuticals and health supplements, and excessive alcohol that poison the microbiota. Consequently, everything introduced into or affecting the body vehicle impacts the microbiome in some way.

Toxic elements, behaviors, and lifestyles that adversely modify the gut microbiome to disturb vital relationships among indwelling gut microorganisms and between the microorganisms and body vehicle intestinal lining barrier and immune cells harm the body vehicle system. Major disruptions of the body vehicle microbiome that occur through any factors can reduce life quality, lead to illness, and shorten life-span. Therefore, behaviors and lifestyles that enhance the health and avoid the poisoning of the body vehicle microbial flora promote body vehicle health and survival.

Increasingly, scientific research inordinately blames intestinal microbes for body vehicle dysfunction and compromised human well-being by linking the intestinal bacteria with excessive weight gain and various other human health disorders including depression, gas, bloating, constipation, diarrhea, inflammatory conditions, allergies, and cancer. Humans, natural crude fuel, whole earth foods, bacteria, and other microorganisms have all coexisted symbiotically for millions of years, long before the dawn of modern living and the emergence of commercial food, pharmaceutical, and health supplement industries, when human nutritional disorders with their attendant suffering and health consequences became rampant and progressive.

What is definitively characterized scientifically is that extraneous human exposures, particularly to environmental agents and orally ingested elements such as food and chemicals including medications and health supplements, shape the balance, composition, diversity, abundance, and activity of bacteria and other indwelling body vehicle microorganisms to impact body vehicle operations, health, and well-being.

Selecting out unfavorable body vehicle microbiomes through poor nutritional, behavioral, and lifestyle choices leads to unhealthier and shorter human lives. As the understanding of the vital importance of the human microbiome in affecting human health and well-being has grown, a new baby has appeared on the scene in the lucrative commercial "health" industry market.

Commercial industries are increasingly emphasizing the relationship of gut bacteria and yeast to human health and longevity to cleverly redirect consumers to develop a new reliance on the rescue industry to rectify self-inflicted human health problems. Profit-hungry commercial industries are heavily marketing commercially designed microbe combinations called **probiotics** or nutrient agents named **prebiotics** that allegedly promote healthier microbiotas to consumers wanting better health.

Meanwhile, humans continue to unwittingly pollute their body vehicles by consuming processed food industry products and using artificially manufactured pharmaceutical agents and health supplements to perpetuate the worsening health plague caused by growing human toxicities. Unfortunately, rescue industries continue to angle toward new horizons of commercial opportunity, manipulating consumers into buying products promoted to purportedly groom body vehicle microbial populations, despite the vast chasms of knowledge existing in understanding the immensely complex worlds of microbe and human interactions.

Artificial manipulation of the internal body vehicle microbial universe is yet another generic megalomaniac industry theme of attempting to dominate the world of human health for profit. The understanding of principles governing even the simplest of body vehicle biological operations and human interactions is significantly limited, and even less is known concerning the intricacies determining complex symbiotic and pathologic interactions between humans and microbial organisms.

Predictable healthy alterations of residing human microbial floras with a few probiotic pills that contain a relatively small variety and number of bacterial or yeast organisms is unlikely to occur in the context of ongoing unhealthy nutritional, behavioral, and lifestyle choices, while fully understanding the consequences of artificially manipulating the indwelling human microbes is even more limited.

Most research on microbial organisms is carried out under scientifically designed and rigorously controlled laboratory conditions at set time points and over finite durations, limiting the generalizations of research findings that can be applied accurately to diversified human populations lively freely over longer time intervals within enormously complex and dynamically changing external world environments.

The immense complexities of vastly integrated human and microbial biological systems that balance delicately within expansive environmental ecosystems create considerable challenges for even the most ardent researchers using the most advanced and sophisticated scientific methods to garner reliably accurate information from their research endeavors.

Commercial industries often thrive financially on the cutting edge of science and misunderstanding, capitalizing on human ignorance and unrealistic consumer expectations to sell health interventions having unproven benefits before truth and understanding restrict or shut down their profit pipelines and opportunities to earn money at consumer expense.

Human stool may be only fecal waste for most but is commercial gold for profit-driven rescue industries that offer stool testing to characterize the bacterial and yeast compositions of evacuated human feces. Fecal microbial testing provides biological information that may be imprecise, inaccurate, or extremely difficult to interpret and correlate usefully with ongoing individual human existences, but unsurprisingly arrives with health advice and product offers to correct supposed fecal microbial imbalances for a fee. Therefore, cultivating a **friendly microbiome** requires feeding the body vehicle with the best Mother Nature–made crude fuel natural whole earth foods, and preventing toxic foods, chemicals, and non-essential pharmaceutical products from accessing the body vehicle as destructive Trojan horses through the sacred "O"-hole fueling portal.

Working harder to make, keep, and support indwelling body vehicle microbial 'friends' that protect and harmoniously coexist with the body vehicle maximizes body vehicle system health and survival. The potential for household cleaners, disinfectants, and personal hygiene products to harmfully impact the body vehicle microbiome is routinely underestimated and understated. Commercial industries manipulate human ignorance and germ phobias to push household and hygiene antibacterial and antimicrobial, antiseptic soaps, disinfectants, sanitizers, and cleansers, which indiscriminately kill microorganisms under the guise of protecting individual and public health and safety but which, in reality, are ineffective in ridding microbes unfairly condemned as unsanitary and dangerous to humanity. Antigerm agents that kill 99.99% of 1 billion germs still leave behind 100,000 live resistant microorganisms that reproduce and multiply rapidly to be unaffected by further applications of the antigerm preparations. The body vehicle internalizes any chemical aerosols, liquids, creams, or powders that contact body vehicle surfaces or membranes. Consumers using antibacterial and antimicrobial hygiene, household, or environmental products unsuspectingly absorb these toxic chemicals through the nasal, mouth, and gut membranes or skin to inadvertently poison the body vehicle system and transform native body vehicle microbial floras in unpredictable ways, predisposing to unknown immediate or future health consequences.

The actual body vehicle detriment and health impact of industrial antimicrobial, disinfectant, and sanitizing products are unknown and undetermined and are likely to remain unknown if powerful industry forces suppress scientific attempts to resolve this subject matter only to continue selling these products to unsuspecting consumers brainwashed to fear germs. In a glimmer of hope, the **Occupational Safety and Health Administration (OSHA)** branch of the U.S. government has instrumentally helped create legislative measures to protect industrial workers from chemical toxicity workplace injuries related to the manufacture of chemicals used in foods or for hygiene, household, and environmental purposes.

15.15 BIOFILM

A crucial thin layer of mucus slime known as **biofilm** superficially coats the internal surfaces of the gut tube membranes and vitally works to separate passing or contained gut materials away from direct physical contact with the intestinal membrane lining cells. Biofilm acts as a sampling medium across which intestinal contents including nutrients, hormones, digestive secretions, and gut microflora, and the cells lining the gut can communicate back and forth to exchange vital chemical and biological information directing body vehicle survival.

As previously discussed, chemical detergents known as **emulsifiers,** which are commonly added to processed foods to allow dispersion and smooth mixing of oil and water-based food ingredients, can dissolve this protective mucus biofilm layer. Without an intact and functional biofilm layer, intestinal contents including gut bacteria and other microorganisms come into direct contact with gut lining cells and membranes, inciting reactive, inflammatory gut immune cell survival responses that lead to the biological breakdown of gut linings to create a "leaky gut" predisposing to numerous health problems.

Another potential source of chemical detergents that may be unintentionally and unknowingly introduced down the gut to disrupt the mucus biofilm layer and adversely impact body vehicle health may come from incompletely rinsed off detergent residues remaining on dishware, cookware, and eating and cooking utensils following detergent washing especially using automatic dishwashers.

15.16 PANCREAS

The **pancreas** is a digestive organ that resides within the posterior abdominal cavity nestled between the spine and the lower back side of the stomach. The pancreas connects with the first part of the small intestine to deliver digestive secretions that neutralize stomach acid and promote the enzymatic chemical breakdown of larger nutrient food particles entering the small intestine from the stomach.

Pancreatic functions additionally include sensing blood sugar levels and then releasing insulin or glucagon hormones as required, which work oppositely to balance blood sugar levels within a biologically safe range for body vehicle existence. Insulin and glucagon hormones work oppositely on the liver and other body vehicle cells to affect the absorption, storage, metabolic processing, and release of sugar molecules to balance blood sugar levels into a normal range.

Modern industrial societies consuming diets substantially in the form of processed and refined food and beverage products that rapidly *flood the blood* with excessive fuel calories are experiencing obesity epidemics with an increasing prevalence of type 2 diabetes. Type 2 or secondary diabetes results from pancreatic burnout or failure of the pancreas gland to adequately keep up insulin production to meet the enormously increased insulin requirements necessary to metabolically process the excessive sugar calorie energy loads delivered repeatedly into the blood.

Cells that are continuously bombarded by sugar calories and insulin eventually develop insulin resistance, conveniently providing pharmaceutical industries with commercial opportunities to design and sell chemical products that can overcome this insulin resistance artificially.

Pharmaceutical agents clear toxic blood sugar levels by forcing the kidneys to dump filtered sugar out through the urine, by stimulating the pancreas to squeeze out more insulin production, by exerting potent insulin-like effects to drive sugar into cells, or by interfering with metabolic, cellular processes producing insulin resistance. Alternatively, administering substantially higher doses of insulin compared to the amounts of insulin that the pancreas releases normally daily temporarily overcomes cellular insulin resistance.

Pharmaceutical diabetes treatments often force-feed more sugar calories into cells already overstuffed with sugar and fat fuel energies and experiencing overwhelmed metabolic capacities to process and assimilate additional sugar fuel energies. Consequently, many individuals pharmaceutically treating type 2 diabetes caused by obesity gain even more weight and develop higher levels of insulin resistance as sugar fuel calories are pounded into energy overloaded cells without reprieve.

15.17 LIVER

The **liver** is a large, solid organ situated in the abdominal cavity against the bottom surface of the diaphragm directly behind the front side of the right lower rib cage. The liver has a dual blood supply and receives both newly oxygenated blood directly pumped from the heart, and all the blood that is returning to the heart for recirculation from the abdominal digestive organs. Sensors in the liver gauge and correctively respond to body vehicle metabolic needs.

The liver receives and filters out virtually all gut products including digested fuel and nutrient constituents and toxins absorbed into the blood for metabolic processing, detoxification, packaging, and storage or export and distribution to all other body vehicle tissues and cells. Metabolic and biochemical liver products release directly into the blood for immediate distribution to all body vehicle cells or are secreted into liver bile down a tube that discharges into the beginning portion of the small intestine alongside the tube that drains pancreatic secretions into the gut.

The liver occupies a strategic crossroads within the body vehicle that ties together body vehicle biochemical and metabolic survival needs with body vehicle nutrition and gut digestive function and microbiome activity. The rich dual blood supply to the liver helps support the many complex biologic and high energy metabolic processes that occur in the liver.

A few of the many essential biologic functions performed by the liver include the following:

> *Body vehicle detoxification*: The liver filters out biochemical toxins generated internally through body vehicle cellular metabolic processes or that externally gain access into the body vehicle through oral ingestion, inhalation, or skin and mucous membrane absorption.

> The liver then biochemically transforms filtered toxins for eventual excretion from the body vehicle through the liver bile into the stool, through the kidneys into the urine, or through the lungs into the exhaled breath.

> *Synthesis, secretion, transformation, and activation of hormones.*

> *Fighting body vehicle infections*: The liver is part of the body vehicle immune system and protectively functions as the killing field where invading infectious microorganisms with their deadly products are cleared from the blood circulation and exterminated.

> *Synthesis, packaging, and distribution of energy, nutrient, and other vital biologic substances that sustain body vehicle metabolic functioning*: The liver stores an emergency supply of ready fuel energy that can be immediately released into the blood for systemic use during times of body vehicle fasting or stress. The production and packaging of cholesterol and fat occur principally in the liver. **Fatty liver disorders** that result from overwhelming the metabolic capacities of the liver with excessive sugar and fat fuel calories are rising in prevalence and rapidly becoming the primary cause of liver failure and death in modern western societies experiencing escalating obesity rates.

> *Production of vital body vehicle life substances*: These include blood clotting elements and essential blood proteins such as albumin, which helps maintain tissue fluid balance and blood pressure and acts as a circulating carrier molecule that distributes hormones, nutrients, and medications throughout the body vehicle to tissues and cells.

15.18 CELLS OF THE BODY VEHICLE

The individual *cells of the body vehicle organ systems* are the destination points for fuel and nutrient delivery and function as specialized units that ultimately perform all the specific genetically assigned biologic roles and metabolic operations that are integrated and combined to maintain body vehicle health and existence. A particularly vital organ system composed of variously functioning cells that disperse throughout the entire body vehicle but function cohesively to monitor the body vehicle intimately against undesirable microbes, noxious agents, and rogue native body vehicle cells is the immune system of defense. The immune system of defense cells and their biochemical weaponry protect the body vehicle against invading microorganisms, disturbances in native microbial communities, mutant cells predisposing to cancer, and toxic corruption of internal body vehicle environments.

Elaborately complex repertoires of energy and nutrient-dependent signaling and communication activities that are acutely sensitive to toxic disruption stringently coordinate the actions of the immune system. The fully intact and operational body vehicle is genetically programmed with innate capabilities to mount immediate immune defense responses against body vehicle incursions and survival threats, or adaptively organize elaborate delayed defenses against hostile body vehicle provocations that arise through harmful environmental interactions. Therefore, immune system properties that are working to ensure body vehicle survival include the capacity to mount immediate or delayed, genetically programmed or learned body vehicle defenses against internal or externally introduced insults; an intimately collaborative communication network among immune and other body vehicle cells; the potential to amplify immune responses and recruit various immune cell lines as necessary to oppose and contain biological, body vehicle assaults; and a capability to form immune system memories for specific body vehicle dangers to allow quicker immune responses in the future.

Formulated chemicals and artificially manufactured food products that biochemically and metabolically stress body vehicle stability may disturb and corrupt delicate naturally programmed and learned immune system of defense survival responses. Maintaining balanced and properly working immune system operations requires that body vehicle nutritional needs be met appropriately to prevent the development of metabolic deficiencies that create immune weaknesses while avoiding excessive fueling and nutrient deliveries that cause immune toxicities.

15.19 BLOOD VESSELS

Body vehicle **blood vessels** combine to form an extensive infrastructure of intricately interconnected branching tubes known as the **vascular system,** which circulates vital blood fluid elements and cells to establish a **liquid communication**

network between the brain, digestive system, liver, and all other body vehicle organs, tissues, and cells.

Complex physiologic sensors densely wire blood vessels to gauge the composition and inherent electrical, physical, and chemical properties of flowing blood contents and then communicate retrieved information throughout the body vehicle system. The dynamic exchange of information between body vehicle tissues carried by flowing blood vessel contents integrates the body vehicle operations that sustain body vehicle viability. Vital body vehicle elements transported, distributed, and delivered by the blood vessel infrastructure include

1. sugar and fat fuels that power cellular energy needs
2. proteins and amino acids utilized to build body vehicle physical structures and metabolically active biologic components
3. mineral, salt, and vitamin micronutrients required for various metabolic, biochemical operations
4. water
5. regulatory hormones that direct and integrate cellular and tissue functions
6. red blood cells
7. blood clotting elements
8. the immune system of defense cells and products that protect against infections, toxicity, and cancer development
9. oxygen necessary to run immune and metabolic processes sustaining body vehicle life
10. warmth for proper regulation of body vehicle temperature-dependent metabolic reactions and physiologic activities

Finally, the vascular system also serves as a conduit to clear away toxins, metabolic waste products, and cellular debris generated during body vehicle cellular injury, repair, disintegration, and metabolic processing.

In summary, the body vehicle is a *life force driven and fuel powered biological machine entity composed of diverse communities of native working cells and microbial passengers,* all integrated to coexist and function together on a unified life journey through the earth.

16 HOMEOSTASIS OR BODY VEHICLE BIOLOGIC EQUILIBRIUM

Whereas inanimate objects rigidly submit to the fundamental laws and forces of nature, the living body vehicle intentionally exploits universal laws to survive and achieve life goals.

Therefore, higher-order, biological life-forms use the laws, forces, and elements of nature with the purpose to accomplish life-sustaining activities. The human body vehicle combines awareness and intellect with purposeful action and physical movement to exist more deliberately than lower biological life-forms.

Homeostasis is a state of body vehicle equilibrium having stable life-sustaining biological balance and function, which is determined by DNA genetic programming and influenced by internal and external body vehicle survival pressures. Complex chemical, physical, and biological body vehicle operations integrate to dynamically drive biochemical functions, physiologic actions, and behavioral routines into a homeostatic balance that attempts to optimize body vehicle existence under various conditions.

Body vehicle sensors carefully gauge all aspects of body vehicle existence and then activate the appropriate effectors to implement the physiologic responses necessary to restore and maintain balanced body vehicle operations with transparent body vehicle functioning. An analogy to preserving homeostasis would be a high-wire act continuously reacting and adjusting balance to keep from falling off a tightrope. Therefore, homeostasis mechanisms work to restore the rhythms and processes of body vehicle physiologic functions into a perfect equilibrium.

Maintaining homeostasis is inextricably intertwined with body vehicle fueling activities and the nutritional effects of ingested foods supplying body vehicle biological requirements. Daily human existence depends on the ability to respond appropriately to internal and external survival challenges while maintaining homeostasis or biological equilibrium. Internal biological signaling continuously alerts the body vehicle of maintenance needs and physiologic disturbances requiring attention, which trigger corrective behaviors or metabolic actions to address alert notifications. For example, hunger is experienced to fuel; a thirst to replace lost water; tiredness to rest and restore depleted energy; warmth to cool off; coldness to warm the body vehicle; and the urge to defecate or urinate to empty the bowel or urinary bladder of accumulated body vehicle wastes.

More significant homeostatic disturbances that imminently endanger body vehicle health and survival insinuate for attention more intensely, with alarms that dramatically interrupt or halt normal routine body vehicle activities and operations to compel more immediate corrective behavioral or biological responses. Interruptive alarms may present as intense cravings, pain, or loss of power, energy, or the ability to carry out usual activities, or may instead produce an overwhelming urge to perform specific body vehicle physical actions.

Homeostasis is a biological state that operationally exists within a representative target range of possibilities established for that state in corresponding human populations studied under defined sets of circumstances or scientific criteria. Unfortunately, the range of possibilities for any state observed for one study population existing under specific circumstances may not always coincide with the range of possibilities observed for that state in other study populations living under alternative conditions. Therefore, the homeostasis target range defined for one study group may not always apply to other similarly studied groups experiencing different environmental influences or social situations.

Biologic parameter values may even vary extremely and differ greatly among individuals having parameters that fall within the homeostasis or derived target range for their population. The imprecise designation of homeostasis results from limitations that emerge attempting to statistically define static optimum ranges for biological parameters measured in complicated biological systems, which are influenced dynamically by a myriad of complex environmental and social factors.

"**Normal**" homeostasis is approximated by making numerous scientifically controlled observations of certain human behaviors or by repeatedly measuring specific biologic properties under a defined set of conditions in various individuals, and then determining the **range of values** or **distribution range** that applies to the 95% majority of observations or measurements. For example, certain **biomarker** substances that indicate the presence of disease, or specific biologic parameters determining blood counts, blood chemistries, or hormone levels are measured in various human populations existing under diverse circumstances, and then grouped for statistical comparison.

Sophisticated scientific observations made on complex human behaviors or anatomical and biological aspects of body vehicle cells can also be assessed and quantified in defined ways for comparative analyses. The operational definition for the "normal" homeostasis range then becomes the *range of measured values* that includes the 95% majority of all measurements taken, having as cutoffs on the low end the 2.5% of measurements falling below the minimum value for the range, and on the high end the 2.5% of measurements falling above the maximum value for the range. Therefore, the "normal" range provides a working *reference* or *target range* with specified limits for any variables studied in populations under defined criteria and approximates the biological ideal for the studied parameters under specific circumstances.

"Normal" is the 2.5%–97.5% statistical range of all measured values for a study population. "Abnormal" only means outside the normal range of values obtained for tested parameters and does not necessarily indicate health imbalance or presence of disease.

When testing assesses individuals as normal or having normal test results, the indication is that test results fall within the statistically derived reference range where 95% of all other obtained test results fall. Conversely, "normal" may not truly be "normal." Parameter values falling within the specified "normal" reference range do not always guarantee the absence of illness states that are statistically more likely to associate with parameter measurements which fall greatly outside the bounds of the "normal" reference range.

Normal health parameters obtained by studying populations existing substantially dependent on commercial industries and uniformly subjected to powerful market forces that promote biologically unhealthy behaviors and lifestyles, may not accurately represent optimal states of human existence that truly maximize health and longevity. Health parameter target ranges that describe and apply to unhealthy populations can erroneously misdirect public health guidelines toward health goals that may not optimize human health, as might otherwise occur by subsisting naturally without any dependence on commercial industry involvement. For example, consider a comparison between two separate behaviorally distinct populations A and B existing under similar sets of societal circumstances, but pursuing different lifestyles.

Population A eats a diet substantially consisting of processed and refined food products; ingests large quantities of animal source foods loaded with hormones and antibiotics; heavily uses artificially manufactured health supplements and other pharmaceutical and recreational chemicals; consumes alcohol in excess; has extensive tobacco and nicotine addiction problems, and is predominantly sedentary and substantially overweight.

Population B exercises regularly; is physically fit; generally carries the appropriate weight for height; subsists predominantly on natural plant-based whole earth foods eaten without preservatives or chemical additives; limits ingestion of animal products while raising animals for human consumption without hormones or antibiotics; avoids environmentally toxic substances; and refrains from using recreational drugs, tobacco and nicotine products, supplemental vitamins, non-essential pharmaceutical products, and alcohol. Consequently, the normal or target reference ranges obtained for various health parameters measured in population A may be significantly different from those for population B, and general health recommendations and guidelines devised for population A may not fit or accurately apply to the actual health requirements benefiting population B.

Defining normal population target ranges for biological parameters involving human health matters leads to enormous social and economic implications that can generate attractive profit opportunities for commercial industries at the expense of society. The designated "normal" homeostasis reference ranges for any measured or observed human biological parameters determine parameter testing and monitoring recommendations, affect screening for health consequences associated with parameter deficiencies or excesses, and drive the sale of commercial products correcting or maintaining parameter levels. For example, consider expenditures related to adjusting "normal" blood levels for vitamin D and cholesterol for the population. Shifting the normal homeostasis target range upward for recommended blood vitamin D levels increases population testing for vitamin D levels, raises the number of individuals having vitamin D deficiency, accelerates demand for vitamin D supplements, and broadly promotes more ancillary studies for various health disorders, such as osteoporosis, that may indirectly result from vitamin D deficiency.

Similarly, moving the recommended cholesterol levels for the population downward leads to more individuals with cholesterol levels that fall above the normal target range, which consequently requires pharmaceutical treatment with cholesterol-lowering agents and more aggressive monitoring of cholesterol levels and triggers more ancillary testing for silent vascular or cardiac consequences associated with "elevated" blood cholesterol counts.

16.1 BODY VEHICLE BIOLOGICAL NOTIFICATIONS

Routine body vehicle existence is substantially automatic and proceeds transparently until the body vehicle experiences significant survival challenges. A healthy body vehicle runs survival programs silently in the background that monitor for body vehicle system malfunction, required maintenance, or developing problems threatening health and survival.

Body vehicle survival programming has surveillance applications that signal internal issues requiring urgent attention. Surveillance applications communicating body vehicle disturbances interrupt transparent body vehicle operations with signals of varying intensities and degrees of urgency. Survival signals may present as high gravity alarms, moderate significance alerts, or lower importance maintenance signals that pervade awareness with various strengths and sustainability to warn or notify of internal body vehicle states demanding attention and corrective actions.

16.1.1 Body Vehicle Alarm Signals

Sensors and detectors protectively equip the entire body vehicle to monitor continuously for disrepair and damage jeopardizing health and survival and then warn of detected dangers that require remedy through alarm signals. Body vehicle alarms signal adverse body vehicle **conditions** with disturbed homeostasis associated with system dysfunction, breakdown, overload, or deficiency states, and inform strongly that the existing state of disrepair or injury imminently threatens body vehicle health and survival.

High gravity biological alarm signals either pervade immediate awareness directly or are determined indirectly by measuring physiologic parameters such as vital signs and weight; by analyzing specific blood elements or body fluids; or by performing radiographic imaging or other diagnostic studies to demonstrate underlying body vehicle compromise. Alarm signals that directly interfere with the transparent operations of body vehicle mental or physical activities and persist unabated require urgent attention. Some examples of body vehicle alarms signaling directly include severe shortness of breath; excessive coughing; intolerable pain; inability to move the body vehicle or a limb properly; pervasive loss of appetite, energy, or weight; difficulty swallowing; active bleeding; abnormal body vehicle tissue growths; and uncontrollable crying, anxiety, or sleep disturbances. Examples of body vehicle alarms indirectly signaling potentially dangerous health disturbances include markedly elevated blood pressure, heart rate, blood sugar, or blood cholesterol levels; abnormal kidney or liver blood chemistry tests; abnormal blood counts; and abnormal findings on radiographic imaging of vital organs or tissues.

Alarm signals demand prompt attention with appropriate measures to correct any ongoing health problems and protect the body vehicle against progressive or irreversible injury or death. Early response to body vehicle alarm signals provides better opportunities to intervene and reduce or reverse damages that may result from an unfolding body vehicle health problem. Ignoring body vehicle alarm signals may numb survival sensor sensitivity toward harmful or toxic circumstances and allow adverse health conditions to progress and cause permanent, irreversible damages or premature death.

Survival sensors can desensitize to dampen alarm signaling in the context of persisting toxicity and abuse as exemplified by the physical acclimation to smoking tobacco, which follows an initial alarm signaling period of unpleasant respiratory symptoms with coughing indicating body vehicle danger and intolerance to inhaling tobacco smoke, followed by the development of tolerance to inhaled smoke.

Pharmaceuticals that modulate brain and nerve function to alleviate pain or treat behavioral health disorders may reduce brain awareness or dull sensory sensitivity to reduce survival signaling and artificially cover-up ongoing body vehicle damages. The loss of survival sensor sensitivity compromises body vehicle capabilities to gauge and appropriately signal concerning body vehicle dangers, predisposing to progressive body vehicle harm and deterioration that risk permanent illness and suffering or premature death.

One vital body vehicle alarm signal is unintentional weight loss, which frequently appears in the context of life-threatening conditions such as cancer; major body vehicle organ failure; severe infections such as AIDS and tuberculosis; metabolic health disorders; or a disturbed body vehicle ability to absorb, process, utilize, or assimilate essential nutrients; and is often associated with severe health compromise and decreased survival. Nutritionally unbalanced weight loss regimens and fad diets that disrupt body vehicle homeostasis to precipitate rapid, large-scale weight reduction without opportunity for the body vehicle to adapt biologically also endanger body vehicle health. During rapid weight loss with inappropriate dieting, initial weight changes substantially reflect dramatic cellular water, salt, and mineral shifts and losses that derange physiologic levels and balances of vital nutrients to threaten the biologic stability and health of the body vehicle. Physiologically unbalanced diets rapidly producing sizable weight losses may deprive vulnerable cells and tissues of essential nutrients to create metabolic stresses toxic to body vehicle functioning.

Attempting to quickly correct chronic metabolic health disorders such as obesity, which develops gradually over time through consistently poor nutritional routines, with unbalanced dieting programs or pharmacologic interventions that severely disturb metabolic homeostatic balances may unintentionally lead to unwanted adverse health and survival outcomes.

16.1.2 Body Vehicle Alerts

Body vehicle alerts are unsustained warning signals of lower intensity than alarms that temporarily raise conscious awareness for potential, underlying or impending body vehicle disrepair, damage, imbalance, or breakdown. Alerts require directed attention and careful consideration of predisposing circumstances prompting alert notifications to ascertain whether any specific environmental, behavioral, dietary, or social factors may be intolerable to the body vehicle and should be avoided or discontinued.

Alert signals present as nondescript symptoms such as fleeting dizziness; occasional muscle cramps, spasms, or twitches; isolated headaches and aches and pains of various body vehicle parts; infrequent cough; minor itching; tolerable self-limited digestive or abdominal symptoms; and numerous other vague physical experiences that are mild, sporadic, short lasting, unpredictable in frequency or regularity, and do not result in significant or sustained body vehicle dysfunction or deterioration.

Many body vehicle alerts are "**one-timer**" or self-limited "**few-timer**" or "**some-timer**" symptoms or findings on biological testing that may come and go and resolve entirely without obvious progression or persistent body vehicle dysfunction, impairment, or interruption of activities. Reoccurring alerts that progress in frequency, duration, and intensity become actual alarm signals that indicate a possible underlying "condition" detrimental to body vehicle health or survival.

16.1.3 Body Vehicle Maintenance Signals

Body vehicle maintenance signals are general body vehicle urges of lower immediate importance to attend to basic health-related survival tasks. Body vehicle
maintenance signals indicate a requirement for routine body vehicle care and
include experiencing hunger to feed, thirst to drink water, an urge to urinate or
defecate to empty the urinary bladder or bowel of accumulated wastes, tiredness
or yawning to rest or to sleep, and coldness or warmth to seek heat or to cool down.
Body vehicle maintenance signals contrast with behavioral craves, which are
strongly irresistible compulsions to carry out learned or conditioned behaviors
that provide intense pleasure or reduce pain or suffering.

16.2 HOMEOSTASIS RECOVERY THRESHOLD

The **homeostasis recovery threshold** is the *biological point of no return* beyond
which accrued body vehicle damages cannot be fixed and reversed to return
homeostasis to preinjury baselines at optimal genetically established set points.
Body vehicle damages exceeding homeostasis recovery thresholds may result in
only partial health recovery at redefined lower function homeostasis set points,
whereby new levels "aren't what they used to be!"

The body vehicle has excellent recovery capabilities for subthreshold injuries
and toxic insults that do not irreversibly reach irreparable levels invoking advanced
repair processes that cause permanent scarring, disfigurement, or loss of function
or that accelerate death. Advanced injuries disrupt delicate architectural frameworks and tissue scaffolding that are necessary to reestablish tissue structures and
destroy progenitor stem cells that can give rise to interdependently functioning
cells composing tissues. Consequently, above the threshold point of no return,
too many cells sustained damage or were destroyed to disrupt tissues beyond
the capability to repair and reverse damages back to genetically programmed
"factory-installed specification" baselines; for example, a trip with a slight fall might
result in contusions with minor bruising that resolve within a few days, whereas
falling out of a three-story window onto the pavement is likely to result in death
or severe tissue damages that cause permanent disfigurement evident for the
remaining body vehicle life-span. Likewise, sunshine is easily tolerated for short
durations until skin acclimation gradually develops, while prolonged, heavy sun
exposures leading to repeated sunburns produce various degrees of advanced
skin injury with wrinkling, scarring, and precancerous skin changes.

The adverse health and survival consequences of repeatedly fueling the body
vehicle excessively over time are frequently not apparent in the short term. If
consuming processed and refined food products immediately provoked dramatic
human illness or body vehicle dysfunction, these food products would stand little
chance of surviving in competitive commercial markets. Instead, low-grade body

vehicle injuries inflicted repeatedly through improper and indulgent fueling unfold below detectable levels necessary to trigger body vehicle alert and alarm signals, allowing ongoing damages to accumulate gradually outside conscious awareness until injuries become advanced.

The body vehicle adequately compensates for isolated dietary indiscretions by protectively redistributing and clearing away excessively ingested fuels and nutrients into temporizing safe zones, reducing metabolic harm inflicted onto cells and tissues following self-limited episodes of excessive fueling. Repeated and persistent dietary indiscretions eventually overcome protective compensatory metabolic responses and lead to more permanent adverse physiologic and metabolic body vehicle adaptations. High-sugar and high-fat diets change brain neurochemical activity to reset healthy homeostasis set points for satiety to hedonistic levels that drive eating behaviors to seek pleasure-reward experiences rather than appropriate nutritional balances. Other adverse effects stemming from unhealthy fueling that proceed undetected until health damages become significant include the transformation of resident microbiota; metabolic and chemical injuries to tissues and cells; resetting of homeostasis set points for blood sugar and cholesterol levels; unfavorable changes to baseline blood insulin levels; and impairment of physical capabilities to perform routine activities of daily living.

Progressive subthreshold body vehicle damages related to fueling disorders gradually build up to eventually produce permanent, irreversible injuries to vital organs such as the heart, kidney, liver, and brain, risking end organ failure that dramatically impairs body vehicle functioning to reduce life quality and shorten life-span. Appropriate body vehicle maintenance behaviors and healthy nutritional and lifestyle choices are consistently the best strategic options to prevent body vehicle injury and toxicity and to avoid the insidious development of body vehicle damages resulting in expensive irreversible health deterioration and premature death.

17 ARTIFICIAL HEALTH MAINTENANCE

Body vehicle homeostasis mechanisms are intensely studied scientifically and heavily targeted for profitable artificial chemical and biological manipulation. Pharmaceutical industries fund homeostasis research expecting lucrative returns on investments through the discovery of unique biological targets that can lead to the development of patentable proprietary drugs that control and regulate homeostasis.

Pharmaceuticals are chemical substances foreign to biological systems that are variously designed to affect biochemical and physiologic actions artificially in living organisms. Designer pharmaceutical effects may strategically modify or interfere with ongoing cellular events through various mechanisms including by altering the levels or activity of cellular regulatory substances, by disrupting cellular signaling, or by changing cellular responsiveness to biochemical triggers that activate or govern physiologic actions. For example, appetite, blood sugar and cholesterol levels, blood pressure, body vehicle salt and water balance and content, and many other biological variables can be artificially manipulated using pharmaceutical chemicals called medicines.

Given the tremendous profit opportunities associated with targeting growing obesity and obesity caused health complications, the pharmaceutical rescue industry continually crafts chemicals creatively modifying native body vehicle metabolic activities and nutritional biology. Pharmaceutical obesity interventions target eating behaviors, disrupt the cellular processing of fuels and nutrients, or artificially alter blood sugar and cholesterol levels signaling overfueling and, more recently, attempt to manipulate the body vehicle gut microbiome found to impact body vehicle energy utilization and harvesting of energies from foods. Potent medications designed to treat overfueling complications such as diabetes chemically trick cells into force-feeding on excess blood sugar to lower blood sugar levels, causing cells to absorb sugar loads beyond biological needs and natural capacities to utilize the high energy sugar.

Other pharmaceutical treatments block the production of cholesterol from sugar in liver cells or interfere with cholesterol absorption by the gut. Potential adverse health effects resulting from the chemical treatment of diabetes include increased appetite and weight gain, while treating excessive blood cholesterol levels with certain medications alters body vehicle sugar processing ironically to cause diabetes in susceptible individuals.

The word *pharma* derives from the Greek root *pharmakon,* meaning "poison." Pharmaceutical agents used to treat health disorders possess the potential for producing dual effects similarly to weapons and electricity, which can provide benefits or cause grave harm if not handled and managed expertly. Since pharmaceutical agents are biologically foreign substances having toxic potential, the body vehicle system continually works to dispose of them. Consequently, medications must be taken into the body vehicle repeatedly at regular intervals to compensate for the activity of detoxification mechanisms that continuously clear out and eliminate foreign chemical substances recognized as having no inherent nutritional or biological value to the body vehicle system.

Body vehicle clearance of nonfood chemicals occurs predominantly through the liver and kidney organs, which act as primary filters to rid the body vehicle of foreign substances serving no natural biological role for sustaining body vehicle health or survival. Sophisticated pharmacologic determinations characterize usual body vehicle chemical clearance and elimination pathways and duration of biologic activity for standard doses of various pharmacologic medicinal agents used to treat health disorders in humans. Medicine dosing schedules are timed to compensate for drug inactivation and removal from the body vehicle, thereby maintaining therapeutic effects and tissue drug levels necessary to predictably engage intended biologic targets regulating body vehicle function.

Excessive reliance on chemical rescue options to treat illnesses caused by adverse health behaviors and lifestyles promotes unnecessary dependence on artificial health maintenance and counters opportunities for individuals to take charge and correct harmful behaviors and lifestyles causing health problems in the first place.

Eating sweets excessively then popping pills to treat the health fallout from making improper nutritional choices provides immediate gratification on both accounts with the temporary pleasure and artificial compensation for dietary indiscretions, but eventually results in poor health accompanied by feelings of guilt for the loss of nutritional control and health compromise.

Pharmacologic manipulation of the body vehicle also risks producing adverse medication effects that compound other consequences arising from unhealthy behaviors and lifestyles. The consolation prize for playing the **Game of Pharmakon** amounts to the development of more complicated health problems unwelcomely combining with increased expenses and suffering.

Furthermore, chemically manipulating or muting body vehicle biological alarm signals such as elevations in blood sugar, blood pressure, or cholesterol counts does not ensure quality survival, restore longevity, promote true health and well-being, or prevent health complications from happening while adverse health behaviors and lifestyles continue unabated.

17.1 DRONES

Industrial chemical meddling with the delicate balance of the human body vehicle and the biosphere immersing the body vehicle is a double-edged sword for human existence fraught with dangers. Chemically manufactured vitamins, medicines, food preservatives, herbicides, pesticides, and antibiotics are designed to target the operations or viability of very limited segments of immensely complicated biological systems. Industry purposely attempts to modify minute elements of vastly interactive, integrated, and interdependent Biosystems selectively without disturbing or affecting other system components.

The ideal objectives of pharmaceutical research are to discover and understand body vehicle biochemical targets that physiologically control complex human biology, and then develop specific chemical agents that can exclusively engage those cellular targets to permit on-demand manipulation of body vehicle operations. Unfortunately, pharmaceutical chemicals once introduced into the complex body vehicle biological system distribute extensively throughout the entire body vehicle *without guaranteed drone target effects.*

Rescue industry chemicals designed to target specific body vehicle operations often fail to restrict their activity exclusively to intended cellular targets within the elaborately integrated and intricately complex human body vehicle system. Pharmaceutical chemicals may even be deliberately devised to broadly target biological master switches that turn a vast array of secondary biochemical reactions on or off, thereby triggering a cascade of cellular events that simultaneously control numerous body vehicle cellular functions across many different cellular levels.

All medications, whether inhaled, injected into the skin or a vein, inserted into a body vehicle orifice or cavity, applied topically to skin or tissue membranes, or ingested orally, disperse generally throughout the entire body vehicle system to exert widespread body vehicle effects, interacting chemically and biologically with both *on-target* and *off-target* cellular elements and biochemical processes. Artificial biochemical manipulation of the body vehicle system with pharmaceutical agents affects and alarms the entire body vehicle system, analogously to how signals reverberate and spread rapidly throughout a giant spider to alert when any part of the web network is disturbed.

Drug information pamphlets and reference sources such as the ***Physician's Desk Reference* (PDR)** manual for pharmaceutical products, which describe intended drug effects for medicinal products provide even greater lists that catalog unintended adverse drug reactions that users of referenced drugs experience. Consequently, pharmaceutical chemicals introduced into the body vehicle unavoidably lead to widespread effects on body vehicle biologic functions which may be by design or by accident.

Unexpected pharmacologic interactions with nontargeted biologic components can precipitate serious "*collateral damage*" injuries to vital body vehicle cellular elements to impact body vehicle health and survival deleteriously. Rescue industry chemicals are scientifically designed and rigorously tested under meticulously controlled "test tube" study conditions that limit chemical drug activities and interactions to carefully isolated biologic cellular targets. Selected cellular targets of interest may be highly specialized and exclusively carry out limited cellular actions, may multitask and control numerous cellular functions, or may serve as backup components that redundantly support critical cellular operations.

After initial test tube laboratory studies, drug efficacy and safety evaluations progress through testing on limited numbers of live laboratory animals, followed by studies on smaller and then larger numbers of human test subjects, before final approval is granted by governmental regulatory agencies to allow drug dissemination into the public domain for general use. Human body vehicle pharmaceutical targets are integrated extensively within the complex body vehicle system and undergo dynamic changes under a multitude of internal and external body vehicle influences. These deeply consolidated pharmaceutical targets may serve numerous body vehicle biologic functions, which may be unrecognized or incompletely characterized under artificially controlled and restrictive laboratory and clinical investigations carried out over relatively short study intervals.

Under complex biologic conditions, rescue industry–designed pharmaceuticals may not entirely behave as anticipated to limit drug activity exclusively to cellular targets and produce desired biological effects but may instead undesirably engage nontargeted cellular elements to various degrees to trigger unanticipated off-target biological consequences.

Diverse nontargeted body vehicle cellular elements that may structurally resemble or function interdependently with pharmaceutical targets are particularly vulnerable to interact inadvertently with designer pharmaceuticals and precipitate unintended drug effects. The observed biological effects of rescue pharmaceuticals may ultimately reflect some undefined constellation of complex interactions involving multiple cellular targets and nontargets that bind pharmaceuticals as designed or unexpectedly. Sometimes, pharmaceutical products cause unintended adverse biologic health consequences termed **side effects** that only become apparent late, after extensive and prolonged use of these agents in large numbers of individuals.

The rescue industry accepts adverse off-target drug side effects that produce unintended collateral damages to body vehicle elements as being part of the cost of doing business using pharmaceutical agents. Repeated consumption of larger quantities or concentrations of various chemical industry creations including pharmaceuticals, food additives, and health supplements over time carries undefined risks for causing unintended side effects that have short and long-term adverse health consequences, which may only be recognized when "aftermarket approval" of products reaches widespread human use and experience. The potential impact of a chemical product that carries a 1% risk to cause an undesirable side effect translates to 10,000 possible adverse events that may occur in 1 million product users, while a 0.1% risk for 100 million users equates to 100,000 potential adverse events.

The federal government has recently teamed up with the commercial interests of chemical, pharmaceutical industries to embark on a new initiative that supports the development and delivery of tailor-made pharmaceutical rescue industry interventions for all human health ailments and maladies. The cooperative "health" initiative forged between the federal government and rescue industries is known as **Precision Medicine.** The Precision Medicine initiative strives to understand the genetic, biologic mechanisms of all human disease states and disease predispositions to target existing or potential health disorders more precisely with rescue industry interventions. Therefore, Precision Medicine attempts to personalize the delivery of health care by identifying and characterizing all prospective biological targets for every human health disorder that might be amenable to pharmaceutical manipulation, dramatically expanding commercial rescue industry opportunities to intervene artificially in human disease states.

The grand Precision Medicine initiative incentivizes scientific drug research to introduce many new and unique pharmaceutical products to humanity, escalating the possibilities for many more unintended adverse drug events to occur. Precision Medicine guarantees the perpetuity of a commercial health care system intent on identifying broken or dysfunctional elements of human body vehicles that may be amenable to commercial interventions and repairs, and virtually ignores the pursuit of opportunities to discover and implement inexpensive and straightforward societal health and behavioral strategies, which can reliably maintain perfectly functioning body vehicle systems at factory specifications without any need for costly commercial health care industry interventions and repairs.

In contrast to the Precision Medicine initiative, a longitudinal survey study in China that followed approximately 500,000 people over four years identified that consuming at least two servings of fresh fruit daily was an inexpensive nonpharmaceutical, noncommercial healthful intervention that reduced cardiovascular events such as stroke and heart attacks risk-free by 40%. Indeed, China can ill afford to provide expensive cardiovascular medications and interventions for a population of 1.3 billion people.

Salient features of the Precision Medicine research and health care initiatives involve exploring the diagnosis and treatment of various human diseases in the context of characterizing DNA genetic, molecular codes, and then biologically manipulating the DNA genetic controls associated with specific illnesses to alter the predisposition or natural history of DNA programmed health disorders. Ongoing Precision Medicine scientific efforts surround linking the entire characterized human genome with active or dormant disease states and disease predispositions, creating ever greater rescue industry commercial opportunities for body vehicle manipulation even preceding the development and onset of active human illnesses. Precision Medicine is bound to create whole new categories of physically, psychologically, and economically captive rescue industry consumer victims, paying industry to diagnose and treat health disorders or protect against illness possibilities that may never materialize under appropriately chosen healthy behaviors, lifestyles, and life circumstances. Therefore, under the Precision Medicine initiative, all body vehicle toxicities, abuse, neglect, and disrepair caused by behavioral and environmental factors conveniently provide industry with welcomed opportunities to study countless human illnesses and disease predispositions indefinitely to allow the tailoring of personalized health care interventions that can be delivered commercially for a fee.

Rescue industry researchers and health care providers will undoubtedly be busy working overtime to discover new scientific ways of targeting human diseases and ailments, while society and health care consumers pay dearly for the initiative with their *lifetimes*. Realistically, if all human health disorders and disease predispositions were targeted individually to be evaluated, treated, and monitored, then carrying out the scientific experiments to assess the feasibility, safety, and efficacy of proposed clinical interventions for every single human condition would be an economically unaffordable herculean effort. Cutting-edge scientific research into human diseases provides invaluable insight into the intricate operations of the body vehicle system and allows for innovative interventions that can stem human biological disrepair, diseases, and suffering,

On the other hand, societal health and finances would likely fare better through intensive study of entirely healthy individuals to ascertain successful behaviors and lifestyle strategies that prevent human illnesses and body vehicle deterioration altogether, which can then be rigorously taught and ubiquitously applied in society to benefit all. Unfortunately, rather than pursuing and implementing strategies that prevent diseases, disasters, and suffering, which are likely to benefit many indefinitely and save money for all, commercial health care industry strategies direct efforts and finances that profit commercial self-interests and the few in the short term at the expense of the many for the long run.

Industry advantageously exploits human curiosity, greed, impatience, need for excitement, fear, uncertainties, and short-sightedness to capitalize and promote what financially rewards industry, especially when human tendencies predictably lead to adverse behavioral choices and unhealthy lifestyles that unleash a Pandora's box of unwelcomed problems for society, which present countless savory financial opportunities for commercial industries to profit.

17.2 ANTIDOTES

Antidotes intercept, block, or reverse the poisonous effects of toxins. Incorporating rescue industry pharmaceutical chemicals to combat health deterioration and illnesses resulting from unhealthy behavioral choices and lifestyles seeks to counteract maladaptive human behaviors artificially with rescue industry pharmaceutical antidotes. Additionally, pharmaceutical interventions used to address various health disorders and illnesses frequently lead toward the use of more pharmaceutical agents to remedy or counteract unintended side effects or toxicities resulting directly from the intended application of therapeutic medicinal interventions. Human dependence on expensive rescue industry chemicals and other health care interventions to serve as antidotes that *compensate* for correctable adverse health behaviors and unhealthy lifestyles is costly to all on many accounts.

Compensating for adverse health behaviors and lifestyles with rescue industry products and services only benefits commercial industries.

17.3 PLACEBO RESPONSE

The **placebo response** refers to the intrinsic healing power inherent to the body vehicle system. Ingesting sugar pills called **placebos** can biologically activate poorly understood self-healing and mending capabilities of the body vehicle system. Placebos fail to generate astronomical commercial industry profits since placebo manufacture, and sale is unrestricted under patent laws otherwise existing to protect proprietary industry products, which confer rescue industries exclusive market rights to produce and sell proprietary pharmaceuticals, allowing pharmaceutical manufacturers to corner commercial markets and deliver proprietary pharmaceutical products for the highest obtainable price.

Many rescue industry services or proprietary pharmaceutical products often provide only limited or no more significant health benefits than placebo interventions. Profit-driven commercial rescue industries routinely advertise placebo-like health remedies that grant various health benefits frequently described vaguely as providing strength and vigor; improved well-being, potency, or stamina; or increased life quality for product users.

Selling the idea that a commercial health product or service with statistically marginal or scientifically unproven health benefits provides users with desirable human attributes or qualities sells the placebo response for the highest possible fees. Through poorly understood mechanisms, the placebo response taps into the relationship between the human power of positive thinking and body vehicle physiologic functioning to activate human survival programs capable of achieving health and promoting healing and recovery from illness. The placebo response possibly underlies the source of internal healing power derived from spiritual meditation, inspirational religious worship, and ritualistic prayers.

Unfortunately, science has neglected to study the placebo response in preference to pursuing more lucrative commercial endeavors that involve the design and creation of exclusive proprietary pharmaceutical products, which reap enormous economic profits and latch societal dependency onto the commercial rescue industry. The placebo response repeatedly underscores the vast chasm of knowledge separating scientific understanding and applications from the actual substance of ongoing human biological existence. Consequently, the placebo response is the "what is unknown and unstudied because it is unprofitable" effect.

Scientific studies that compare the effects of expensive pharmaceutical products on human health disorders with cheap placebos often only demonstrate marginally better health benefits derived from employing the considerably costlier proprietary industry medicines and health care interventions than from utilizing placebo treatments.

Clinical therapeutic responses to medical interventions for digestive health disorders such as inflammatory bowel disease and irritable bowel syndrome serve as illustrative examples of the inherent power of the poorly understood placebo response. Individuals with inflammatory bowel disease may clinically improve with expensive commercial medications costing thousands of dollars per treatment in only 30%–45% of instances while using cheap placebos can achieve similar clinical responses sometimes up to 15%–20% of the time.

Pharmaceuticals commonly used for irritable bowel disorders and comparatively costing hundreds of dollars monthly may provide symptom relief 60% of the time, while placebos can work equally well in up to 40% of users. Consequently, since inexpensive placebo treatments achieve respectable treatment response rates at minimal costs compared to using expensive designer pharmaceuticals, which coincidentally predispose to sometimes life-threatening drug side effects, it would seem rational, economically feasible, and societally advantageous to study and understand the placebo response intensively to improve societal health more naturally and at lower health care delivery costs.

Unfortunately, pharmaceutical drug trials are not designed to undermine or derail the potential profitability from precious **rescue industry money maker drugs,** especially those in widespread use for poorly understood human health disorders. More commonly, commercial rescue industries use aggressive media and marketing campaign strategies to generate health care provider and consumer excitement surrounding the impending release and availability of expensive newly patented commercial chemical remedies for health disorders, which often provide unimpressive and only marginally better treatment response rates than their placebo counterparts.

17.4 LIBERATION AND FREEDOM

Daily living poses dangers to body vehicle survival, and often these dangers are seductively packaged in small pharmaceutical containers promising great health benefits.

Cures in vials deliver health claims, not health.

Pharmaceutical health product claims are curiously often delivered with product disclaimers and warnings containing long laundry lists of potential adverse health effects associated with product usage. Consequently, seek liberation from gratuitous exposures to potentially dangerous drug side effects and from unnecessary reliance on pharmaceutical industry chemicals to compensate for dodging the personal responsibility to maintain body vehicle health optimally naturally.

Behavioral compromises and unhealthy lifestyle choices are substantially responsible for causing many human health disorders and much of the suffering affecting modern societies. Appropriate dietary, activity, and behavioral choices can properly maintain and often naturally restore optimal body vehicle function and homeostasis to substantially reduce or eliminate the need to use artificially manufactured chemicals to improve personal health and life quality. Therefore, protect the body vehicle system from avoidable chemical exposures delivered through processed foods; nonessential pharmaceutical, medicinal agents; and unnecessary health supplements.

Trim and strip away personal dependence on commercial industries for artificial sustenance and health maintenance that negatively affect natural body vehicle operations. Avoid using manufactured rescue industry products without established health benefits when simply making better behavioral, and lifestyle choices would best optimize personal health. Choose natural, healthy living over artificial maintenance when modifying behaviors and lifestyle can predictably promote and restore health.

Seek liberation from rescue industry dependency in the pursuit of health and happiness.

Artificial maintenance is the reserve option to treat disease and relieve suffering when appropriate behaviors and lifestyle modifications inadequately suffice to achieve body vehicle health and survival goals.

17.5 ESSENTIAL ARTIFICIAL MAINTENANCE: THE BACKUP PLAN

In modern society, advances in health care undeniably contribute to the health and survival of humanity. Indisputably beneficial opportunities exist to use rescue industry interventions appropriately. Available rescue bail-out interventions serve as appropriate backup alternatives to recover lost health and maintain survival when natural options for doing so are too slow, nonexistent, or failing.

A few practical, not all-inclusive considerations to help discern whether artificial rescue interventions are being utilized appropriately include whether interventions

1. maintain survival, which would otherwise deteriorate rapidly and end prematurely (e.g., certain heart medications, specific cancer treatments, and various autoimmune health disorder interventions)
2. restore critical body vehicle biologic function or balance (e.g., promote movement in Parkinson's disease; correct blood mineral, salt, or sugar imbalances imminently threatening body vehicle function or survival; rebalance behavioral health in conditions impairing daily living)
3. replace vital biologic substances no longer sufficiently produced or absorbed by body vehicle tissues (e.g., thyroid hormone, insulin, iron, vitamin B_{12})
4. supply critical metabolic agents to compensate for acquired body vehicle deficiencies or hereditary production limitations
5. manage debilitating or intractable pain adversely impacting life quality and ability to function physically
6. treat severe or life-threatening infections with appropriate antibiotic agents confirmed by susceptibility testing to definitively target responsible microorganisms undermining health

18 AGING

No matter what humans do, this much is true:
No one gets out of life alive.
Aging is the number one cause of human death and disability.

Collective body vehicle expiration time, or **life-span,** is likely programmed into DNA genetic software codes possibly to make room for newer body vehicle models to be introduced on earth. Body vehicle programming appears to lead inevitably to human aging with progressive loss of function and eventual death. Currently, human life-span is ostensibly finite and not significantly longer than 100 years. A delicate balance exists between body vehicle cellular growth and death, which maintains normal body vehicle existence and proper functioning of body vehicle tissues and organ systems.

Cellular survival balance is affected by numerous intrinsic body vehicle and extrinsic environmental factors, some of which are evident or scientifically characterized and many more of which are poorly understood, undefined, or unknown. Under suitable biological triggers, cellular programs become activated to direct orderly biological events producing irreversible deterioration and the terminal expiration of body vehicle cells.

Aging reflects the cumulative degradative transformation of body vehicle cellular and tissue components interacting with physical, chemical, and biological life challenges, which lead to the progressive biologic dysfunction, decline, and eventual death of the entire body vehicle system.

Numerous factors influence the pace of body vehicle aging and onset of body vehicle death. Genetic mutations and evolutionary changes propagated through species reproduction and affected by innumerable extraneous environmental pressures and survival stresses over individual and species lifetimes influence body vehicle expiration times. DNA genetic codes running cellular reproduction, growth, maintenance, and repair are prone to make detrimental reprogramming errors during repair and regeneration of body vehicle cells and cellular constituents. Aging cells progressively lose the capability to carry out critical housekeeping functions that cleanup and clear out cellular biological debris produced and accumulated through daily wear and tear, predisposing aging cells to become increasingly cluttered and progressively poisoned with their accumulated wastes, eventually leading to loss of cellular function and cell death.

Burning fuel to run body vehicle metabolic processes to generate energy, detoxify the body vehicle system, eliminate wastes, and repair and regenerate body vehicle system components generates heat along with metabolic, biochemical waste by-products and reactive chemical elements, which in turn may secondarily harm the body vehicle system biologically.

Fighting the forces of friction and gravity also burns energy, further producing toxic metabolic by-products, and continuously causes progressive, accumulating, and eventually permanent and irreparable mechanical wear and tear and disrepair to body vehicle components. Breathing oxygen in the air, being exposed to sunlight, maintaining a balanced symbiotic existence with the internal microbiome, and fighting off opportunistic infections are other biological processes continually stressing the body vehicle system which gradually deteriorate cellular and tissue integrity. Maximal body vehicle component and global expiration times are eventually reached directly as a consequence of living and are unlikely to be lengthened beyond personal DNA genetic program code limits anytime soon.

Aging is something to be successfully achieved healthfully and not accelerated or prematurely interrupted with death by making incorrect behavioral or lifestyle choices.

Life-span and longevity can be shortened by failing to maintain the body vehicle properly and by stressing the body vehicle system with toxins and harmful behaviors and lifestyles, which produce excessive and irreparable body vehicle wear and tear and interfere with homeostasis and health recovery mechanisms to cause debility, disability, and premature death. Eventually, the culmination point of all accumulated irreversible body vehicle injuries and disrepairs becomes the body vehicle expiration time leading to the death of the entire body vehicle system.

Continuous attention to fulfill body vehicle maintenance requirements and survival needs appropriately and avoid behaviors toxic to the body vehicle system maximizes lifetime to anticipated body vehicle timelines and functional milestones to present many more opportunities for greater personal accomplishment.

18.1 THE GOLDEN YEARS

It is never too late to start living healthfully.

The **golden years** of aging are the final stretch of human existence that provide final opportunities and the last hurrah to reap and enjoy any rewards earned from a life well lived but also represent the last chance for commercial addictification and rescue industries to squeeze out that last bit of human *lifetime* to profit from declining human health.

During a human lifetime, end-of-life health care to sustain any semblance of well-being and slow the demise of an aged, physically deteriorating, and shutting-down body vehicle can be one of the most physically and emotionally taxing and financially expensive endeavors imposed upon individuals as well as society, especially within the United States.

Elderly health care consumers are mined like gold by commercial rescue industries to fuel growing industry opportunities for profitability with human aging reaped through older adult wellness and end-of-life health care spending.

The golden years can impose tremendous financial and emotional burdens on individuals, families, and society when continued spending to recover lost health or attempts to slow down approaching death proceed without significant progress or meaningful breakthroughs, and ultimately, fail to provide real lifetime returns on expended efforts and incurred costs.

The development of numerous health conditions that layer and combine adverse health effects during a lifetime can multiply the costs of health care with aging many-fold. Annual U.S. per capita health expenditures costing less than a few thousand dollars during younger and middle-aged years can rise by as much as $1000 yearly between the ages of 60 and 85, translating into a possible 1000% or more increase in annual health care costs to care for elderly as compared to younger individuals, and totaling several hundred thousand dollars overall in health care expenses to finance the health care needs for aged individuals surviving through their golden years into their nineties.[9]

The addictification food industry is a pipeline that cultivates unwary future customers for the rescue industry with unhealthy food products that progressively deteriorate the body vehicle until ripe for future rescue industry picking later in life. Consumers are continuously brainwashed during their lifetimes to unwittingly indulge in unhealthy behaviors and lifestyles that profit industry, and which prime individuals to later develop health disorders that make them victims dependent on costly health care. The rescue industry then persuades older adults to spend finances futilely on products and services that offer unrealistic opportunities to regain a sense of youthfulness or to extend a diminishing life-span.

Elderly health care consumer victims, frequently suffering from prior behavioral and lifestyle indiscretions, often live out final days dependently navigating complex health care mazes and paying for costly rescue industry care ordered by well-intentioned health care providers. The golden years often culminate in a progressive flurry of increasing financial spending for health care services and products by individuals having little energy, motivation, or recourse to stop or refuse to partake in the expanding spiral of their rescue industry driven health care consumption.

End-of-life care can wring out that very last bit of human *lifetime* to profit industry. During end-of-life care, anticipated human death can become expensively

---

9. https://www.forbes.com/sites/danmunro/2012/12/30/2012-the-year-in-health
    care-charts/#34d8e1b46c8c; https://jamanetwork.com/journals/jama/fullarticle/2661579; https://
    jamanetwork.com/journals/jama/fullarticle/2594716.

delayed by aggressive rescue industry forces attempting to extract any remaining *lifetime* value from a dwindling human life force, often to sacrifice the last shreds of quality human existence.

With a lifetime spent being inattentive and neglectful toward properly meeting body vehicle nutritional and health maintenance needs, any monies painstakingly scrimped and saved to enjoy the benefits of retirement are vulnerable to being diverted into the possession of rescue industry elements. *Lifetime* spent working to earn a "living" then becomes the sustenance voraciously consumed by rescue industry feeders.

19 FUELS, FRAMEWORK, AND FRIENDS

19.1 CALORIE

The energy supplied by earth fuels that power body vehicle operational needs and existence is expressed scientifically in **calorie** units. **Food calorie content** denotes the approximate payload of available energy delivered within a designated single serving size weight of food when converted by the body vehicle into the energies powering cellular functions.

A **small calorie** is the quantity of thermal or heat energy necessary to raise the temperature of 1 g of water 1 °C from 14.5°C to 15.5°C. A **big calorie** is the energy unit used for quantitating the fuel energy delivered by food and equals 1,000 small calories, being the amount of thermal or heat energy needed to raise the temperature of one kilogram (1,000 g) of water 1°C.

The **caloric density** of foods expresses the compactness of fuel energy concentrated within the designated serving sizes of food and equals the *number of calories contained per unit weight of food substance*:

CALORIC DENSITY = calories per gram weight of food

Therefore, a 1 ounce or 28 g serving size of food delivering 112 calories would have a caloric density of 112 calories per 28 gm (112 ÷ 28) or 4 calories per 1 g of food.

Caloric energy in natural, unprocessed particularly plant source crude fuel whole earth foods is diffusely scattered typically embedded within complex predominantly water-based matrices, which dilute the calories to lower caloric density and require considerably more digestive work energies to release the bound-up food energy calories for body vehicle utilization.

The caloric density per serving size of unprocessed crude fuel, whole earth foods tends to be substantially lower than that of processed foods and often measures less than two calories per gram of food. Food processing removes water from solid natural whole foods to extend shelf life, which consequently concentrates calories to increase caloric densities commonly well above four calories per gram weight of processed food product. Adding noncaloric fillers or moisture to processed food products artificially reduces caloric densities to fool consumers concerning caloric energies and nutritional benefits delivered per serving sizes of processed foods.

Although different foods may contain equal numbers of calories, the ease and rate of delivery of available food calories into the body vehicle may vary considerably according to the physical form and composition of the foods in which the calories exist. Some foods release energy calories more slowly to manageably supply body vehicle nutritional needs and benefit health, while other foods release calories more rapidly to overwhelm body vehicle metabolic and utilization capacities and harm health.

Processed and refined food products require comparatively less body vehicle work energy to release food calories for body vehicle utilization since the chemical and mechanical food processing steps artificially free up and concentrate natural crude fuel whole earth food calories to facilitate caloric energy extraction by the body vehicle.

Foods that densely deliver caloric energies not immediately utilized for body vehicle metabolic purposes create body vehicle energy surpluses that become deposited for future use into fat cell energy storage banks. Food caloric density measures can help with sorting out the health value of foods.

Approximate caloric requirements to power basic body vehicle survival operations for average-sized (100–200 lbs.) adult humans are as follows:

> 25–35 calories per kilogram (2.2 lbs.) of ideal body weight for height (IBW) per day (25–35 cal/kg/d) and depends on the intensity of physical activity as follows:
>
> **Sedentary activity** requires approximately 25 calories per kilogram of IBW per day
>
> **Moderate activity** requires approximately 30 calories per kilogram of IBW per day
>
> **Intense activity** requires approximately 35 calories or more per kilogram of IBW per day

Daily **caloric requirements** range roughly between 1,200 and 3,200 calories for average-sized adults, with 1,200 calories necessary for a sedentary person weighing 100 lbs. and up to 3,200 calories or more needed for an intensely active individual weighing 200 lbs., which translates to approximately 50–130 calories per hour required to power basic existence for most average-sized adult humans.

19.2 PROTEIN

Proteins comprise the larger operational and structural molecular units within animal and plant cells and tissue fluids that diversely perform vital life-sustaining biologic functions. Dietary proteins contain the basic chemical elements carbon

(C), oxygen (O), hydrogen (H), nitrogen (N), and sulfur (S) bound together within simple smaller building block units called **amino acids,** which couple together to create the larger and more complex protein structures.

Amino acids chemically link to create the larger conglomerate cellular and tissue protein entities that ultimately carry out specific biochemical and physiologic assignments maintaining life in living organisms. Humans build all existing body vehicle proteins entirely from *20* basic amino acid building blocks. The body vehicle can synthesize *11* of the necessary amino acids from simple nutrients but *cannot manufacture nine* other amino acids termed *essential amino acids,* which must be supplied externally from animal, plant, or insect sources.

Proteins exist in the meat component of natural crude fuel, whole earth foods such as fish, seafood, poultry, red meats, nuts, beans, and seeds and in insects and direct animal products, such as milk and eggs. Intrinsic body vehicle or dietarily ingested proteins not biochemically used for body vehicle operational purposes become metabolically broken down to supply energy calories to the body vehicle system. When the body vehicle metabolizes proteins, the protein nitrogen is initially released substantially as **ammonia,** which is toxic to the body vehicle and requires biochemical conversion in the liver to a less toxic substance called **urea** that is removed from the body vehicle through the kidneys in urine.

Protein inefficiently delivers approximately *four calories of energy per gram weight* when utilized as a fuel energy source. Typical protein requirements for average-sized adult humans are **0.8–1.5 g of protein per kilogram (2.2 lbs.) of ideal body weight (IBW) for height per day (0.8–1.5 gm/kg/d)** and depends on body vehicle age, health status, kidney and liver function, and specific needs for growth, tissue healing, illness recovery, and ongoing immune and metabolic activities. *Daily* protein requirements range roughly between 40 and 140 g or 1.5 and 5 ounces of protein across the spectrum of protein needs for average-sized adult humans.

19.3 FAT

Fat represents the most concentrated and structurally compact form of packaged biological fuel energy that maximally conserves storage space to deliver the highest metabolically available energy payload per unit weight of substance. The body vehicle produces fat to store excess unused fuel energy calories efficiently.

The main basic chemical elements that make up fat are almost exclusively carbon (C) and hydrogen (H), with a relatively small proportion of oxygen (O) that serves to link smaller fat molecules together to create more massive conglomerate chemical structures. Fat densely supplies approximately *nine calories of energy per gram weight.* Fat is a potently reactive nutrient fuel toxic to the body vehicle in large amounts. Fat administered into the body vehicle directly through a vein at quantities exceeding 2 g/kg of ideal body weight risks suppressing immune system function to increase infection risk.

Daily intake of fat calories is best limited to approximately no more than 30% of the total calories required to appropriately supply the ideal body weight caloric needs for specific intensity levels of physical activity. For example, consider a moderately active adult male with an IBW of 70 kg (154 lbs.) that requires 30 calories of energy per kilogram of IBW daily to total 2,100 calories:

(70 kg × 30 calories / kg for moderate activity = 2,100 calories)

For this adult male, fat calories are preferably limited to 630 calories = 2,100 calories × 30% maximum fat. Since fat delivers nine calories per gram, the maximal daily fat intake should be limited to 70 g:

(630 calories ÷ 9 calories/g of fat = 70 g)
70 g of fat = 2.3 ounces of fat
(1 ounce ≈ 28 g; so, 70 g ÷ 28 gm/ounce = 2.3 ounces)

Fats are a subgroup within a broader category of biomolecular structures possessing similar chemical properties termed **lipids.** Lipids comprise fats and various fatty element derivatives including vitamins, hormones, waxes, cholesterol, and structural cellular components, which maintain cellular integrity and function and play key roles in cellular signaling and body vehicle immune and inflammatory activities.

Linoleic acid (omega-6 fatty acid) and **linolenic acid** (omega-3 fatty acid) are **polyunsaturated fatty acid (PUFA)**-type lipids *essential* for body vehicle cellular development, growth, and inflammatory operations, which body vehicle metabolic processes cannot manufacture and consequently must be supplied externally from environmental seed, nut, seafood, or plant sources.

Fish oils refer to various combinations of essential omega fatty acids that are derived artificially from natural sources of omega fatty acids and then sold commercially as health supplements.

Natural sources of essential omega fatty acids include flaxseed, chia seeds, walnuts, spinach, kale, collard greens, Brussels sprouts, broccoli, cauliflower, and tissues of oily fish such as mackerel, salmon, tuna, and halibut. Fats in nature substantially exist in the fatty portions of animal tissues; within direct animal products such as milk; in nuts and seeds and "meaty" plants such as avocados and coconuts; and in plant oils.

Not all fats are created equal.

Unprocessed plant- and seafood-based fats naturally deliver excellent health benefits to lower health risks, while fats from certain animal sources or those that are modified chemically to artificially increase fat stability and shelf life for commercial purposes, increase health risks if consumed in excess. Certain chemically modified fats known as **trans fats,** created to prolong the shelf life of artificially manufactured food products, lead to blood vessel injury to produce serious cardiovascular health consequences, such as heart attacks and strokes, over time.

Appropriate ingestion of fat nutrients is necessary to maintain the correct balance of the immune system of defense mediators that control immune cell signaling and competence to protect against infection, cancer, and autoimmune disorders. Detrimental body vehicle health consequences result from excessive fat ingestion either from naturally fatty foods or from commercial products containing large amounts of chemically altered fats added to modify food product taste, texture, or shelf life.

Adverse body vehicle health consequences following repeatedly excessive fat ingestion include

1. corruption of body vehicle inflammatory activities to compromise the immune system of defense actions to increase risks for infection, autoimmune disorders, and cancer
2. breakdown of intestinal membrane barrier functions to produce a leaky gut, which allows environmental toxins and microorganisms normally restricted to the gut compartment to access protected blood circulation and harm vulnerable cells
3. injury to blood vessels carrying excessive fat loads and gut leaked toxins and microorganisms, which create vascular inflammation to deteriorate blood vessels and cause blockages resulting in secondary damage to vital organs and cells depending on adequate blood flow to remain viable and functioning properly
4. alteration in the biological integrity of various organs and tissues such as the brain, heart, and liver that assimilate, utilize, and store high energy fat, predisposing to numerous adverse health consequences such as food addictions, strokes, heart attacks, and liver failure following continual bombardment with excess fat
5. development of obesity with all its attendant health complications
6. desensitization of brain sensors toward protective stop eating regulatory signaling by hormones such as leptin, when continuously produced by body vehicle fat cells packed excessively with stored fat

19.4 SUGAR

Sugar is a body vehicle **fuel** existing in the simplest energy delivery form, which requires limited biochemical handling for blood absorption from the gut for cellular utilization to power life functions that make body vehicle existence possible. Sugar is composed exclusively of the basic chemical elements carbon (C), hydrogen (H), and oxygen (O) combined in relatively fixed proportions.

Individual body vehicle functional and genetic capabilities may limit intestinal processing and absorption of certain types of sugars such as lactose and fructose to create dietary intolerances for these sugars. Pure sugar typically supplies approximately *four calories of energy per gram weight* of sugar substance.

All sugars are not alike!

The rate of sugar fuel energy delivery from the gut into the blood from foods for cellular energy utilization depends on the biochemical complexity of the foods containing the sugars and the biological capacity of gut barrier membranes to pass the sugars through into the blood. Sugars firmly assimilated within natural crude fuel, whole earth foods, such as fruit or real, natural, whole grains, require more extensive digestive work to release and, consequently, access the blood more slowly than sugars loosely packed within refined food products that require minimal digestion to pass sugars essentially straight into the blood.

Gut linings readily accommodate the transport into the blood of reasonable loads of simple sugars, such as fructose and glucose, released from foods without significant delay. Ingestion of larger quantities of fructose-sweetened food and beverage products saturates the capacity of sugar transporters in gut membranes and traps the chemically reactive fructose awaiting transfer into the blood within the intestines. Large fructose loads dwelling in the gut for significant periods of time toxically react with intestinal cells to damage gut linings and transform residing gut microbes in adverse ways. Following gut absorption, the subsequent trafficking of the larger, chemically reactive sugar loads through blood vessels and tissues additionally harms exposed cells handling the excessive sugar energies.

A **high "flux"** or **heavy trafficking** of reactive energy molecules such as sugar throughout the body vehicle not only harms vulnerably exposed tissues and cells but also chemically disrupts cellular constituents involved with the programming and expression of DNA to increase cancer risks.

One useful clinical, biological marker for monitoring health status in diabetics is the **hemoglobin A1C level,** which reflects the extent to which body vehicle red blood cells have chemically reacted with elevated blood sugar levels over time. The hemoglobin A1C biomarker relates measurements of a red blood cell component that has been chemically altered by sugar to the average blood sugar levels for the preceding three months, with higher hemoglobin A1C levels indicating higher average blood sugar levels during the previous three months.

Body vehicle components that sustain damage when battered repeatedly by excessive sugar loads include the intestinal linings processing and transporting sugars into the blood; blood vessels carrying and distributing sugars throughout the body vehicle; liver cells packaging and exporting sugars to other tissues; and organs such as the brain, heart, kidneys, and nerves dependently receiving and utilizing sugars to energize metabolic operations. In fact, dense caloric energy deliveries into the blood from any sources containing concentrated reactive sugars and fat fuels cause immediately identifiable changes to red blood cell membranes that can predispose to adverse health consequences, giving fresh meaning to the phrase "heart attack meals."

Liquid sugars such as juices; blender-made smoothies; rehydration, sports, or soda pop beverages; and alcohol products require minimal gut work to *mainline calories* through intestinal membranes directly into the blood, overwhelming cellular fuel energy processing and utilization capacities with surplus sugar loads toxic to cellular membranes and tissue components.

Solid sugars, which comprise heavily processed and refined food products often made from grains and fruit, are formulated to dissolve with limited digestive work and behave like liquid sugars (e.g., pasta, cookies, bread, and candy). Humans are biologically incapable of breaking down certain raw crude fuel, whole earth foods through chewing or intestinal digestion, especially natural whole grains, such as wheat and rice, which require preparatory steps, such as cooking, for body vehicle utilization.

Commercial food industry preparation of indigestible natural foods for human consumption involves processing steps that not only physically and chemically break down whole food structures but also separate out and remove vital food nutrients. During the quest to create tasty powder fine flours and other easily mass consumed commercial food items, modern industrial food processing routinely refines and separates commercially "desirable" from "undesirable" food constituents.

Commercially "desirable" natural food derivatives dissolve readily into sugar to feed human pleasure craves and are cheaply formulated into numerous tasty commercial food products such as bread, pizza crusts, pastry goods, and pasta to leverage enormous profit margins for commercial food enterprises. Consequently, terms such as "whole grains" or "all natural" are misnomers since food processing disrupts and unbalances "natural" grain "wholeness" and artificially compounds dismantled grain components into enticing shapes desirable for human consumption using binding **food glue** substances.

Natural whole grain processing and refinement into flours, which are then formulated with artificial additives and shaped with food glue substances, not only disturb the nutritional value of natural foods but also deliver unwanted hitchhiker substances within final food product preparations. Suspected grain sensitivities in humans may instead be intolerances to artificial food formulations that unbalance and concentrate individual whole food components or possibly be reactivities to unwanted hitchhiker food additives and contaminants included through processing within formulated food products.

19.5 GLUTEN

Gluten is a protein component found almost exclusively within the seed portion of wheat, rye, and barley grains and a cross grain between wheat and rye called triticale, which provides valuable nourishment for seed germination. Gluten is one type of natural food glue substance commonly utilized to bind powdered grain flour ingredients together to create various processed food products. Commercially, gluten from whole grains is extracted, refined, and condensed, then artificially added in unnaturally high concentrations to processed foods and beverages to enhance taste, add body and texture, prolong shelf life, and bind other processed food ingredients into appealing shapes.

Individuals genetically predisposed to gluten sensitivity that are exposed continually to gluten-containing processed food and beverage products may lose their gut immune tolerance to further gluten exposures and develop immune-mediated gut reactions toward gluten, which destructively attack the gut lining to cause severe and sometimes life-threatening adverse health consequences. Consequently, commercial industries have opportunistically created an entire "gluten-free" food industry in a marketing strategy aimed at capturing vulnerable segments of the population experiencing or having concerns about gluten sensitivity, who are reluctant or unable to abuse themselves any further with gluten-packed processed foods and beverages. Similarly, excessive consumption of any highly processed and refined grain, nut, or seed food products made from wheat, soy, peanut, and chocolate can predispose genetically susceptible individuals to develop immune, digestive, or general health intolerances for these foods, as is more evident within modern societies substantially subsisting on processed foods and beverages.

Notably, natural crude fuel, whole earth foods, such as fruits; vegetables; raw nuts; nonwheat, nonrye, nonbarley, and nontriticale real whole grains and seeds such as whole corn, quinoa, brown rice, oats, and flax; unprocessed poultry, seafood, fish, meat, and eggs; natural spices; and dairy products such as milk, plain yogurt, and aged fermented hard cheeses are all completely gluten-free, unless gluten is an inadvertent contaminant or has been added surreptitiously.

19.6 CARBOHYDRATES AND STARCHES

Carbohydrates are sugar fuel energy substances exclusively containing the chemical elements carbon (C), hydrogen (H), and oxygen (O) proportionately combined within basic "hydrated carbon" (CH_2O) units composed of one carbon (C) atom bound to one water (H_2O) molecule. *Simple carbohydrates* are termed *sugars* or *saccharides* and combine only 5 or 6 CH_2O units into a *single* ring structure (*monosaccharide*) that may additionally bind to another 5 or 6 CH_2O unit ring to form a *double* ring structure (*disaccharide*). Basic monosaccharides are glucose, fructose, and galactose, while common disaccharides are sucrose (ordinary table sugar), lactose (milk sugar), and maltose. **Complex carbohydrates** called *poly-saccharides* form by chemically linking *many* 5 or 6 CH_2O unit ring structures together. Complex carbohydrates require more work energy to assemble and, consequently, disassemble or dismantle for body vehicle needs than simple carbohydrates require.

All living earth plant, animal, insect, and microbe organisms biochemically weave simple sugar carbohydrates into larger, more complex sugar-based structures, which perform diverse biologic functions. Some of the roles played by complex polysaccharide carbohydrates in living organisms include: linking with proteins and lipids to provide cellular adhesion, identity, and structural membrane support; operating as energy storage units; and acting as constituents of secretions such as mucus and tears.

Two main energy-storing polysaccharides are **starch** and **glycogen,** while structural polysaccharides include **cellulose,** which makes up plant cell walls, and **chitin,** which composes the external armor of insects and shellfish. Starch stores energy by binding together and condensing multiple individual glucose sugars into larger polysaccharide units.

Complex carbohydrates substantially comprise the skin and pulp or flesh of fruits and vegetables and the matrix of whole grains such as brown rice, barley, quinoa, oats, and corn, while nuts and seeds contain approximately equal proportions of protein and carbohydrates and at least twice as much fat (mainly unsaturated) as carbohydrates. The food industry manufactures *artificial polysaccharide-type substances* such as carboxymethyl cellulose, carrageenan, maltodextrin, and xanthan gum to act as food product thickeners, emulsifiers, dispersants, binding agents, and preservatives.

The body vehicle must chemically break down starches in the mouth and gut to release individual starch sugars for intestinal absorption and blood distribution to energize cells. Starches exist along a vast continuum of biochemical sizes and complexities having varying work energy requirements to disassemble into individual sugars. Industrial food processing uses mechanical and chemical means to artificially break down complex food starches into simpler forms requiring less digestive work to separate further into free sugars easily absorbable into the blood.

Extensive processing and refinement of whole fruits, vegetables, and grains produce simple carbohydrate juices, syrups, jams, jellies, soft drinks, candy, and table sugar, all of which use relatively minimal energy for rapid blood delivery of contained sugar energies. Complex whole grain starches are also extensively processed to make refined flours consisting of simple carbohydrates that dissolve readily in the mouth and require relatively minimal digestive work to complete sugar release for blood absorption. Consequently, processing of natural whole food starches allows starch sugars to pass faster and more directly into the blood after ingestion.

Resistant starches are more complex carbohydrates that escape digestion during normal gut transit, because the body vehicle either lacks the necessary digestive enzymes to break these starches down into simpler forms or the carbohydrate structure is too large, complex, or firmly rooted within the natural whole food matrix and therefore would demand more work energy and time to break down and release bound sugars than available during routine digestive processing. For example, starches found in natural whole grains, legumes, vegetables, and fruit require more oral and gut work with chewing, mashing, squeezing, agitating, and chemical digestion to break apart and, consequently, uncouple individual sugars more slowly while using more energy during body vehicle digestive processing. Resistant starches that entirely escape small intestinal digestion deliver starch components known as **fiber** into the colon for further digestive processing and energy extraction by gut microorganisms.

Body vehicle metabolic processes "combust" carbohydrates ($-CH_2O-$) to generate cellular energy by reacting each carbohydrate carbon (C) atom with two oxygen (O_2) atoms inhaled from the air to produce carbon dioxide (CO_2) and release water (H_2O) along with energy:

$$CH_2O + O_2 = CO_2 + H_2O + Energy$$

The body vehicle lungs then exhale the carbon dioxide (CO_2) into the air to be taken up by earth plants, which use **sunlight** and **water** (H_2O) in a biochemical process called **photosynthesis** to recover the bound carbon (C) atom to rebuild plant carbohydrates and discharge the oxygen (O_2) back into the atmosphere:

$$CO_2 + Plants + Sunlight + H_2O = Plant\ Carbohydrate\ (-CH_2O-) + O_2$$

Carbohydrates supply approximately *3–4 calories of energy per gram weight* depending on the degree of carbohydrate complexity (simple vs. complex), which determines the amount of digestive work energy necessary to dismantle whole carbohydrate structures into simple sugars for cellular usage. The more complex the carbohydrate structure, the more the carbohydrate resists digestion and the higher are the work energy demands to digest the carbohydrate, proportionately reducing the amount of fuel energy that the carbohydrate delivers into the body vehicle to power metabolic operations. Basically, simpler carbohydrates utilize less energy being digested than equivalent weights of complex carbohydrates utilize for digestion.

19.7 CHOLESTEROL

Cholesterol is a vital lipid that critically functions as a backbone or building block component for body vehicle cellular membranes, hormones, constituents involved with cellular signaling, and numerous other structural and operational body vehicle components. Body vehicle components built from cholesterol provide membrane and cellular shape and maintain proper body vehicle development, growth, and cellular operations.

The body vehicle can completely meet cholesterol needs by manufacturing cholesterol from dietary fats and sugars through complex multistep biochemical processes within the liver, intestines, and specialized glandular tissues such as the adrenal glands. The liver is the primary producer of cholesterol for body vehicle needs. Liver cells release cholesterol directly into the blood or out into liver bile, which flows into the small intestines to assist the chemical digestion of ingested fats and help maintain proper gut microflora composition and function.

Body vehicle cholesterol needs drive cholesterol production from the metabolic breakdown of stored fats and sugars, while ingested fats, sugars, and carbohydrates also stimulate cholesterol manufacture in the liver, with higher consumption pushing the liver to make more cholesterol. Heavy alcohol consumption can also lead to higher body vehicle cholesterol production indirectly through complex metabolic effects on the liver, until the alcohol destroys enough liver function to produce liver failure which then causes blood cholesterol levels to fall.

The manufacture of each cholesterol molecule utilizes the equivalent of four glucose sugar molecules. Consequently, blocking cholesterol production in the liver with medicines such as statins can elevate blood sugar levels and cause diabetes in susceptible individuals, typically those who are already obese and have fuel energy overloaded cells. The gut additionally absorbs cholesterol from dietary sources, with fatty diets high in cholesterol leading to higher blood cholesterol levels.

The primary dietary sources of cholesterol are animal products, as plants are essentially cholesterol free but contain key healthy fats that may be indirectly converted biochemically into cholesterol in small amounts. Cholesterol is chemically reactive with various cellular membranes especially that line blood vessels, which transport and distribute cholesterol to supply cellular needs and are susceptible to develop inflammatory injuries leading to vascular occlusion following repeated exposures to high blood cholesterol concentrations. Therefore, diets high in animal fat or processed food calories raise blood cholesterol levels either through increased cholesterol absorption from the gut or stimulated cholesterol manufacture in the liver, causing numerous health consequences such as gallbladder disease with gallstone formation from cholesterol-rich liver bile, and heart, kidney, or brain injuries precipitated by cholesterol damages to vital blood supplies.

Since cholesterol intimately comprises structural and functional components of cells and is not readily used as an energy source to supply cellular energy needs, cholesterol is not easily burned away by increasing physical activity when excessive cholesterol ingestion and body vehicle manufacture exceed metabolic utilization. Consequently, control of body vehicle cholesterol levels responds better to dietary management that reduces excessive cholesterol ingestion and lowers consumption of processed and refined sugars and fats driving cholesterol manufacture.

19.8 **ALCOHOL**

Alcohol (ethanol) forms by fermenting sugars derived from fruit and grain carbohydrates with yeast and is a potent fuel that provides approximately *7 calories of energy per gram weight of alcohol.* The quantity of "pure" alcohol (alcohol/volume) contained equivalently in 5 ounces of wine (12% alcohol), 12 ounces of average strength beer (5% alcohol), or 1.5 ounces of hard liquor (40% alcohol) is approximately 14 g, which provides 98 calories of alcohol fuel energy that does not include additional calories delivered from sugars and other ingredients mixed into alcoholic beverages.

Consuming large quantities of alcohol regularly to provide calories beyond immediate body vehicle energy needs and overwhelm the liver capacity to metabolize the alcohol produces a fatty liver and increases risks for developing advanced liver disease including cirrhosis while predisposing to obesity as excessive alcohol calories become stored as fat.

In addition to delivering large caloric payloads, alcohol is a potent toxin that threatens body vehicle health and survival with regular consumption. Regular alcohol drinkers have shorter life-spans and greater risks for developing cancer compared to nondrinkers. The liver and gut are intrinsically equipped with metabolic capabilities to detoxify alcohol, which is naturally produced in minute quantities by the gut microbiota during digestive fermentation of ingested foods. Alcohol consumed in excess potently redirects body vehicle energy producing and fuel burning metabolic activities toward clearing toxic alcohol from blood, which may temporarily drop blood sugar levels down to cause problems in diabetic individuals already taking medications that lower blood sugar levels.

Additionally, alcohol dissolves well into both oil and water to make alcohol a biological poison that can chemically disrupt cellular membranes and protein structures, which is a useful "sanitizing" property that allows alcohol to kill microbes, but which also predisposes alcohol to harm vital body vehicle cells and tissues. Heavy alcohol consumption dramatically impacts the composition and balance of the oral and gut microbiota, likely by eliminating vulnerable microbes and promoting the existence of resistant microbes while altering the function of immune cells and barrier membranes, and coincidentally injures protective intestinal barrier membranes to allow toxins and dangerous microbes to migrate through gut membranes into the blood, compounding other alcohol poisoning effects on the body vehicle system.

Since alcohol delivers concentrated fuel energy and possesses toxic chemical properties predisposing to numerous adverse biologic and metabolic effects, living organisms including body vehicle cells and microbes have evolved complex biochemical, survival mechanisms to protect against alcohol exposure that become overwhelmed with higher alcohol levels.

19.9 WATER SOLUBILITY TEST

The **water solubility test** is a simple procedure illustrating the relative work energies necessary to break down natural solid crude fuel whole earth foods compared to the work energies that processed and refined food products use up during digestive preparation for blood absorption. Natural solid crude fuel, whole earth food structures change minimally to remain substantially intact when immersed in water for relatively long periods of time. Fresh fruit, vegetables, nuts, seeds, and meat fail to fall apart and disintegrate, sometimes even after soaking in water for days or even weeks. In contrast, processed food products, such as cookies, cakes, pasta, bread, and candy bars, soften, disintegrate, and dissolve after water immersion for minutes or only a few hours without requiring much additional work to break down original solid food structures completely into simpler nutrients. Likewise, processed and refined food products dissolve rapidly in the mouth with saliva to release concentrated simple sugars and food additives for immediate gut absorption and blood delivery, whereas naturally complex crude fuel, whole earth foods require extensive mechanical and chemical body vehicle work to extract usable nutrients that are integrated tightly fastened within intact crude fuel whole food structures.

19.10 MAINLINING CALORIES

The direct infusion of pharmaceutical formulations of concentrated simple sugars, lipid fats, and protein amino acids into the bloodstream through a vein to provide nutritional sustenance to individuals incapable of using their gut for nutrition, can produce nutrient imbalances, metabolic disturbances, immune impairment, and liver toxicity from nutrient and energy overload.

The continuous delivery of large quantities of concentrated nutrients through the gut into the blood by consuming processed and refined food and beverage products repeatedly risks causing similar body vehicle toxicities as if nutrients were being mainlined directly into the blood through a vein.

The toxic metabolic effects that result from consuming concentrated calories and other nutrients excessively to overwhelm cellular biological capacities for energy and nutrient utilization predispose to body vehicle disrepair inciting immune repair responses and causing illness and premature demise.

Eating excessive flour dough and fatty foods can make one go extinct like the dodo bird.

19.11 **HUMAN SUSTENANCE REQUIREMENTS**

The body vehicle has specific nutrient and fuel energy requirements for powering cellular operations that maintain the structural and functional integrity of the body vehicle system to carry out life activities and withstand the stresses of daily existence. Carbohydrates, proteins, fats, vitamins, and minerals compose the mainstay of biochemical body vehicle biochemical nutrients providing fuel energy calories and the building blocks required for the body vehicle to exist physically.

Numerous factors determine actual daily body vehicle protein, calorie, and fat needs including body vehicle age, size, activity level, kidney and liver function, state of health with underlying illnesses, and rate of energy metabolism governed by genetics, blood hormone levels, and the composition and balance of indwelling gut microbiota. The body vehicle tightly regulates energy utilization so that all absorbed fuel calories are either burned to supply immediate energy needs or stored for later usage. Excess protein, fat, or carbohydrate delivered into blood beyond immediate body vehicle metabolic needs and utilization capacities are processed and repackaged to store unused energies as fat in liver and fat cells, or as compacted sugars called **glycogen** in liver and muscle cells, which can readily supply cellular energy needs later on-demand.

Certain individuals are born with **"thrifty" genes** to be *metabolically lean energy burners.* **Lean burners** use fewer calories per hour to run metabolic operations to power usual body vehicle activities compared to the number of calories normally used by average individuals for similar activities, possibly as a primitive adaptation to survive famine conditions. Gut microbiota composition, balance, and metabolic activity are additional factors affecting the actual caloric energy harvested from ingested foods and ultimately supplied to drive body vehicle cellular functions.

Prolonged intake of unutilized surplus calories increasingly deposits excess fuels into body vehicle energy storage banks eventually to cause obesity. Therefore, regularly consuming processed food and beverage products that rapidly flood the blood with excessive calories to exceed body vehicle metabolic utilization predisposes to obesity, especially in individuals possessing metabolically thrifty genes or certain gut microbial compositions; which creates major challenges to reverse obesity under circumstances where processed food and beverage products are abundant, cheap, easily accessed, and consumed excessively without restraint for pleasure and convenience.

19.12 **FAST-NOW FUELS**

Fast-now fuels are extensively processed food and beverage products predominantly containing simple sugars and fats compacted into high caloric densities, which digest rapidly (*fast*) and absorb immediately (*now*) soon after oral ingestion to *flood the blood* with chemically reactive caloric energies. Commercial food processing and refinement accelerate the gut transfer of food energies into the blood so that fast-now fuels behave as **caloric energy bombs,** which require minimal digestion after oral ingestion to absorb quickly through gut membranes to deliver large fuel energy payloads into the blood at once.

Most **fun junk foods** artificially made of refined flours, sugars, and oils are fast-now fuels, as are many purportedly healthy foods such as various breakfast cereals and blender-made fruit smoothie beverages. Fast-now fuels digesting in the gut have **high immediate caloric extraction ratios** with proportionately more food calories absorbed sooner in initial gut segments compared to the relative number of calories delivered further down the gut for later absorption. Intestinal absorption of fast-now fuels is analogous to mainlining or injecting food calories directly into the blood through a vein. Fast-now foods *push* calories and other contained nutrients into the blood often beyond existing body vehicle metabolic needs and handling capacities.

Alcohol is an additional fast-now type fuel energy substance densely packed with calories that readily penetrates intestinal barrier linings to access blood immediately and pummel cells with toxic alcohol energy payloads. Rapid deliveries of large sugar or fat energy shipments into the blood to raise blood sugar or fat levels dangerously high disturb homeostasis and metabolically stress the body vehicle system. Reactive sugar and fat fuel energies dispersing throughout the blood in high concentrations are chemically toxic to directly exposed blood vessels and cells.

High blood sugar levels especially activate body vehicle alarms that trigger protective compensatory homeostatic responses such as the release of insulin from the pancreas gland to lower high blood sugar levels quickly. Insulin released from the pancreas gland clears high blood sugar levels by shuttling sugar excesses into cells, forcing water to follow the sugar into the cells to rebalance water concentrations across cellular membranes which leads to swelling of energy stuffed cells. Ballooning cells filling up with excessive sugar energies and water may then burst and disintegrate immediately or after similar events are repeated to cause progressive cellular dropout that adds up over time to deteriorate the function of vital organs and tissues.

Clearing sugar rapidly from blood to drop blood sugar levels precipitously signals danger to the body vehicle that excites survival alarms triggering corrective metabolic responses which release storage sugars and stimulate eating to counterbalance plummeting blood sugar levels, leading to a vicious cycle of blood sugar energy swings creating metabolic pressures that compound other body vehicle overfueling stresses.

Frequent high and low swings in blood sugar levels eventually reset baseline homeostatic activities of compensatory body vehicle hormonal and metabolic stress responses at abnormal levels, adversely impacting nutritional behaviors and cellular fuel energy handling to compromise body vehicle health and longevity.

Consequently, consuming excessive fast-now fuels that heavily traffic chemically reactive high energy sugar and fat molecules through blood produces toxic metabolic disruptions predisposing to permanent body vehicle cellular, tissue, and organ damage.

Diets high in fast-now refined sugars and fats contribute toward the development of diabetes, high blood pressure, and high blood cholesterol levels to accelerate vascular wear and tear eventually manifesting as atherosclerosis or hardening of the arteries, which interrupts critical blood flow to vital organs to precipitate strokes, heart attacks, and kidney failure. Therefore, fast-now fuels deliver excessive energy and nutrients into the body vehicle at rates exceeding metabolic tolerances and utilization capacities, activating compensatory responses that may become maladaptively sustained to the detriment of body vehicle health and survival.

19.13 SLOW-LATER FUELS

Slow-later fuels are whole natural foods in crude unprocessed, and unrefined form with low caloric densities, which have prolonged (*slow*) digestion and delayed (*later*) absorption following oral ingestion to pass caloric energies and other nutrients further down the gut before eventual delivery into the blood. Slow-later fuels require more extensive mechanical and chemical work by the mouth, gut, and other digestive organs to release bound-up nutrient ingredients and energy for blood distribution to power cellular operations. With higher resistance to digestive breakdown, slow-later fuels have **lower immediate caloric extraction ratios** with proportionately fewer calories absorbed earlier in initial gut compartments to allow relatively more calories to pass farther along down the gut to be absorbed later.

The gradual gut passage of slow-later fuels prolongs gut retention and stretches out digestive processing over longer gut segments to pace the release and blood delivery of fuel energies and other nutrients to match cellular metabolic needs and utilization capacities better. Extending slow-later fuel transit further down the gut allows the body vehicle to *pull* calories and nutrients gradually from digesting foods to regulate body vehicle nourishment safely. Longer digestion of slow-later fuels in the temporary gut holding tank prevents flooding the blood with excessive fuel energies and nutrients as occurs with fast-now fuels.

The body vehicle conveniently possesses all required hardware and capabilities to biologically process and transform natural crude fuel whole earth foods into basic life-sustaining nutrients and energy essential for body vehicle existence. The body vehicle ultimately consumes proportionately more of the initially ingested caloric energy payloads to process slow-later crude fuels to power the body vehicle than to process the same caloric payloads of fast-now fuels.

The energy costs attributed to break down and store ingested foods for body vehicle metabolic usage is known as the **specific dynamic action** of foods. Slow-later fuels have a much higher specific dynamic action than fast-now fuels since the body vehicle expends more energy to digest and ready slow-later fuels for cellular use than to prepare the equal number of fast-now fuel calories for body vehicle energy needs.

19.14 COMPARING FAST-NOW AND SLOW-LATER FUEL DELIVERY

Consider two calorically equivalent foods, one being a medium-sized apple with skin that contains approximately 50 slow-later fuel calories and the other an average-sized cookie that delivers 50 fast-now fuel calories. The artificially manufactured cookie is formulated with refined flour, sugar, and fat and laced with chemical additives to create an enticing, recognizable, and commercially appealing appearance, smell, taste, and texture. The cookie crumbles easily and dissolves in the mouth with minimal chewing to immediately release simple sugars and fats that do not require much additional digestive work for the gut linings to absorb the delivered fuel calories directly into the blood.

Rapidly absorbed sugars and fats then surge calories into the blood to biochemically scorch blood vessels transiting the concentrated sugar and fat fuel energies for cellular distribution. The cookie has a low specific dynamic action, so the body vehicle expends minimal work energy digesting the cookie to conserve nearly all 50 original cookie fuel energy calories which absorb rapidly into the blood possibly within 20 minutes; proportionately supplying the equivalent of 150 calories per hour of fuel energy to exceed estimated average adult human fuel energy requirements of approximately 50–130 calories per hour. Consequently, cookie calories delivered into the blood at rates above cellular fuel energy needs are shuttled protectively into body vehicle energy storage banks for later use to clear the blood of biochemically reactive fuels that are toxic to exposed cellular and tissue constituents.

Nutrients contained in processed and highly refined food products, such as cookies, which have a high immediate caloric extraction ratio, are substantially absorbed within initial segments of the small intestines, depriving lower-gut microbiota of essential energy and nutrient deliveries necessary to sustain a healthy microbiota responsible for maintaining body vehicle health. Furthermore, toxic chemical food additives and preservatives having no body vehicle nutritional value are digestively separated from cookie nutrients and swept down the intestines to kill susceptible gut microorganisms, injure intestinal lining cells, and distress resident gut immune cells exposed to cookie toxins.

Cookies are sold in one-size-fits-all serving sizes to be consumed equally by 30-pound children as well as 300-pound adults and frequently are eaten in multiples complemented by additional fast-now fuels such as skim milk or juice to wash cookies down into the gut. The potential for body vehicle toxicity amplifies when high potency fast-now fuels are consumed in combination especially by younger children who ingest relatively huge proportions of fast-now fuel energies into correspondingly tiny body vehicles sizes.

A medium-sized apple that includes the skin also contains approximately 50 calories of potential fuel energy. Apples require more extensive chewing and mechanical manipulation using the tongue and mouth muscles to break down to the proper consistency for swallowing into the gut for further digestive processing. Despite laborious mouth work, swallowed apple fragments require additional digestive effort from the stomach and intestine with mechanical agitation and chemical breakdown, before apple nutrients fully release and are available for blood absorption through gut linings.

Since the apple has a higher specific dynamic action, the body vehicle may expend 10%–20% of originally contained apple calories to process and prepare apple nutrients for final systemic utilization, which in this case equals approximately 5–10 calories. The apple spends more time trafficking down the gut temporary fuel holding tank while being gradually digested for absorption and consequently is carried longer and further down the gut to produce more extended feelings of satiety and fullness to curtail craves for additional eating.

The slow digestive release of fuel calories and nutrients from the apple synchronizes better with body vehicle energy demands and utilization capacities to reduce accumulation of energy surpluses requiring storage in fat cell energy banks for later use. Additionally, human digestive enzymes and intestinal processing may be incapable of completely digesting certain apple skin and pulp constituents, which then pass down into lower portions of the intestine to feed the gut microbiota. Therefore, the original 50 apple fuel energy calories might reduce to only 40 calories absorbed slowly over 4 hours, amounting to a blood delivery rate of 10 calories of fuel energy per hour to fall well below levels toxic to blood vessels and cells or predisposing to obesity. Consequently, digestive activities slowly release apple fuel energy and nutrients for blood absorption to match systemic delivery with cellular metabolic utilization and processing capabilities while maintaining energy and nutrient blood levels below concentrations harmful to the body vehicle.

The **Glycemic Index** nutritional food ranking system analogously expresses the concept of fast-now and slow-later fuel energy deliveries into the blood, and ranks foods on a scale of one to 100 (minimum to maximum) according to the extent that the foods increase blood sugar levels, with pure glucose sugar rated at 100 and many nonstarchy raw vegetables rated below 20–30.

19.15 FIBER

Fiber is a complex carbohydrate component of plants composed of tightly bound sugars resistant to separation by human oral and gut enzymatic and mechanical digestive processing. Plant fibers such as cellulose and pectin act as structural scaffolds that bind or support other vital plant fuel and nutrient ingredients and provide the roughage and dietary bulk found in vegetables, fruit, beans, legumes, nuts, seeds, and whole grains. Consumable fibers are commonly categorized based on their ability to dissolve in water. **Soluble fibers** dissolve readily in water to form a gel, whereas **insoluble fibers** do not dissolve in water and require extensive mechanical, chemical, thermal, or gut microbial processing to separate into simpler elements that can mix into water.

The digestive apparatus of the human gut does not possess the necessary enzymes and digestive capabilities to dismantle and chemically break down resistant plant fibers into absorbable nutrients. Plant fibers that resist chemical and mechanical digestion following oral and intestinal processing can still be converted into nutrient and energy molecules by indwelling gut bacteria, which feed on undigested plant fibers to secondarily produce nutritional elements termed **short-chain fatty acids (SCFA)** that directly nourish the intestinal lining cells and help modulate gut immune activity. SCFA help intestinal barriers remain intact and critically influence gut immune development and function to prevent gut microbial overgrowth and translocation across the gut lining and protect against body vehicle infection and cancer.

Fiber also binds and carries water down the gut to moisturize and dilute intestinal contents, providing an aqueous medium in which digestive juices and gut microbiota can mix with consumed foods to chemically and enzymatically release nutrients bound within whole plant food structures. Indigestible plant fibers such as cellulose and pectin are commercially used as fillers in many low-calorie food products to provide moistness, texture, thickness, and bulk, while another common soluble commercial fiber **psyllium** serves as a laxative to moisturize stool and promote easier expulsion of colonic feces to regulate bowel movements. Soluble plant fibers are found more commonly within watery fruit and vegetables, legumes, and whole grains that ripen quickly or dissolve with simple cooking. Bananas, plums, peaches, oranges, tomatoes, cucumbers, and various beans, peas and oat, barley, and brown rice grains serve as typical sources of soluble fiber. Insoluble plant fibers usually compose the hard, nutty, crunchy, or chewy roughage of plant skins and shell components, or the internal matrix of whole grains, seeds, nuts, and beans, which require extensive cooking to break down and fail to liquefy or dissolve into a paste in the mouth despite extensive mechanical chewing with saliva.

19.16 COLON SCRUBBERS

Colon scrubbers are the unabsorbed indigestible nutrient components of slow-later fuels, such as soluble and insoluble fibers, and other plant source substances that make their way down into the colon. Natural crude fuel, whole earth food digestive waste by-products transiting down the gut bind and carry water and sweep along gut debris and other ingested or metabolically produced toxins for eventual expulsion out of the body vehicle in feces.

Water consumed alone unescorted by a fiber vehicle to drive the water down into the colon is substantially absorbed within the small intestines and diverted through the kidneys to increase urination, as opposed to being delivered directly into the colon to increase stooling. Driving water down the gut into the large bowel dilutes fecal toxins to reduce their concentrations and toxic potency and moistens stool to facilitate the evacuation of accumulated fecal waste stored by the colon.

Colon scrubbers also provide nourishment for the vast population of gut microbes and help keep the microbes "friendly" and working with and for the body vehicle to protect against illness and invasion by undesirable microorganisms that threaten to compromise health. Diversified plant-based diets that incorporate a large daily intake of various fruits, vegetables, beans, legumes, nuts, seeds, and real natural whole grains provide a variety and generous supply of colon scrubber type substances to promote more diversified, abundant, and healthier gut microbial floras optimizing intestinal barrier and immune functions that translate into body vehicle health and well-being.

19.17 PROBIOTICS

The **World Health Organization (WHO)** defines **probiotics** as *live microorganisms* which, when administered in adequate amounts, confer a health benefit to the host. Probiotics are biological products commonly manufactured industrially, which may initially be wholly or substantially viable, but usually lose viability progressively with storage following manufacture.

Commercial probiotics are selective combinations of a few or several varieties of variously live or dead bacterial or yeast microorganisms and their products, which are delivered as pills, liquids, or specialized food products for ingestion into the gut to confer some assumed health benefits. Probiotic preparations are speculated to affect the diversity, composition, abundance, or activity of native gut microbial communities and possibly impact the function of gut barrier membranes and residing intestinal immune cells to influence body vehicle health in beneficial ways. Actually, anything introduced into the mouth such as food or other substances is contaminated unavoidably with environmental microbes that travel down the gut ultimately to combine and interact with the internally contained native body vehicle microbiome. Classic probiotics generationally passed down from ancient times include natural yogurt, kefir, and fermented hard cheeses. The definite biological activities and health effects of probiotics introduced into the body vehicle remain poorly understood and mostly undefined.

19.18 PREBIOTICS

Commercial **prebiotics** are industrial formulations of indigestible nutrient food substances for oral delivery into the gut, which are postulated to nourish the microbiome. Prebiotics are presumed to feed gut microbes selectively to enhance their growth, metabolic activity, and function or increase their proportion within their microbial communities to benefit the health, well-being, or function of the body vehicle host.

Quintessential ubiquitously available and timeless old-world prebiotics are all existing natural crude fuel, whole earth foods, which provide the ideal nutritional sustenance to optimize the existence, function, and health of both the body vehicle and all symbiotic indwelling microorganisms. Mother Nature crude fuel, whole earth foods maximally deliver the nutritional variety that is indeed the spice and essentiality of human and indwelling microbial life.

19.19 GUT FLORA MANIPULATION

The merchandising of industrially formulated probiotic and prebiotic products to manipulate the gut flora reaps enormous profits for rescue industries. Heath benefit claims for artificial gut flora manipulation rest on a scientific knowledge base existing in a very primitive stage that possesses a limited understanding of human and microbial interactions.

Ingestion of generically formulated prebiotic substances to selectively affect the growth or activity of the immense and intricately complex body vehicle gut microbiota is analogous to delivering certain food supplies into a vast, uncharted, and ostensibly chaotic tribal nation with poorly understood governance and organizational infrastructure and expecting to feed select inhabitants and influence tribal behaviors and national activities predictably.

Similarly, ingesting probiotic preparations containing relatively small quantities of a few commercially selected strains of microorganisms with the intention of materially altering the general makeup and function of an enormously large and diversified gut microbial community is equivalent to emigrating a small family from a foreign country into a vastly pluralistic society with millions of inhabitants possessing tremendous ethnic, racial, intellectual, and economic diversities in an attempt to appreciably transform societal operations.

The unproven assumptions behind probiotic use are that oral ingestion of relatively limited numbers of very few strains of commercially selected bacterial or yeast microbes presumably drops an adequate and viable load of microorganisms or their products precisely into desired gut locations to exert predictable effects on native gut floras and confer specific health benefits to the host. Before producing any potential health effects, commercially selected probiotic organisms must traverse 20–30 feet of intestines and survive stomach acid, liver bile, harsh digestive enzymes, and innumerable immune system interactions while encountering trillions of other diverse and competing microorganisms, any of which can modify, disrupt, or destroy original probiotic formulations.

Notably, one predictable commercial probiotic action includes consumer money extraction. Predictable delivery of commercially available probiotics into the colon can be more reliably accomplished through the direct administration of probiotic formulations as a rectal enema, which is unlikely to become popular for the public or probiotic manufacturers and suppliers that coincidentally produce and sell tasty commercial food products and orally ingested health supplements. Consequently, probiotic products that are commonly regulated similarly to foods and dietary health supplements are unlikely to be offered in enema form to be prominently displayed on grocery store shelves directly competing for consumer attention alongside yogurt, cheese, and other commercial snack food items such as cookies and chips.

Ancient probiotic-type substances that possibly render users some health benefits with regular consumption include natural yogurt, kefir, and old-time fermented hard cheeses available to humanity throughout many generations, long before industry got wise to the immense profit potential of this previously untapped and relatively unregulated commercial opportunity. More importantly, dramatic dietary alterations are known to drastically modify the composition, abundance, richness, and activity of gut microbiota within as little as a few days. Consistent adherence to specific nutritional behaviors and dietary routines over a few weeks leads to more sustained changes in the makeup and function of indwelling gut microbial communities. Therefore, a healthy diet that avoids poisoning gut microbes with processed and refined food products and their additives, and incorporates consumption of diversified natural crude fuel, whole earth foods with a greater variety of unprocessed plants and fresh animal flesh, cultivates healthier gut microbiotas and produces innumerable other health benefits more predictably.

Limited roles exist for rescue industry attempts to repopulate, repair, and rebuild healthier gut microbial floras using formulated commercial-grade probiotic and prebiotic products. For instance, the use of prebiotics, probiotics, and their combination termed **synbiotics** possibly may be beneficial temporarily following aggressive antibiotic or cancer chemotherapy treatments, which exert chemical warfare on the body vehicle system to kill vulnerable gut microbes indiscriminately and deplete protective colonic microbial inhabitants to allow opportunistic microorganisms to invade and attack the body vehicle.

Fecal microbial transplantation (FMT) is a medical procedure that involves the direct delivery of large volumes of fresh stool harvested from presumably healthy donors into the gut of sick recipients through nasally, orally, or rectally inserted tubes or with numerous pills to transfer entire populations and communities of diversified gut microorganisms immediately into the colon. FMT is life-saving in circumstances where native colonic bacterial populations are wiped out or over-run by pathologic microorganisms in immune compromised individuals following antibiotic or cancer chemotherapy, which allow deadly antibiotic-resistant opportunistic microbes to proliferate wildly in the compromised gut to threaten body vehicle survival. Unfortunately, FMT also transfers unwanted microbes and adverse microbe-driven health effects from FMT donors to recipients.

The universal body vehicle system encompassing all native body vehicle cells and indwelling microbial inhabitants is exquisitely designed to work symbiotically in concert to purposely promote body vehicle life on earth. The body vehicle system additionally integrates intimately into a complex interdependent ecosystem of planet earth plant and animal domains. Long before commercial food processing and manufacturing enterprises existed, humans adaptively evolved to physically and functionally survive and thrive exclusively and entirely on unprocessed, natural whole earth foods. The body vehicle is optimally equipped to proficiently perform and accomplish all necessary work to extract and utilize energy and nutrients from crude fuel whole earth foods to properly sustain body vehicle and indwelling resident microbial life.

Predicting the biological health effects of gut microbe manipulations with one-size-fits-all fixed formulations of commercial-grade prebiotic and probiotic preparations is virtually impossible, given the extreme heterogeneity of internal body vehicle environments and external environmental influences, and the diversity in composition and complexity of actions and interactions among indwelling gut microbial inhabitants. In contrast, a healthy diet and lifestyle predictably confer numerous health benefits on many accounts to reduce lifetime suffering and health care expenditures significantly.

20 ENERGY MATTERS AND ENERGY EXCESS: THE ORDER AND CHAOS OF CHEMICAL REACTIONS AND ENERGY MOVEMENT

Body vehicle biological existence is entirely energy dependent and energy driven. Biological existence involves harvesting and utilizing chemical energies from fuel sources known as food. The energies delivered by foods vary considerably in magnitude. Humanity progressively exists artificially in a chemically engineered world. Understanding some basic chemistry and physics principles governing food energy content and release will highlight the importance of adhering to appropriate nutritional behaviors to fuel the body vehicle system to maximize health and survival.

An appreciation for the dangers existing in using artificially engineered chemicals known as medicines to remedy health disturbances created through improper body vehicle fueling comes from possessing a rudimentary knowledge of basic chemical and physical reactions, particularly which occur between the body vehicle system and any extraneous substances introduced into the body vehicle.

20.1 MATTER

All physical earth substances, including the body vehicle, other earth life-forms, and crude fuel whole earth foods *are composed of matter having a specific mass or quantity that occupies a certain space at any given time.*

All physical matter contains energy, as described by physicist Albert Einstein in the famous equation

$$E = mc^2,$$

where E = energy, m = mass or quantity of substance, and c = speed of light.

Based on Einstein's equation, a 1 g quantity of ordinary earth matter being approximately the size of a small sugar cube contains the energy equivalent of 21.5 kilotons (21,500 tons) of TNT, which is enough to wipe out an entire city the size of Chicago, Illinois, if all the contained energy were somehow released instantaneously. Therefore, the careful pacing of energy release from matter allows energy power to be harnessed controllably for safe utilization.

Energy in physical matter is carried predominantly within oppositely charged positive and negative forces or particles that attract each other and combine in enormous numbers to make up all known earth elements and substances.

Larger, positively charged energy particles are called **protons.** Smaller, negatively charged energy particles are called **electrons.** Electrons are fundamental energy particles in the known universe and serve as the currency of energy transactions in nature.

Oppositely charged particles attract each other while same charge particles repel. Additional large, neutral, uncharged energy particles called **neutrons** combine with protons and electrons to *balance energy forces* among all combined energy particles.

Natural earth elements form when the larger protons and neutrons cluster in equal numbers and firmly secure within nuclear energy cores, while smaller electrons collect in numbers equaling the number of protons and distribute more freely in specific energy cloud domains which surround and are secured in place by these nuclear energy cores. In the universe, electrons seek to exist in pairs within their energy cloud domains surrounding the nuclear cores.

Protons, neutrons, and electrons variously combine in specific numbers to balance positive and negative charges into an equilibrium of electrical neutrality and form basic elemental sets called **atoms** or **atomic elements.** Atomic elements in the known universe exhibit specific chemical properties and physical behaviors according to the number of protons contained in the nuclear energy cores and the number and activity of surrounding electrons.

The number of protons defines the **atomic number** of an element, and the combined number of protons and neutrons designates the **atomic weight** or **mass** of the element. A chart known as the **Periodic Table of the Elements** lists scientifically known chemical elements with their specific combination of protons, neutrons, and electrons according to an increasing number of protons, and ranges from 1 through 118 with elements grouped based on exhibiting similar chemical properties.

Individual atoms aggregate and combine in various numbers and assortments to form larger chemical entities called **molecules.** Atoms and molecules are energy clouds that carry various combinations of oppositely charged proton and electron energy particles and uncharged neutron particles, which unite in the appropriate numbers balancing energy forces into electrical neutrality to form known physical matter.

All earth life-forms, consumable food, and water are entirely made up of energy containing atoms and molecules combined in immense numbers on a massive scale to create readily identifiable physical earth substances and entities. Chemical reactions in the known universe are collisions and interactions occurring between massive numbers of atomic and molecular energy clouds obeying repulsive and attractive, electrical and physical fundamental forces of nature. Therefore, the body vehicle and all other earth life-forms and physical substances are massive multiatomic and multimolecular energy cloud events, concentrated and bound together in space and time into characteristically recognizable forms.

The unique biological nature of individual living earth organisms is essentially a complex material rearrangement and consolidation of elemental earth substance energy clouds guided by fundamental physical principles that universally govern energy movement and distribution. All biologic events that occur in living matter are mega-scale atomic and molecular energy cloud chemical interactions, describable physically using chemical formulas of kinetic reactivity that are governed dependently by time, temperature, electrical charges, and concentrations of chemically interacting entities. The whole living body vehicle energy cloud is held fastened together into its characteristic biologically animated physical shape by energy and some complex binding life force. Within the body vehicle, atoms and molecules acquire energy charges that create attractive or repulsive forces for oppositely charged entities, which on larger scales result in currents of energy flow. Energy flowing in currents results in the chemical reactions and biochemical events that transfer around energy and direct the movement of biological entities within the water mediums of body vehicle cells, tissues, and organs to sustain body vehicle life.

Good health and a long life depend on consistently maintaining favorable atomic and molecular interactions and the proper flow of energy currents within body vehicle cells and working biological structures. Body vehicle membranes are restrictive barriers that line organ structures, separate and compartmentalize fluids and cellular and tissue components, or act as scaffolding and shelves to support working biological elements. Barrier membranes that envelop cells and tissue structures or line the walls of the gut or other hollow organs such as the urinary bladder are composed of atomic and molecular energy clouds that link biochemically to form electrically charged sheets or globular collections, which exert repulsive or attractive forces on passing atoms and molecules.

Collections of specialized molecules embed within barrier membranes in special arrangements to create pores, channels, or gates that serve as access points where various atomic or molecular particles pass through to balance chemical and electrical forces across barrier membrane surfaces. Particles can biologically penetrate through membrane access points by streaming across while propelled by electrical or concentration differences between particles across the membranes, or by being actively transported by structures that physically rearrange shape to carry and transfer particles through the membranes.

The ability of barrier membranes to control and restrict passage of crossing particles is known as **permeability.** Permeability through barrier membranes depends on various factors including membrane integrity, particle size, particle concentrations on either side of membranes, and the strength of interacting repulsive or attractive electrical forces between membrane components and particles passing through.

Compromised barrier membranes become **leaky membranes** that act like sieves incapable of restricting and controlling the passage of membrane crossing biological and chemical entities, including microorganisms and chemical toxins. Additionally, high chemical concentrations of particles existing on either side of a membrane or strong electrical forces operating between particles and barrier membranes can disturb membrane capabilities to regulate the passage of crossing particles. Therefore, chemical and electrical forces guide the movement of life-sustaining atoms and molecules as well as toxic substances within living organisms, and ultimately govern all metabolic processes involving the utilization, transformation, and production of energy in the body vehicle system.

The body vehicle requires food to resupply the atomic and molecular energy clouds that are depleted, utilized, transferred, dissipated, and lost maintaining body vehicle system structure, function, and existence. Excessive ingestion of fast-now calories containing various chemical additives to deliver large concentrations of reactive energy clouds into the gut can exert powerful chemical and electrical forces on gut compartment linings and across cellular membrane surfaces.

Concentrated energy cloud surges across intestinal barrier membranes occurring from any source including foods, chemical toxins, and pharmaceutical agents, may directly cause barrier cell injury or death to disrupt gut membrane integrity and barrier function leading to **leaky gut** conditions. Exposing any cells and tissues throughout the body vehicle to reactive chemicals especially at greater loads predisposes to the development of numerous adverse health consequences.

Scientific investigations that study the permeability of various human barrier membranes demonstrate that chemical substances cross through gut linings into the blood and may possibly penetrate gut and urinary bladder linings directly to leak into the surrounding abdominal or pelvic cavity to produce untoward health effects. Therefore, pharmaceutical products, environmental toxins, and chemical food additives that pass directly down the gut or indirectly gain access to the gut or urinary bladder through blood circulating through the liver or kidneys can potentially leak into the abdominal and pelvic cavities to exert toxic effects locally that compound any systemic toxicities.

20.2 THE MOLE: AVOGADRO'S NUMBER

The individual atoms and molecules that make up visible earth matter including living organisms, food, and other natural earth substances are extraordinarily tiny and combine in astronomical numbers and infinite variations to create identifiable physical earth structures and entities. Even the smallest microscopic sized earth substances are composed of immensely staggering numbers of individual atomic and molecular constituents.

The concept of the **mole** has made quantifying the enormous numbers of contained and interacting constituents of physical matter easier.

The mole, known as Avogadro's number, equals 602 billion trillions and enumerates exceedingly large numbers of objects.

The mole, or 602 billion trillion by definition, is the number of atoms found in precisely 12 g of the chemical element carbon-12.

The number 602 billion trillion (1 mole) happens to be huge when numerically written out as 602,000,000,000,000,000,000,000,000, so the mole is expressed shorthand mathematically as 6.02×10^{23}.

A mole is a unit of measurement that conveniently represents 602 billion trillions of anything, similarly to how a dozen designates 12 of anything. Chemical reactions occurring in the known universe between vast numbers of atoms and molecules are conveyed scientifically in simplified form by expressing only the specific mole amounts of reacting atoms and molecules. For example, H_2O (water) is made by chemically reacting 2 moles of the atomic element hydrogen (H) with 1 mole of the atomic element oxygen (O) forming 1 mole of the aggregate water molecule (H_2O),

$$2H + O = H_2O,$$

which is alternatively expressed in longer form as 2 × 602 billion trillion hydrogen atoms + 1 × 602 billion trillion oxygen atoms = 602 billion trillion water molecules.

The **atomic weight** of basic chemical elements such as hydrogen (H), oxygen (O), nitrogen (N), carbon (C), and sulfur (S), which determines the unique chemical properties for that element, designates the weight in grams of that element containing exactly one mole or 602 billion trillion atoms.

The Periodic Table of the Elements lists scientifically known earth elements sequentially according to increasing atomic weights in grams containing precisely 1 mole (602 billion trillion) of atoms for listed elements. For example, in the Periodic Table, the atomic weights of 1 g of hydrogen, 12 g of carbon, 14 g of nitrogen, 16 g of oxygen, and 32 g of sulfur are all listed in order of increasing atomic weights that equally contain one mole of atoms, with each element displaying completely different chemical properties based on their particular atomic weight.

The **molecular weight** of chemical compounds designates the number of grams of an aggregate compound that contains one mole, or 602 billion trillion molecules of that compound formed by combining various mole amounts of individual atomic elements.

The human body vehicle is estimated to be made up of approximately 4 trillion native individual cells and carry between 10 and 100 trillion bacterial microbial inhabitants, without counting other poorly itemized body vehicle inhabitants such as yeast, fungi, archaea, and viruses.

Native body vehicle cells are biologically grouped and categorized according to various organ systems responsible for executing similarly specialized biologic functions. Organ systems are found either physically confined to fixed locations to make up solid organs and tissues, or are widely dispersed to distribute throughout the body vehicle system.

The brain and other solid organs, such as the liver, heart, lungs, and kidneys, perform more centralized biological functions, while other more diffuse organ systems, such as the nerves, blood vessels, and various blood elements, extensively infiltrate or freely circulate throughout the body vehicle and the solid organs to perform monitoring, delivery, modulatory, or protective roles. For example, the intestines and liver are aggregate cellular structures localized to fixed locations within the abdomen, but also internally contain various blood elements flowing freely throughout along with various nerves and blood vessels that originate from external sources and course through to connect in an elaborate network within these structures.

Each body vehicle cell also carries only a single set of 23 separate pairs of DNA chromosomes (23 chromosomes acquired from each parent), which function as blueprints containing a unique pool of genes that drive all individual body vehicle cellular characteristics, growth, development, reproduction, and survival functions.

Humans are estimated to have 20,000–25,000 working genes actively programming body vehicle existence and working at various times, which incidentally amounts to less than 2% of the entire DNA genetic component of which the other 98% is yet to be fully understood.

DNA chromosomal genes dictate virtually every actual and potential human body vehicle physical and behavioral feature, trait, and action, and contain a coded repertoire of body vehicle susceptibilities and responses to toxic environmental, biologic, or emotional body vehicle insults. Any foreign substances introduced into the body vehicle including foods, pharmaceutical agents, health supplements, and various other chemicals such as food additives or environmental contaminants interact with body vehicle metabolic operations and DNA genetic programming.

Toxic foreign substances delivered into the body vehicle not only affect cellular, biologic and metabolic activities but may also assimilate into body vehicle cellular membranes and react with DNA if not expeditiously detoxified, cleared, and eliminated from the body vehicle system.

All food and other nonfood chemical entities introduced extraneously into the body vehicle, including food additives, environmental contaminants, and pharmaceutical substances such as medicines, health supplements, and vitamins, deliver atoms and molecules in mole percentage quantities.

Typically, nonfood chemical agents of various sorts are taken into the body vehicle in fractional mole quantities of substance while foods are ingested in multiple mole quantities of nutrient atoms and molecules. The potential biologic impact of introducing any foreign material into the body vehicle can be appreciated better by determining the actual number of atoms or molecules delivered into the body vehicle and distributed proportionately to each body vehicle cell.

Usual doses for commonly prescribed medications range approximately between 1 and 1,000 mg (0.001–1 g) by weight. One milligram (1 mg) is roughly the size of a tiny grain of sand and, therefore, requires added chemical fillers to create pharmaceutical vehicles and increase medication size to be appropriate for oral drug administration, whereas 1 g approximates the size of a small sugar cube and more frequently amounts to medication dosages delivered as large pills or oral liquids, or as solutions that are infused directly into a vein through an intravenous line.

The molecular weights of common medications delivering 1 mole or 602 billion trillion molecules range typically between 100 and 1,000 g. Consequently, the approximate mole amounts and the number of molecules of medicinal agent delivered into the body vehicle per usual medication dosages are calculated as follows:

> **Lower range:** 1 mg medicine/1,000 g molecular weight = 0.000001 moles
> *0.000001 moles = 602 thousand trillion molecules of medicine delivered into the body vehicle by this tiny 1 mg dose.*

Since the body vehicle contains approximately 4 trillion cells, this 1 mg medication dose delivers

> 150,000 molecules of medicine to every single body vehicle cell (602 thousand trillion molecules ÷ 4 trillion body vehicle cells)
> **Higher range:** 1,000 mg medicine/100 g molecular weight = 0.01 moles
> *0.01 moles = 6 billion trillion molecules of medicine delivered into the body vehicle by this 1,000 mg (1 g) medication dose, equaling approximately 1.5 billion (1,500,000,000) molecules of medicine delivered to each body vehicle cell (6 billion trillion molecules ÷ 4 trillion body vehicle cells)*

Many medications are commonly introduced into the body vehicle at 0.01 mole (1/100th or 1% of a mole) dose quantities, equaling approximately 1.5 billion molecules of medicine provided to every single body vehicle cell. Unfortunately, there can be no false sense of security or safety for even the smallest doses of medications administered into the body vehicle. Even a tiny 1 microgram (1 mcg) or one-millionth of a gram (0.000001 g) quantity of a medication or chemical taken into the body vehicle, which is invisible to the naked eye and can occupy the sharp point of a very fine pin can still send enormous numbers of molecules to each cell when considered on a mole basis, for example,

1 mcg = 0.000001 g medicine/1,000 g molecular weight = 0.000000001 moles
0.000000001 moles = 602 trillion molecules delivered into the body vehicle, equaling approximately 150 molecules of medicine provided to each body vehicle cell.

These seemingly minuscule quantities of chemical substances pummeling body vehicle cells typically fall within the range found for potently active biological hormones, vitamins, as well as extremely toxic environmental contaminants.

Standard pharmaceutical medication dosing regimens deliver drugs repeatedly on various time schedules to achieve stable **steady state** tissue concentrations or blood levels of chemical agents that produce sustained levels of desired pharmacologic activity, but which also create a continuous exposure of all body vehicle cells to potential drug toxicities. The steady state drug level is the balance point between the introduction of chemical molecules into the body vehicle through various routes, and the removal through protective chemical detoxification, clearance, and elimination pathways. Consequently, the repeated bombardment of all body vehicle cells with foreign substances as during medication dosing regimens or through frequent ingestion of processed foods laced with additives, metabolically stresses the tissues and cells saturated chemically without interruption; which include the liver and kidney organs pressured continuously to filter and clear toxic chemical substances from the body vehicle system.

Introducing a mixture of numerous pharmaceutical agents, vitamins, health supplements, chemical food additives, and environmental toxins simultaneously into the body vehicle, exposes all body vehicle cells to vast numbers and combinations of variously reactive chemical substances, which combine to affect vital body vehicle cellular metabolic functions and genetic DNA expression unpredictably.

Some chemicals introduced into the body vehicle preferentially concentrate within specific cells or tissues to increase the potential for exerting detrimental biological effects. Chemical substances have various binding affinities for body vehicle cellular and tissue elements, which frequently are based on the inherent capacities of the substances to dissolve in oil and water. Additionally, chemical substances may be designed specifically or possess inherent biological properties to enable preferential binding in a kind of lock and key configuration to matching components or receptors of select body vehicle cellular constituents.

The chemical and biological tendencies of substances to gravitate toward, sequester, and concentrate within specific body vehicle cellular and tissue compartments predisposes to unbalanced accumulation and uneven distribution of the substances within the body vehicle system.

The **volume of distribution (VOD)** is a pharmacologic principle that describes the extent to which pharmaceutical and chemical agents introduced into the body vehicle will distribute once absorbed. The VOD for various chemical substances including medications, vitamins, health supplements, food additives, and environmental toxins substantially depends on the oil and water solubility of the chemicals, and on any selective binding and special handling of the substances within specific cellular or tissue compartments.

Volumes of distribution within the body vehicle for various medicinal products or chemical agents can range from as little as a few liters to hundreds of liters. The average volume of the human body vehicle varies approximately between 50 to 100 liters to coincide with the body vehicle mass in kilograms that roughly estimates the body vehicle volume in liters.

The blood volume of an adult is approximately five liters. Therefore, substances having a small 5-liter VOD remain restricted primarily to the blood compartment, while substances with a very high 500-liter VOD disperse throughout the body vehicle to concentrate heavily in specific tissue compartments such as bone, muscle, or fat. Consequently, the potential for toxic biologic effects amplifies dramatically when drugs and chemicals introduced into the body vehicle accumulate preferentially within specific cellular compartments.

Although the previous mole calculations for pharmaceuticals delivered into the body vehicle assume that molecules distribute evenly across and within all body vehicle cells, this is not necessarily the case when molecules collect for various reasons within specific body vehicle compartments. For example, considering the dose calculations for the one mcg of medication evenly distributing 150 molecules of medicine into every single body vehicle cell, if the volume of distribution for that same medicine is high at 500 liters, then the medicine will exert enhanced pharmacologic and potential toxic effects associated with the cellular compartments of preferential accumulation.

Body vehicle cellular growth, development, and function are controlled predominantly by genetic programming coded into the 23 pairs of chromosomes found within each body vehicle cell. Cancer may develop when cellular biological programming behaves aberrantly, and sometimes occurs after only a single gene or a limited number of genes in chromosomal DNA within an individual cell become mutated or biologically disrupted. When millions and billions of foreign chemically reactive atoms and molecules flood every single body vehicle cell repeatedly, the probability of injuring strategic chromosomal DNA genes to induce abnormal cellular behaviors which lead to cancer development or metabolic disturbances that impact health adversely rises precipitously. Therefore, medication dosing considered on a chemical Mole basis points out how even tiny amounts of medicine and other chemical substances infrequently introduced into the body vehicle can cause large-scale disrepair, dysfunction, or injury to vital body vehicle cellular components and biochemical, metabolic processes to result in body vehicle illness, cancer, or death.

An additional caveat within the broad spectrum of potential adverse effects that foreign chemical substances can exert on body vehicle cells involves the unpredictable interaction of foreign substances with the body vehicle immune system of defense. The immune system of defense cells continuously survey, scout, and monitor all elements of the body vehicle for microbial intruders and undesirable foreign substances. Once activated, immune cells aggressively mobilize and biologically recruit additional immune system elements to amplify protective body vehicle immune responses to neutralize identified body vehicle intrusions or threats. Additionally, immune system cells have memory capabilities and learn to remember agents of harm, which then stimulate even greater reactive immune system responses upon subsequent body vehicle exposures. Consequently, even a few harmful molecules may incite tremendous immediate, delayed, or ongoing body vehicle immune responses that can impair body vehicle health and endanger body vehicle survival, as exemplified by the life-threatening immune reactions exhibited by penicillin or peanut allergic individuals and the persistent immune reactivity experienced by the gluten intolerant in modern societies.

While various chemical contaminants and pharmaceutically manufactured products are introduced into the body vehicle as only fractions of mole quantities, food nutrients are often ingested in multiple mole amounts, since consumed food servings weigh many ounces to provide hundreds of grams of nutrients at one time (1 ounce = 28 g). For example, 8 ounces of meat (224 g) + 4 ounces of grains (112 g) + 4 ounces of vegetables (112 g) + 6 ounces of dessert (168 g) = 22 ounces of food (616 g). Despite the total weight of food equaling 616 g, the actual dry weight of nutrient molecules delivered into the body vehicle depends on the state in which foods are consumed.

Processing of solid crude fuel whole earth foods reduces natural water content, thereby concentrating food nutrients to various extents. Crude fuel whole earth foods naturally contain different percentages of water and deliver nutrient and fuel molecules as some proportion of the total food weight.

Approximate natural water and dry nutrient content *by weight* for some general food categories are as follows:

> *Raw fruit and vegetables*: water, 70%–95%; nutrients, 5%–30%
>
> *Raw nuts* (macadamia, cashew, almond, filbert, peanut, hazelnut): water, 1%–7%; nutrients, 93%–99%
>
> *Fresh beans* (kidney, navy, pinto, black, pink, white, fava): water, 10%–13 %; nutrients, 87%–90%
>
> *Dried seeds* (pumpkin, safflower, sesame, chia, flax): water, 4%–6%; nutrients, 94%–96%
>
> *Fresh animal flesh* (chicken, turkey, pork, beef, seafood, fish): water, 50%–75%; nutrients, 25%–50%
>
> Approximate molecular weight (MW) ranges for common nutritional elements that deliver 1 mole, or 602 billion trillion nutrient molecules follow:

simple sugars = MW 180–340 g, contained in grains, fruit, and vegetables (e.g., fructose, glucose, galactose, lactose, sucrose, maltose)

amino acids = MW 75–205 g, comprising proteins in meat, seafood, nuts, and dairy

fatty acids = MW 150–300 g, making up the animal and plant fats (e.g., palmitic, stearic, oleic, linoleic, linolenic)

Full meals estimated to weigh approximately 600 g (21 ounces) and contain 50% water and 50% nutrients by weight provide roughly 300 g of nutrients. Assuming the average molecular weight for the combined food nutrients in the meal to be approximately 300 g, then 300 g of food delivers 1 mole of nutrients or 602 billion trillion nutrient molecules to provide 150 billion trillion nutrient molecules to nourish every single body vehicle cell:

300 g of food ÷ 300 g molecular weight of food = 1 mole of food
(602 billion trillion nutrient molecules (1 mole) ÷ 4 trillion body vehicle cells)

Since nutrient molecules carry energy into cells to power life functions, cells become overloaded with energy when receiving too much energy rapidly to exceed cellular energy utilization capacities, as occurs when processed and refined food products that carry concentrated fast-now fuel nutrients are dumped into the body vehicle in excess.

20.3 THERMODYNAMICS

Human existence and interactions are life energy transactions.

Human biological existence and social interactions are entirely energy dependent and energy driven, making energy transactions central to human life. Powering the entire body vehicle energy cloud to remain alive and function within the known world requires energy to be supplied continually and utilized purposefully by the body vehicle system. Body vehicle diseases such as cancer, autoimmune disorders, and infection divert body vehicle energies away from sustaining routine body vehicle operations.

Earth matter known as food provides the energy source that powers the body vehicle. Energy in food matter must be released and transferred to the body vehicle system for utilization. Fundamental laws of physics govern the chemical reactions that release and transfer energy within biological systems. A simple understanding of some of the underlying physical laws of nature that dictate life energy transactions provides insight into the importance of appropriate body vehicle fueling.

Thermodynamics describes *energy* or *heat* (thermos) *flow* or *movement* (dynamics) in the known universe. Laws of physics state that all energy in the universe is conserved and remains constant by transforming between various forms. The physical laws of nature that govern energy flow specify that concentrated energy spontaneously dissipates to flow downhill from higher and more concentrated energy states to lower and less concentrated energy states to level out energy balances across the energy continuum, whereas additional energy inputs are required to maintain or raise the base energy level of an already energized state.

Batteries losing charge or power over time are one example of concentrated energy stores spontaneously dissipating or losing energy into surrounding lower energy environments. Most can appreciate how stored heat (higher energy) escapes into cold (lower energy) in winter from a warm house through open doors or windows. Additionally, few ever forget that touching live electrical wires storing an energy charge (higher energy) will shock and burn the skin (lower energy) when electrical energy flows downhill from live electrical wires full of energy into lower energy flesh.

The living body vehicle exists in a high energy state continuously requiring and utilizing energy to function as an exceptionally complex working biological system. The body vehicle has to continually reenergize with food to recharge energies lost to drive metabolic operations that power physiologic functions and maintain structural integrity to sustain life, or death occurs if life-sustaining energies drop below a critical threshold level. Thermodynamic laws of nature predict that without continually energizing the life force that cohesively binds the body vehicle physical elements into a characteristically recognizable and biologically functional living state, the highly ordered body vehicle energy cloud would spontaneously dissipate all concentrated energy into a lower energy form, like a plume of dense smoke disperses into thin air, causing body vehicle life to end. Consequently, upon losing the life force preserving the organized body vehicle structure and function, the complex body vehicle system dies and physically disintegrates into elemental dust matter that scatters chaotically back into the universe for recycling.

Energy stored within physical matter can be transferred or converted into other energy states including heat, as illustrated when natural gas or coal burns or nuclear fuels generate electricity to cook food or warm a house, or similarly when the body vehicle biologically metabolizes foods to release stored energy to keep the body vehicle warm and operating correctly. Body vehicle energy utilization is continuous, orderly, and highly regulated, proceeding systematically within tightly integrated metabolic, biochemical reactions that strategically harness, transfer, and interconvert energy supplied by food into various forms necessary to sustain vital body vehicle life functions. Body vehicle metabolic fuel processing also continuously generates heat as a chemical reaction byproduct, which then dissipates into surrounding tissues to maintain the core body vehicle temperature at an optimal homeostatic set-point or radiates out from the body vehicle to be lost externally into the surrounding environment. Consequently, utilized or lost body vehicle energy must be continually replaced by eating food to sufficiently reenergize and sustain vital metabolic, biochemical life reactions and maintain the appropriate body vehicle working temperature.

The fundamental currency of energy flow within living biological systems is the electron charge transferred between atomic and molecular elements of living matter.

The body vehicle is essentially a large conductor of electricity that strategically shuttles around electrons in metabolic processes that progressively expend electron energies to drive body vehicle physical existence and social interactions and internally generate heat energy to live. Food provides the body vehicle with the necessary electrochemical electron energy pulses that power metabolic life processes and keep the body vehicle warm. The body vehicle biochemically unravels and harvests energy from crude fuel whole earth foods by systematically peeling off electrons that ultimately drive ongoing biologic functions.

Sugar, fat, and protein substrate molecules deposited into the fluid matrix of body vehicle cells are biochemically broken down to progressively release electrons that are shuttled in an orderly manner within designated cellular energy powerhouses named **mitochondria,** which then channel the electron energies to generate power to run cellular operations.

Mitochondrial cellular energy powerhouses possess a complex system of folded membranes containing complementarily arranged enzymes that cascade electrons down an **electron transport chain (ETC),** which is an orderly energy gradient that sequentially harnesses and then stores usable electron energies into a carrier molecule named **ATP (adenosine triphosphate). ATP** then distributes the harnessed energy throughout the cell to power various metabolic reactions.

20.4 OXIDATION

Energy extracted from foods to power living biological systems flows tightly regulated within highly integrated metabolic, biochemical, cellular reactions. As noted above, the currency of energy transfer within living biological organisms is the electron, which is the freely mobile negatively charged subatomic particle that is an integral part of all atoms and molecules.

Larger positively charged protons embed deeply within the nuclear energy core of atoms and molecules to be anchored immovably, while smaller negatively charged electrons remain freer circulating within atomic clouds that distribute around and remain held in place by forces emitted from the nuclear core.

Atoms and molecules chemically interact to balance electrical energy forces and dissipate any positive or negative energy surpluses. Loosely held electrons are more easily dislodged and transferred between reacting chemical entities to neutralize existing charge differentials and balance charge quotas among inter-acting elements into an electrochemical equilibrium.

Oxidation refers to the process of transferring electron energies downstream from atoms and molecules possessing relative electron surpluses and higher energy states to atoms and molecules with relative electron deficiencies and lower energy states. Therefore, oxidation is removal of electrons from atoms or molecules that have electrons available to give up or lose. Shifting electron energies from domains of energy surplus to areas of electron deficiency dissipates concentrated energy surpluses while charging up lower energy states, driving downstream energy transfers to continue further along toward the lowest balanced energy state attainable between interacting chemical entities.

The movement of electron energies from higher and more concentrated energy states toward lower energy states releases work energy that runs cellular biochemical reactions and generates heat energy in the process. The *reverse upstream process of acquiring or gaining electrons* to raise base electron energies from relatively lower or less concentrated energy states toward higher or more concentrated energy states is termed **reduction** and requires electron energy infusions that are conveniently provided by complementary oxidation reactions which reciprocally release electron energies for metabolic utilization.

Reduction-oxidation electron transfer reactions between atoms and mole-cules are termed **redox** reactions and form the basis of all life-sustaining metabolic, biochemical reactions that power living biological systems. Biological entities strategically align complementary redox systems in complex energy flow cascades such as the **electron transport chain** in mitochondria to carry out life-sustaining metabolic operations faster and more efficiently. Therefore, within living biological systems, interacting life molecules acquire surpluses or run deficits of electron energies, and then strategically align to drive life-sustaining metabolic, biochem-ical redox reactions purposefully.

Chemically reacting molecules then gain or lose electrons as necessary to redistribute and balance energy forces and power body vehicle life. Cellular chem-ical entities that carry electron surpluses relative to the number of protons are considered negatively charged and have electrons available to share or give away. Cellular entities carrying a deficiency of electrons relative to the number of protons are considered positively charged and have electron deficits that require filling.

Biochemical entities that actively carry negative or positive charge surpluses are called **ions** and will attract and combine with oppositely charged ions to balance overall ionic charges into an electrically neutral equilibrium for the combined interacting entities. Within biochemical reactions involving ions, electrons may be wholly given up and transferred away or only be shared to satisfy individual ion electron energy needs.

The chemical reactions that occur between cellular atomic and molecular energy clouds and induce electron energy flow from higher, electron excess energy states downstream into lower, electron deficient energy states produce work and release heat energy in the energy transfer process. The greater the electron energy differential between entities having electron surpluses and entities with electron deficiencies, the greater the flow of energy and level of oxidation generated during ensuing chemical reactions that balance electron energies.

Electrons flowing downstream to balance electrical forces between reacting cellular entities generate work energy and release heat analogously to how water cascades down a waterfall, over a dam, or onto a waterwheel to create hydropower work energy or heat. The higher the cascade or dam, or the larger the quantity of water falling over the dam, the greater the energy power generated.

Electrons also compose the energy force of electricity that flows within electrical currents to power electrical gadgets and similarly animate biological life. Living, biological organisms obtain electrons to power individual life existences and functions by consuming energy delivering foods and then carefully peeling off electrons to run vital metabolic operations. Too many electrons surging at once through living cells imparts excessive electrochemical energies that overload delicate metabolic circuits and disrupt biologic operations to affect body vehicle function, integrity, and health adversely.

Therefore, the body vehicle uses up electron energies to remain alive and function. Foods are the electron rich **reducing substances** that the body vehicle oxidizes metabolically to supply more electron energies to power body vehicle life.

Fast-now fuels are electron dense and rapidly release excessive electron energies into the body vehicle to cause cataclysmic biochemical oxidation reactions in cells, tissues, and energy storage banks, which essentially overcharge and burn out delicate biological circuit breakers and fuses not gauged to withstand major power surges from massive fuel energy deliveries.

Mitochondria cellular energy powerhouses that may be functionally compromised by toxic food additives, pharmaceutical drugs, and excessive vitamin, herbal, and dietary health supplement effects and are overworked processing excessive fuel energies, may burn out to precipitate cell death when pulsed with additional caloric energy infusions.

Overfueling energy-taxed mitochondria is analogous to striking an older, weather-beaten power station working at maximal capacity with a lightning bolt to blow out overloaded power station circuits with more energy, causing the power station to shut down and cease to function resulting in massive power outages in energy-dependent communities.

Body vehicle cells and tissues damaged by excessive food energy infusions activate inflammatory repair responses that generate further energy surges by cells performing repairs at damage sites, which compound initial degrees of harm induced by infusing too much energy into the body vehicle system. Oxidative stress injuries from overfueling and damages from corrective repairs combine to deteriorate, disintegrate, scar, and shrivel affected tissues, eventually to manifest recognizably as body vehicle disrepair, loss of function, health impairment, aging, and premature death. Consequently, excessive consumption of processed foods made from refined grain flours, oils, butter, margarine, shortening, and sugar, which deliver concentrated, pure sugar and fat energy pulses to body vehicle cells and tissues, overloads and blows out delicate metabolic circuits leading to adverse health consequences. Therefore, highly processed and refined food and beverage products such as soda pop, bread, cake, bowls of pasta, cereal, candy, ice cream, fatty salad dressings, and mayonnaise are energy dense, and pound heavy electron energy loads into the body vehicle to create electron energy surpluses that charge up biochemical circuits and energy stores beyond cellular electron energy handling capacities.

Sizable electron energy infusions that cannot be safely contained, harnessed, and distributed appropriately in a regulated manner disperse freely to rampantly trigger widespread oxidation reactions, which detrimentally scorch and deteriorate susceptible body vehicle constituents exposed to extreme electron energy loads.

Tactical cellular structures such as blood vessels and nerves that vitally sustain other working tissues burn out when encountering excessive deliveries of fuel energy, causing dependent tissue elements to deteriorate faster and exacerbate other overfueling injuries. Oxidation thermodynamics governs body vehicle heat generated by combusting ingested foods and fuel energies held in fat cell energy storage banks. Excessive storage fat as with obesity undergoes continuous metabolic oxidation, generating surplus heat energies that add to the heat insulating effects of fat to overheat the body vehicle and accelerate other oxidative heat-producing biochemical reactions damaging to the body vehicle system. Consequently, an overheated body vehicle activates protective cooling responses such as excessive perspiration to evaporate water vapor from the skin and release high energy water particles that carry heat energy away from the body vehicle. Therefore, excessive cellular oxidation that overheats body vehicle cells and tissues as occurs with obesity and overfueling causes progressive metabolic meltdown of delicate life circuits to harm and deteriorate the body vehicle, compounding other structural and functional damages from the daily wear and tear of transporting around excessive weight, all of which combine to increase the propensity for illness, accelerate aging, and shorten survival.

20.5 ESSENTIAL ELEMENTS OF LIVING MATTER

Known biological life-forms on earth are predominantly composed of six basic chemical elements of matter which are carbon (C), hydrogen (H), nitrogen (N), oxygen (O), phosphorus (P), and sulfur (S). These six atomic elements combine and interact with other chemical elements such as sodium (Na), potassium (K), calcium (Ca), and magnesium (Mg), and trace mineral elements such as iron (Fe), zinc (Zn), copper (Cu), and selenium (Se) to create living biological organisms.

All organic matter by chemical definition contains the basic chemical elements carbon (C) and hydrogen (H).

The various food industry representations of organic conveyed commercially to consumers differ considerably from the actual chemical definition of *organic*. The food industry uses *organic* as a crafted legal term that indicates compliance following a defined set of rules and protocols during the growth, procurement, and processing of certain food commodities. Food industry usage of the term *organic* is often distinct from the chemical definition of *organic,* which broadly applies to all biological life-forms as well as diverse natural and commercially manufactured products such as oil, coal, plastics, rubber, furniture, paper, and innumerable other substances of matter that simultaneously contain the basic chemical elements carbon and hydrogen.

20.5.1 Carbon

Carbon (C) is an abundant earth element that forms the working backbone and fundamental chemical basis of essentially all structural and functional biological components of living matter including sugars, carbohydrates, protein, fat, DNA, and numerous other metabolically operating life molecules.

Physical matter is not organic without carbon. Familiar, carbon-containing compounds other than intact living organisms and plants include crude oil, coal, graphite, and diamonds, which are all produced naturally from high-pressure compression and heating of decayed organic plant and animal matter densely packed underneath many layers of earth dirt for millions of years. Carbon is also found ubiquitously dispersed throughout the earth atmosphere combined with oxygen as **carbon dioxide (CO_2),** produced by oxygen-respiring biological organisms or by combusting organic earth fuels with oxygen.

Plants absorb carbon dioxide (CO_2) from the air and use sunlight and water to release the carbon to reform plant carbohydrates while liberating oxygen back into the earth atmosphere. Carbon is a biological fuel element possessing free electron energies, which can be oxidized readily to power metabolic, biochemical reactions or shared through chemical bonds with other atoms and molecules to create the framework of cellular constituents.

Powerful oxidation reactions occurring in biological systems can disrupt carbon backbones in organic matter to destroy vital biological components. The extreme potency of oxidation reactions that consume organic carbon compounds is apparent when carbon-rich fuels such as crude oil and coal burn with oxygen to generate heat or power mechanical or electrical devices.

Likewise, controlled combustion of carbon-containing biologic fuels such as sugars, carbohydrates, and fats within the body vehicle gradually releases energy to safely power metabolic life functions and warm the body vehicle.

20.5.2 Hydrogen

Hydrogen (H) is the lightest chemical element and contains only one proton in its nuclear energy core and one solitary electron orbiting in a shell surrounding the atomic nucleus and is the most abundant universal element making up 75% of the entire mass of the universe. Hydrogen is readily oxidized to freely donate its lone electron to stronger oxidizing substances such as oxygen or instead can share its single electron to fill electron energy needs of other atoms or molecules such as carbon, which binds hydrogen to create the chemical basis of all organic earth matter. Therefore, both carbon and hydrogen are jointly required to form truly organic matter.

Hydrogen is lighter than air and extremely combustible and was used to float blimps until the *Hindenburg* blimp catastrophically ignited and exploded in a massive oxidation reaction in 1937 known as the *Hindenburg* disaster, killing many passengers on board and ending the use of hydrogen to float blimps. Hydrogen also combines with oxygen to form water as H_2O, which incidentally composes more than 50% of body vehicle volume and covers over 70% of the earth surface.

20.5.3 Nitrogen

Nitrogen (N) is an essential life element that makes up approximately 78% of the earth atmosphere and integrally assimilates within the protein and DNA molecules of all living earth organisms. Within living matter, nitrogen strategically composes part of the linkage arm that helps individual amino acids interconnect to form larger working protein structures and constitutes integral components of DNA genetic codes.

Nitrogen is an electron-rich energy donor that helps drive key metabolic oxidation reactions which maintain biochemical, cellular functioning. Nitrogen-containing biological molecules such as amino acids, proteins, and DNA are metabolically broken down in body vehicle tissues to produce toxic **ammonia (NH3)** that the liver converts into **urea,** which is less toxic and excreted safely from the body vehicle through the kidneys in the urine.

20.5.4 Oxygen

Oxygen (O) is an abundant earth element that exists as a gas comprising approximately 21% of the earth atmosphere and binds hydrogen atoms to form all the water (H_2O) found on earth and within the body vehicle. Oxygen is a potent oxidizing chemical element that easily rips away electron energies from weaker electron donating elements such as carbon, hydrogen, nitrogen, phosphorus, and sulfur to fill its own electron energy needs.

The potent oxidizing property of oxygen conducts strongly attractive forces toward electron-rich chemical elements and allows oxygen to form electrochemical bonds within the various oxygen-containing life molecules such as amino acids, proteins, sugars, carbohydrates, and DNA.

Oxygen is integral to all biological life on earth. The metabolic processing and burning of fuels by the body vehicle to produce work energy and generate heat energy requires oxygen. Body vehicle clearance and elimination of toxins heavily depend on metabolic reactions that utilize oxygen. Body vehicle cellular and tissue injury repair processes involve oxygen dependent biochemical reactions. Repelling and killing foreign microorganisms invading and infecting body vehicle tissues and fluids exploit oxygen-derived by-products as immune system defense weapons. Destroying defective and cancerous type cells produced in the body vehicle during cellular regenerative and reparative processes requires oxygen and oxygen generated by-products.

20.5.5 Phosphorus

Phosphorus (P) is an electron-rich earth element having abundant loosely held electrons that are easily oxidized or chemically shared with other biological life elements. Up to four electron hungry oxygen atoms can simultaneously bind to one phosphorus atom, creating a sphere of electron energy that is transferable between body vehicle molecules to power metabolic reactions that drive physical functioning.

Phosphorus is diversely incorporated into various body vehicle structures including cellular membranes, muscle, bone, teeth, and DNA, and combines with oxygen to form **ATP** (adenosine triphosphate) and **NADP** (nicotinamide adenine dinucleotide phosphate), which are vital energy-carrying molecules that transfer around electron energies necessary to power cellular operations in living organisms.

Phosphates are potent oxidizing chemical substances formed by variously combining phosphorus with oxygen, and are utilized extensively to manufacture soaps, detergents, pesticides, nerve gas, and matches; make phosphoric acid which is added to soda beverages to provide flavor tartness; and formulate food preservatives that kill microbes to extend the shelf life of processed food products. Therefore, chemical phosphates can potently disrupt and destroy living organic matter.

20.5.6 Sulfur

Sulfur (S) contains many freely mobile electrons and is an ambivalent earth element that can function as an electron donor or electron acceptor to work as a vital constituent in numerous body vehicle metabolic reactions. The freely mobile sulfur electrons form the basis of many of the useful chemical properties of sulfur-based compounds.

Sulfur occurs in some vitamins and a few amino acids, within body vehicle biochemical detoxification enzymes, and as a structural component imparting stiffness to hair and feathers, and incidentally produces the characteristic pungent odor of rotten eggs and matches. Sulfur variously binds oxygen to form **sulfates** and **sulfites,** commonly comprising preservatives for processed foods such as dried fruit and beverages particularly wines and forms the basis of strong inorganic acids such as sulfuric acid. Commercial sulfur compounds are potently toxic in minute quantities to delicate organic cellular components.

Sulfites have been implicated in immune response reactivity, causing allergic reactions in hypersensitive individuals and provoking asthma attacks in vulnerable asthmatics. Artificially manufactured polysaccharide-type food additives, such as carrageenan which is used as a processed food thickener and emulsifying agent, incorporate sulfates to accomplish desired chemical food additive effects.

Certain gut bacteria metabolically thrive on sulfur and remove sulfur from foods, and other sulfur-containing molecules delivered down the gut to produce **hydrogen sulfide (H_2S),** which shuttles around electrons in bacterial redox reactions to drive metabolic operations used against the body vehicle or other bacteria.

20.6 OXYGEN FREE RADICALS AND REACTIVE OXYGEN SPECIES

Body vehicle metabolic oxidation-reduction (redox) reactions involving oxygen generate toxic chemical by-products known as **oxygen free radicals** and **reactive oxygen species (ROS).** Free radicals and ROS are atoms or molecules that have unpaired electrons and can remove electrons from or donate the electrons to other chemical entities having electrons available for pairing. Under normal biological circumstances, cellular metabolic operations purposely generate ROS and oxygen free radicals to be used protectively as weapons of defense by immune system cells or to operate as electrochemical currency that drives intricately complex biological reactions involving cellular signaling and homeostasis functions.

Reactive oxygen species (ROS) and oxygen free radicals contain unstable electron energy surpluses and must be carefully managed by body vehicle metabolic cellular processes to maintain a delicate, restrained balance between optimal cellular function and cell death.

Generated oxygen free radicals and ROS are highly chemically reactive with cellular biological constituents, and excesses are scavenged continuously and cleared away through protective body vehicle oxygen free radical scavenging mechanisms.

Maintaining appropriate tissue balances between creation and clearance of toxic oxygen reaction by-products is essential for preserving body vehicle integrity, homeostasis, and health. Excessive cellular and tissue production of highly reactive oxygen free radicals and ROS risks disrupting orderly biochemical reactions and metabolic operations to deteriorate strategic body vehicle biological components, inducing body vehicle dysfunction, illness, premature aging, and possibly death. Alternatively, deficient production, defective function, or excessive clearance or neutralization of body vehicle produced reactive oxygen free radicals, and ROS may shift protective body vehicle oxygen free radical and ROS balances to increase risks for infection, cancer, autoimmune disorders, and death.

Artificially manufactured antioxidants in the form of vitamins or food preservatives ingested in large quantities can excessively and indiscriminately clear and neutralize purposefully generated body vehicle ROS and reactive oxygen free radicals.

20.7 NITROGEN FREE RADICALS

Nitrogen is also amenable to biochemical conversion into more reactive chemical forms. **Nitrogen free radicals** are chemical by-products generated from metabolic redox reactions involving nitrogen. Chemical oxidation reactions occurring between reactive nitrogen molecules, reactive oxygen species (ROS), or oxygen free radicals, and amino acids and proteins which make up native body vehicle cellular and tissue elements or ingested foods can produce reactive nitrogen free radicals that carry excessive electron energies.

Nitrosamines are one category of chemically reactive nitrogen species associated with causing cancer. Nitrosamines are generated chemically in acidic environments such as the stomach through chemical reactions involving nitrogen-containing substances called nitrites. Nitrites are food preservatives commonly added to processed meats such as ham, lunch meats, and hot dogs which give the processed meats a characteristic pink color.

In the acidic environment of the stomach, nitrites react with the protein nitrogen of the processed meats or stomach lining to form nitrosamines. Generated nitrosamines then react with DNA material of gut barrier lining cells to produce genetic mutations leading to cancer development. Additionally, increased body vehicle generation of ROS and excessive dietary consumption of nitrogen-rich, protein-containing foods may likewise lead to harmful nitrogen reactions within the body vehicle that alter strategic structural, functional, or genetic body vehicle constituents to compromise health.

Chemically reactive nitrogen free radicals are also neutralized and cleared through body vehicle free radical scavenging mechanisms, which protect against aberrant chemical interactions between high energy nitrogen free radicals and metabolically vulnerable lower energy cellular biomolecules. Therefore, consuming processed food products that contain chemical additives and deliver excessive energy loads in the form of highly refined sugars, fats, carbohydrates, and proteins risks generating reactive chemical substances that metabolically damage the body vehicle to cause illness, premature aging, and shortening of life-span.

20.8 EXCESS

Excessive fueling chemically harms the body vehicle to cause adverse health consequences in numerous ways.

Overfueling the body vehicle floods cellular energy stores with high energy sugar, fat, and protein molecules to produce metabolic disturbances and dangerously reactive chemical by-products, which destabilize body vehicle homeostasis to challenge body vehicle function and viability. Consuming excessive sugar and fat fuels that carry excessive electron energies to donate greatly augments the body vehicle burden of chemically reactive substances including reactive oxygen species (ROS).

Mitochondrial cellular energy powerhouses produce more oxygen free radicals and ROS harmful to internal cellular environments when overloaded with excessive dietary sugar and fat energies. Overindulging on calorie-rich fast-now food products especially if already experiencing diabetes or cholesterol disorders, markedly elevates blood and tissue sugar and fat levels which can react with ambient oxygen to generate toxic free radical by-products injurious to cells.

ROS deliberately produced by the body vehicle to maintain cellular homeostasis may also react with excessively ingested sugar and fat to generate ROS surpluses damaging to cells. Sugar and fat energies heavily concentrated within overfueled body vehicle cells can undergo **autoreactive redox chemical chain reactions** that uncontrollably produce chemically reactive products destructive to cellular constituents. For example, excessive lipid fat stored in body vehicle fat cells can enter self-sustaining redox chemical chain reactions termed **lipid peroxidation** [lipid(fat) per("petual") oxidation], which produces large quantities of ROS and other oxidation reaction by-products that can overwhelm protective removal by neutralizing cellular ROS scavengers and predispose to cellular harm.

Similarly, large gut loads of ingested fat undergoing digestion can also spontaneously undergo lipid peroxidation chain reactions to produce excessive ROS that break down gut linings to weaken protective barriers and create a leaky gut unable to contain toxins and dangerous microorganisms from migrating through to blood. Additionally, overfueling the body vehicle considerably beyond energy utilization capacities leads to excessive production of toxic metabolic and oxidation by-products that can escape body vehicle detoxification and clearance mechanisms to damage cells.

High levels of reactive sugar and fat nutrients and oxidation reaction chemical by-products continuously bathing cells and tissues may chemically degrade cellular biomolecules to undermine the structure and function of vital body vehicle components. Excessive oxidation stresses prematurely age the body vehicle and increase the probability for cancer development.

ROS scavenging by the immune system of defense cells reduces with aging to lower protection against ROS generated through environmental, chemical, and dietary factors, raising the likelihood for detrimental tissue oxidation to occur at lower levels of ROS.

Diets limited to processed and refined sugar, fat, and protein products may favor the growth of less desirable gut microorganisms that can adapt and survive on restricted nutrients, while less adaptable gut microorganisms that may optimally maintain body vehicle health and gut function and feed on diversified nutrients provided through natural crude fuel whole earth foods may starve when deprived of nutrient varieties.

Large sugar or fat caloric energy loads regularly delivered down the gut may alter gut microbe communities or their metabolic activities to drive nutrient fermentation into producing alcohol, which then becomes absorbed into blood predisposing to alcohol type liver damage. Therefore, processed and refined food and beverage products deliver heavy payloads of energy-dense chemically reactive simple sugars, fats, and proteins, which unpredictably modify gut microorganisms and overwhelm body vehicle metabolic capabilities and protective clearance mechanisms to deleteriously react with and oxidize intestinal membranes, blood vessel structures, and cells vulnerably exposed to these concentrated nutrient deposits. Eventually, all accumulated body vehicle injuries including from overfueling combine with body vehicle repair processes compounding original injury effects to predispose to body vehicle dysfunction, illness, cancer, accelerated aging, and premature death.

In contrast, natural, unprocessed crude fuel whole earth foods that sparsely distribute nutrient sugars, fat, and proteins deeply embedded within complex substantially water-based matrices require extensive digestive work to dismantle; slowing nutrient gut transit, digestive break down, and blood absorption to safely synchronize nutrient deliveries with cellular fuel energy metabolic and utilization capacities to lower production of chemically reactive oxidation by-products.

20.9 OIL AND WATER

Many toxic chemical substances termed **carcinogens** that are known or suspected to cause cancer are industrially synthesized and manufactured organic compounds (contain both carbon and hydrogen) that dissolve more readily in oil as opposed to water.

Fat is essentially a solidified form of oil. Except for seeds and nuts, plants are predominantly composed of water and quantitatively contain negligible or limited fat stores compared to the amounts of fat proportionately found in animals. Since animals carry substantially more fat than plants carry, animals can correspondingly store more fat-soluble cancer-causing chemical substances within their fat-containing cells and tissues.

Fats contained in animal tissues and cells are also in a state of dynamic chemical and biological flux continuously being added, removed, or exchanged based on cellular metabolic needs, whereas fats composing nuts and seeds remain relatively static chemically until seeds begin to germinate into plants. Therefore, plant seed and nut fats remain relatively stable and more resistant to accumulating fat-soluble toxins.

Animal source food products deliver proportionately larger payloads of fat-soluble cancer-causing substances carried within fatty components, which upon ingestion into the body vehicle redistribute into body vehicle fat stores to become ticking time bombs that raise lifetime risks for developing body vehicle cancer. Therefore, possessing overly abundant body vehicle fat stores not only causes oxidative toxicities leading to more body vehicle inflammatory responses but also heightens lifetime cancer risks by increasing the cumulative body vehicle burden of cancer-causing toxins that become stored in body vehicle fat.

Consequently, processed and refined food products delivering excessive nutrient and caloric fuel energy payloads impair health and shorten life-span through numerous mechanisms, including by causing obesity with all its attendant consequences, by creating metabolic toxicities that damage vital cellular elements, by promoting inflammatory responses, and by increasing lifetime risks for cancer development.

20.10 ABDOMINAL VISCERAL FAT OR "BELLY FAT"

Belly fat is a body vehicle stress and heater organ.

Abdominal visceral fat termed **belly fat** is a highly, metabolically active body vehicle organ system. Visceral fat may function as an *adaptive primordial survival organ* that supplies other vital organs with immediate fuel energies during stress and fight or flight survival threats and, additionally, burns fat energy to maintain an appropriate body vehicle core working temperature, particularly within dangerously cold environments.

The dense fat energy stores and high metabolic activity within belly fat increase the propensity for generating excessive oxygen free radical oxidation by-products and ROS as well as inflammatory chemical mediators.

Excessive belly fat with abdominal obesity increases risks for illness and premature death. Reactive inflammatory chemical mediators produced within visceral fat are capable of precipitating cardiovascular events such as heart attacks and strokes or triggering immune dysfunction to increase risks for developing an infection or autoimmune disorder. Inflammation, immune dysfunction, and infection additionally predispose the body vehicle to the development and progression of cancer. Therefore, obesity and excessive visceral fat stores disturb immune function and effectiveness while promoting body vehicle inflammation and ROS generation, which compromise body vehicle health and survival.

Fueling the body vehicle excessively to increasingly expand a metabolically active abdominal visceral organ already packed with concentrated fuels, dissolved toxins, and reactive biological mediators disrupts homeostasis even further to escalate risks for illnesses that threaten body vehicle existence. Excessively stored electron energies in belly fat in effect cook the body vehicle system from the inside to progressively deteriorate health and accelerate body vehicle demise. Consequently, humanity has fewer worries about going extinct from heating up the planet to cause disastrous climate change, than about disappearing from the face of the earth due to suffering deadly consequences from obesity pandemics in modernizing societies, which burn humans from the inside to cause death from overfueled metabolic heater organs working overtime.

Waist circumference provides an indirect measure of abdominal visceral fat. Waist circumference is measured above the hip bone at the level of the naval after exhaling, preferably while fasting on an empty stomach and after urine and stool elimination. Various definitions exist for abdominal obesity or excessive belly fat according to the scientific institutions assessing risks for associated health disorders.

The American Heart Association and National Heart, Lung, and Blood Institutes define abdominal obesity as a waist circumference for males greater than 102 cm (40 inches), and for females greater than 88 cm (35 inches). The International Diabetes Foundation defines abdominal obesity as a waist circumference for males greater than 90 cm (35.5 in) and for females greater than 80 cm (31.5 in), with cutoffs for maximal waist circumferences modified accordingly for various ethnic groups. The World Health Organization defines abdominal obesity using waist-to-hip measurement ratios as being for males greater than 0.9 and females greater than 0.85.

A protruding abdomen that interferes with the ability to see the toes when standing erect and looking straight downward toward the feet infers the presence of excessive belly fat.

Excessive belly fat reduces health and longevity.

The risks of developing diabetes and cardiovascular events more than double by having abdominal obesity even for an acceptable body mass index (BMI). When waist circumference measurements combine with body mass index (BMI) calculations, predictions for suffering various metabolically related health disorders such as diabetes, cholesterol elevations, hypertension, fatty liver, heart attacks, strokes or premature death become more reliable and certain. As for other health risk factors, as abdominal obesity combines with rising BMI levels, illness and death risks multiply. Consequently, illness and death risks increase as the BMI rises for specific waist circumferences or the waist circumference expands for certain BMI levels. Therefore, lose excess belly fat to improve health and longevity.

In addition to eliminating the intake of excessive and unhealthy fuel calories and increasing physical activity, another potential strategy to get the belly fat organ working to burn excessively stored fat calories is to make the ambient room temperature chilly to stimulate the body vehicle heater organ function. Chronic illnesses and aging reflect the accumulated burden and fallout of all body vehicle cellular and tissue injuries and repairs, toxicities and detoxifications, and magnitude of fuel burning, storage, and reactivity experienced over time.

The cumulative consequences of many years of excessive body vehicle energy deliveries and oxidative metabolism resulting in repetitive metabolic damages and reparative responses, visibly manifest as costly body vehicle dysfunction with progressively deteriorating health and accelerated aging. The prospects for health, youthfulness, and a more prolonged survival increase by reducing body vehicle fat stores and avoiding excessive intake of concentrated high potency calories and fat to decrease oxidative body vehicle toxicities.

Shrink body vehicle fat, stay lean, look better, and live healthier longer.

Regularly fueling only sufficiently to power the body vehicle and utilize fuel energies promptly maximizes longevity. Pacing body vehicle fueling to equal fuel energy demands and utilization capacities minimizes activating metabolic oxidation reactions that generate toxic chemically reactive oxidation by-products; and reduces the need for the body vehicle to store and accumulate reactive fuels to produce obesity and predispose to cancer and other health problems.

Eating a crude fuel natural whole earth food diet with slow-later fuels that require extensive digestive processing before blood absorption better paces body vehicle fueling to allow intestinal caloric deliveries to meet cellular energy needs more safely and efficiently, whereas dumping excessive reactive fast-now fuel energy loads into the gut to race calories into the bloodstream creates oxidative stresses when fuel energy deliveries exceed biologic capacities for timely metabolic fuel processing and assimilation. Therefore, all aspects of the body vehicle including the gut benefit and thrive when efficiently and appropriately nourished and put to work.

Consumption of highly processed and refined food products reduces opportunities for the entire length of the gut to participate in digestive work to extract vital food nutrients that sustain gut membrane and microbiome integrity and allow the body vehicle system to thrive. Daily body vehicle energy demands depend on body vehicle size, age, state of health, and intensity and duration of physical and mental activities.

The number of energy calories delivered down the gut and passing into blood per unit of time impact nutritional health. Advertised low-calorie processed food products can still deliver calorically dense fast-now fuel energy calories into the gut that quickly access the blood.

Three hundred fast-now fuel energy calories dumped down the gut to pass immediately into the blood, metabolically shocks the body vehicle system with excessive fuel energies that dramatically exceed usual immediate fuel energy demands, whereas passing 500 slow-later fuel calories gradually down the gut to seep into the blood slowly over 5 or 6 hours metabolically suits typical physiologic body vehicle energy needs approximating 70–100 calories per hour.

Eating like a snake to predominantly consume natural crude fuel whole earth foods that "stick to the gut" and remain longer within the gut temporary fuel holding tank compartment to digest slowly before energy calories pass through to blood, better matches fuel consumption with body vehicle fuel energy utilization.

20.11 ANTIOXIDANTS

Antioxidants are the cleanup crew chemical scavengers that neutralize the excessive free electron energies of oxygen and nitrogen free radicals, reactive oxygen species (ROS), and other oxidation reaction by-products, which otherwise can indiscriminately react with vital cellular biomolecules. Antioxidant sources include: some of the vitamins found naturally in crude fuel whole earth foods such as fruit, vegetables, nuts, seeds, beans, legumes, and animal flesh, or produced internally by residing body vehicle microbiota; metabolic constituents generated through body vehicle biochemical, cellular reactions; and agents synthesized artificially using industrial chemical processes.

A vast commercial market exists for synthetic antioxidants. Industrially manufactured antioxidants are added routinely to various commercial products including processed and refined food and beverage products and organic hydrocarbon compounds such as plastics to slow product spoilage and deterioration and prolong shelf life for eventual product sale and consumption.

Relatively large quantities of artificially produced antioxidants are commonly delivered into the body vehicle either intentionally or unknowingly from various sources. Familiar sources of synthetic antioxidants ingested deliberately into the body vehicle are the commercial vitamin and health supplements, and vitamin-fortified processed food and beverage products.

Antioxidants inadvertently introduced into the body vehicle include processed food and beverage product preservatives, and container vessel chemical stabilizers that migrate into food and beverage products during storage to be ingested unsuspectingly along with container-stored foods and beverages.

Excessive intake of antioxidants into the body vehicle may saturate tissues and cells and predispose to indiscriminate clearance of cellular oxygen free radicals and ROS, some of which may have been purposely generated to work strategically in various metabolic and protective cellular roles. Unnatural saturation of body vehicle tissues and cells with antioxidants unpredictably disturbs delicate homeostatic balances of metabolic redox reactions that biochemically carry out complex health and survival operations. For example, ROS are produced intentionally by the body vehicle immune system of defense cells to work protectively in numerous immune-mediated biochemical reactions, which destroy aberrantly developing cancer type cells or neutralize foreign or invading pathologic microorganisms attempting to infect the body vehicle system. These purposefully generated ROS immune system of defense weapons may themselves become neutralized and cleared away by antioxidants.

Antioxidants saturating body vehicle tissues and cells may interfere with the activity of these strategically generated ROS weapons of defense to compromise immune system operations and shift immune balances to increase susceptibility for developing cancer, infection, and autoimmune diseases. Additionally, body vehicle cells purposefully produce electron charged ROS to work as metabolic triggers and switches, which activate or suppress the function of critical enzyme chains that align in orderly cascades to carry out numerous complex life-sustaining biochemical actions.

Hindering the production or activity of biologically generated ROS with anti-oxidants may, therefore, hamper crucial enzyme systems from executing vital biologic roles within the body vehicle system. No guarantees exist that saturating the body vehicle with antioxidants will restrict antioxidant effects exclusively to neutralize and clear out only the harmful oxidation by-products. Consequently, artificial saturation of body vehicle tissues and cells with antioxidants can interfere unpredictably with native metabolic processes and cellular functions to disrupt the homeostatic operations and balances required for maintaining cellular integrity and health.

20.12 VITAMINS

Vitamins are vital micronutrients that assist strategic body vehicle life-sustaining metabolic operations involving cellular development, function, growth, and energy utilization. Vitamins are essential cofactors that work as catalysts to increase the speed and efficiency of body vehicle biochemical reactions and are required in very minute quantities since vitamin molecules are repeatedly reutilized to activate numerous metabolic cellular reactions.

Human cells are incapable of manufacturing vitamins, which consequently must be externally supplied through the diet or internally produced by resident indwelling body vehicle microbiota. Therefore, plant and animal crude fuel whole earth foods and residing body vehicle microbial organisms are the principal natural sources that supply vitamins required to keep the body vehicle system operating correctly.

The vital nutrient content of food diminishes with cooking time, extended food storage, and environmental or microbial food decomposition, and eating foods raw and when fresh preserves a higher content of vital nutrients.

Some of the many vital roles served by vitamins in the body vehicle system include

1. assisting metabolic, biochemical reactions in breaking down, processing, and utilizing nutrient fuels efficiently to energize body vehicle operations
2. facilitating chemical detoxification processes
3. functioning as antioxidants to scavenge excess reactive oxygen species and oxidation reaction by-products generated through assorted body vehicle metabolic processes

4. possessing hormone-like properties to perform actions ensuring the proper assimilation of nutrients to maintain appropriate cellular and tissue development, function, and growth
5. helping body vehicle cells synthesize biologically active constituents essential for cellular immunity, inflammatory responses, tissue repair, and fighting cancer

There are *13 vitamins* essential for proper body vehicle function that are grouped according to chemical ability to dissolve in oil or water.

Fat-soluble vitamins A, D, E, and K dissolve only in oil or fat.

Water-soluble vitamin C and eight B vitamins dissolve only in water.

The entire human body vehicle is composed of oil (fat) and water compartments, which intimately intermingle but distinctly separate to carry out designated life functions without mixing as sugar dissolves and mixes into the water.

Vitamins distribute within body vehicle compartments based on their oil or water solubilities and then essentially remain within those compartments to perform vital biologic roles. A little bit of vitamin goes a very long way since individual vitamin molecules are catalysts which work in multiple biochemical reactions to accomplish cellular duties repeatedly until being chemically dismantled or eliminated from the body vehicle system. The catalyst functions of vitamins are analogous to the roles played by a few stadium ushers that seat and monitor entire stadiums of spectators or the strategic utility provided by a small number of tools used for various construction projects.

Natural crude fuel whole earth foods are the ideal source of vitamins for the body vehicle system. Serving sizes of fruits, vegetables, nuts, seeds, legumes, beans, whole grains, dairy products, eggs, and animal flesh naturally supply significant portions of total daily body vehicle vitamin needs. Gut microorganisms that also feed on ingested crude fuel whole earth foods additionally manufacture certain vitamins to satisfy body vehicle needs.

The slow digestion of natural crude fuel whole earth foods in the gut paces the release and delivery of essential vitamins and other micronutrients to suit body vehicle physiologic and metabolic needs more optimally. Therefore, the best ways to deliver vitamin C are through kiwis, strawberries, and oranges; omega-3 fatty acids through fish, nuts, and seeds; B vitamins through leafy green vegetables and fruit; and calcium through kale, milk, and dairy products.

Fat-soluble vitamins absorb better from the gut when dissolved in dietary fat as with meals. Following gut absorption, fat-soluble vitamins distribute throughout the body vehicle to concentrate within fatty membranes and tissues and fat cells, making fat-soluble vitamins more prone to accumulate excessively within fatty compartments and predispose to vitamin toxicities. Water-soluble vitamins absorb from the gut to dissolve into cellular water compartments or circulate freely in blood to filter continuously through the kidneys for urinary excretion and, consequently, require dietary replenishment daily to keep up with ongoing body vehicle elimination and losses.

20.13 COMMERCIAL-GRADE VITAMIN AND HEALTH SUPPLEMENTS

U.S. government health agencies devised specific guidelines outlining the recommended average daily intake of essential nutrients such as vitamins to *adequately or sufficiently satisfy the essential nutrient needs for 98% of the healthy general U.S. population.* The **Dietary Reference Intakes (DRI)** document provides essential nutrient intake guidelines and includes the **Recommended Dietary Allowance (RDA)** that specifies average daily requirements for well-studied micronutrients, and the **Adequate Intake (AI)** that advises daily intake for micronutrients having insufficient scientific data to establish an RDA.

Governmental recommendations for vitamin and other micronutrient requirements derive from scientific studies that study relationships between various vitamin and micronutrient levels in humans and the probabilities for humans to experience normal or impaired health and development.

Huge markets exist to sell artificially produced vitamins and health supplements by industries that intentionally skew the consumer perception of healthy behaviors to generate enormous commercial profits. Industry advances the all too familiar rationale that supplementation completely satisfies daily body vehicle vital micronutrient needs inadequately met through usual nutritional choices and dietary routines to promote the widespread use of vitamin and health supplements.

RDA "satisfies daily essential micronutrient needs for 98% of the general U.S. population."

Therefore, "supplementing" daily nutritional sustenance with the standard commercially available high potency vitamin supplements that provide and often exceed 100% of the RDA for *all* vital micronutrients contradicts healthy nutritional wisdom.

The irrationality of excessive vitamin supplementation is highlighted by considering the medical principles that guide the restoration of health during treatment of specific health disorders. For example, the goals of pharmacologic treatment of mildly elevated blood pressure or an underactive thyroid under routine circumstances are to reestablish a healthy balance to normal blood pressure and normal blood thyroid hormone levels. Consequently, aggressive medical regimens that markedly lower blood pressure below physiologic needs or raise thyroid hormone levels far above normal lose health benefits and potentially jeopardize body vehicle survival.

Similarly, vitamin supplementation that substantially exceeds the scientifically estimated RDA or AI for body vehicle needs risks affecting body vehicle health and survival adversely. Additionally, if artificial supplementation of essential vitamins and other micronutrients is necessary to meet nutritional health needs, then dietary choices inadequately provide real nutritional value.

Since industrial food processing strips away nutritional value including vitamins and minerals from crude fuel whole earth foods, manufactured food products are routinely artificially **enriched** or **fortified** to replace some of the micronutrients lost or removed during food processing. If certain foods fail to supply body vehicle micronutrient needs naturally, then why eat those foods, and why not alter dietary choices to satisfy micronutrient requirements appropriately naturally?

Alternatively, if dietary choices are healthy and naturally supply the essential micronutrient needs fully, then why supplement nutrients artificially especially in amounts far exceeding the RDA or AI? Additionally, if most essential micronutrient requirements are met adequately through a proper diet, then no sound health rationale exists to justify artificially supplementing *all* essential micronutrients daily at or above the maximum RDA.

The obvious nutritional maneuver to execute when diets fail to satisfy essential vitamin and mineral needs naturally is to improve the diet to supply body vehicle micronutrient requirements correctly, and not resort to taking commercial supplements to compensate for a nutritionally deficient diet. When a healthy diet meets essential nutrient requirements, then additional nutritional supplements create micronutrient excesses that may toxify the body vehicle system.

Nature fails to set a precedent and supply natural food sources or nutrient systems that behave like **nutrient bombs,** which chemically discharge to rapidly release mega doses of an individual or multiple vitamins and minerals crammed into a single shipment entity devoid of any complementary nutritional value. Therefore, artificially manufactured commercial-grade vitamins and health supplements act like **chemical grenades,** which blast out high concentrations of artificially made active nutrient and inactive filler ingredients that behave like biological shrapnel to deleteriously pierce and saturate body vehicle system membranes and cellular compartments upon ingestion.

The body vehicle carefully regulates the absorption and utilization of vitamins according to metabolic needs. A nutritionally well-stocked body vehicle may biologically limit additional micronutrient assimilation. Consequently, commercial-grade vitamin and health supplements taken in amounts far exceeding immediate body vehicle needs provide no additional biological benefits and go unutilized to be eliminated from the body vehicle or stored within tissue compartments to accumulate and possibly exert harmful biochemical effects.

Protective body vehicle mechanisms divert and stockpile large surpluses of vitamin, mineral, or other essential nutrient payloads that flood the body vehicle system in quantities greatly exceeding immediate biological needs into tissue storage compartments, or pressure the liver and kidney filtering organs to clear and eliminate nutrient excesses into the stool and urine to reduce the potential for body vehicle toxicities.

Micronutrient surpluses shuttled into body vehicle storage compartments may gradually migrate out to distribute throughout the body vehicle and exert delayed toxicities, or minimally produce expensive urine and stool when protectively dumped out of the body vehicle. Therefore, **Naturalists** attempting to optimize personal health by ingesting commercially manufactured pills, which routinely deliver essential micronutrients in quantities greatly exceeding body vehicle biological needs and utilization capacities, are **artificialists** who more likely are physiologically stressing and toxifying the body vehicle than obtaining health benefits through artificial supplementation.

The vast spectrum of biological activities for many essential vitamins and other micronutrients and the entire expanse of health benefits or risks derived from artificial micronutrient supplementation are incompletely understood and frequently unknown. On the other hand, numerous body vehicle toxicities that occur through excessive intake of various vitamins and nutrients are well characterized and described in medical literature sources easily accessed online through internet search engines. Consequently, commercial industries promote and sell artificially manufactured vitamins and health supplements to fulfill the Recommended Dietary Allowance (RDA), enhance health in obtuse ways, or vaguely meet consumer health expectations.

Under more profitable commercial settings, frequent testing of blood or body fluids combines with micronutrient supplementation to achieve and maintain micronutrient levels within desirable reference ranges established for tested human populations, as commonly occurs when vitamin D supplementation is monitored by repeatedly measuring blood vitamin D levels.

One crucial variable that affects the disposition and utilization of ingested vitamins and other health supplements in unknown ways is the vast gut microbiota that is also shaped by the gut micronutrient environment. Scientific studies on the impact of micronutrient supplementation on the gut microbiota, which functions as a metabolic machine to interact intimately with body vehicle nutrition, biologic operations, and nutritional behaviors, are only in the very early stages.

20.14 SALTS, MINERALS, AND ELECTROLYTES

Salts and minerals are vital chemical elements that serve strategic functional and structural roles within the molecular framework of biological fluids, enzymes, and cellular membranes. Common salts and minerals that the body vehicle utilizes in bulk or trace quantities include sodium (Na), potassium (K), chlorine (Cl), calcium (Ca), phosphorus (P), magnesium (Mg), iron (Fe), selenium (Se), chromium (Cr), zinc (Zn), copper (Cu), iodine (I), manganese (Mn), and nickel (Ni). Calcium and phosphorus comprise 2–3 % of the body vehicle mass mainly composing the bones and teeth, and activate cellular metabolic processes, while sodium, potassium, and chlorine constitute less than 1% of body vehicle mass and help to maintain the shape, fluid balance, and electrical properties of body vehicle cellular compartments.

For many of these essential chemical elements, apart from scientific measurements that quantitate their body vehicle content and descriptions of their mechanistic involvement identified within specific cellular enzymes and metabolic processes, there is insufficient experimental data to define the entire scope and importance of their body vehicle actions.

Salts and minerals dissolve within body vehicle cellular water compartments and acquire surpluses or deficiencies of electron energies to activate into charged ions called **electrolytes.** Charged electrolytes attract and associate with oppositely charged ionic salts, minerals, and other cellular biomolecules to balance electrical forces for the combined ionic aggregates and carry out biochemical operations.

Salts, minerals, and their charged electrolytes ultimately provide much of the electron energy currents that drive biochemical reactions within biological systems, or they may act strategically as docking stations within vital enzymes and molecules that transport essential life elements such as oxygen. For example, the mineral iron is a potent redox agent that carries around and transfers electrons in various cellular metabolic and detoxification reactions, and vitally composes the oxygen docking station within circulating red blood cells that distribute oxygen to all body vehicle cells.

The body vehicle circulates a particular carrier protein in the blood that picks up and shuttles around the iron for distribution to various cells for metabolic utilization and maintains another vital protein within cells to protectively store iron and reduce the potential for iron to cause oxidative cellular injuries. Because of the critical role that iron plays in body vehicle homeostasis, the body vehicle tightly regulates iron absorption by intestinal cells based on body vehicle iron needs.

Additionally, gut bacteria utilize iron functionally for growth and in metabolic processes directed against other gut bacteria or body vehicle intestinal cells, and, consequently, gut cells protectively compete against bacteria to absorb and utilize free iron passing down the intestines. Therefore, excessive iron ingested through mineral supplements and iron-fortified foods, which the body vehicle cannot use when iron stores are well stocked, passes unabsorbed down the gut to undesirably promote the growth of gut bacteria that may compromise body vehicle health.

Natural crude fuel whole earth foods contain only trace quantities of sparsely dispersed salt and mineral elements such as sodium, potassium, calcium, magnesium, phosphorus, sulfur, iron, copper, zinc, and selenium, with actual levels determined by soil, water, and other environmental factors existing where foods are grown and cultivated. The trace salts and mineral elements within natural crude fuel whole earth foods embed within the complex fuel and water matrices that require substantial work energy to release the vital micronutrient elements for body vehicle utilization.

Factors that affect the availability and release of salt and mineral elements from foods include food ripeness; food preparation and cooking methods; food combinations consumed; eating technique including thoroughness of chewing; fluid type and quantity ingested during meals; digestive gut work; and activity of gut microbial organisms that aid digestion and also feed on nutrients in the gut.

The body vehicle system stringently balances salt, mineral, and water levels to maintain appropriate body vehicle concentrations necessary for homeostasis and metabolic operations. The body vehicle meticulously manages the absorption of salts, minerals, and water from the gut to fulfill body vehicle biological needs. Providing the body vehicle with excessive dietary salts and minerals such as described above for iron may pass unabsorbed nutrient portions down the gut into feces to exert untoward effects on gut microbial activities predisposing to adverse body vehicle health consequences.

Body vehicle requirements for various salts and mineral elements are better met physiologically by ingesting natural crude fuel whole earth foods since artificially processed food products contain artificially added salts and minerals in quantities and concentrations that significantly exceed those found in natural foods or are required for immediate body vehicle needs. The body vehicle employs various homeostatic mechanisms to regulate blood levels of circulating salts and trace mineral elements. The absorption and elimination of micronutrients are controlled predominantly by the gut and kidneys. The kidneys strategically maintain body vehicle salt and mineral concentrations within narrow exacting ranges. The kidneys detect any salt and mineral deficiencies or surpluses in blood continuously filtering through, and then avidly reabsorb or vigorously excrete filtered salts and minerals as necessary to correct identified imbalances. Additionally, the skin sweats out, and gut membranes secrete certain salts or water to affect body vehicle salt and water balances.

Processed and refined food products, artificial health and dietary supplements, and pharmaceutical agents are not only artificially laced with toxic chemical additives, fillers, and preservatives, but are commonly loaded with sugar, salt, and mineral elements to stabilize product formulations and enhance taste experiences.

Concentrated chemicals and salt and mineral elements from processed foods and beverages biologically force their way through gut membranes into the blood to saturate body vehicle fluids, tissues, and cells, and tax homeostatic countering responses that must protectively filter out and clear substance excesses through urine and feces.

Excessive dietary ingestion of salts such as sodium chloride, which distributes throughout the body vehicle, pulls water into cellular and tissue compartments that accumulate the salts to cause fluid retention and swelling that stresses blood flow dynamics and predisposes to high blood pressure conditions such as **hypertension.**

Minerals and salts commonly enter and exit body vehicle cells through cellular membrane transporters, which often co-transport other salts, minerals, sugars, or water in the same or opposite directions to strategically balance the movement of various elements across membranes to maintain cellular homeostasis.

Processed and refined food products that are laden with readily available salts and concentrated fuel energies and are fortified excessively with vitamins and minerals deliver large payloads of micronutrients that saturate membrane transporters and unbalance internal cellular microenvironments, leading to cellular distress that provokes compensatory cellular survival and recovery responses. Cells experiencing excessive flux of reactive micronutrients across membrane surfaces may dangerously swell or shrivel following micronutrient accumulation or depletion to disturb cellular homeostasis and body vehicle health.

20.15 TAXI SERVICE

Manufactured or artificially prepared chemical substances that are biologically active such as medicines and herbal, mineral, and vitamin dietary health supplements require pharmacologic carrier systems to deposit active ingredients into the body vehicle system. Pharmaceutical industries engineer special chemical *vehicles* that act as *drug carrier systems* to taxi bioactive substances into the body vehicle.

Drug carrier systems exist as pills, gels, liquids, powders, mists, or patches to be ingested orally; applied topically onto skin or nasal mucous membranes; injected into skin, muscle, or veins, or inserted into vaginal or rectal cavities to deliver "the active goods." The chemical constituents formulating the *coatings, casings, fillers, dispersants, or solution liquids* of pharmaceutical vehicles that transport bioactive ingredients into the body vehicle are presumably *biologically inactive.*

In the real world of chemical reactivity, drug carrier system ingredients that accompany their bioactive constituents to enter the body vehicle as *hitchhikers* are *not chemically inert or nonreactive* with body vehicle biological and biochemical constituents. Package listings for the presumptively inactive carrier ingredients of artificially manufactured health and pharmaceutical products are often longer and more complex than for the active ingredients themselves. Names such as colloidal silicon dioxide, fumed silica gel, titanium dioxide, magnesium stearate, microcrystalline cellulose, cellulose acetate, hydroxypropyl cellulose, crospovidone, dibasic calcium phosphate, glycerin, gelatin, polyethylene glycol, propylene glycol, "edible" ink, **Federal Food, Drug and Cosmetic Act (FD&C)** Blue#'s, Red#'s, and Yellow#'s food colors and dyes, calcium lake, aluminum lake, lactose monohydrate, hypromellose, polydextrose, dextrose excipient, maltodextrin, carnauba wax, mineral oil, gum arabic, sodium starch glycolate, red iron oxide, croscarmellose, sorbitol, mannitol, sucralose, and aspartame specify only some of the chemicals listed under pharmaceutical agent "inactive" ingredients lists, which form the carrier systems that taxi artificially manufactured biologically active substances into the body vehicle.

The greater the quantity and mix of pills and other pharmaceutical vehicles that artificially transport biologically active substances into the body vehicle system, the higher the amount and assortment of nonnutritive foreign chemicals deposited into the body vehicle that require detoxification, clearance, and elimination from the body vehicle system.

Both the **bioactive pharmaceutical agents** and their presumably **inactive hitchhiker chemical carriers** are **xenobiotics** that are extraneous substances foreign to body vehicle metabolic processes, which combine effects to pose undefined health risks to the body vehicle system, especially following repeated, high-dose, and long-term body vehicle exposures.

The body vehicle works to eliminate and excrete all extraneously introduced bioactive and inactive xenobiotic substances foreign to body vehicle biological requirements for existence. Xenobiotic substances are metabolically inactivated and cleared by body vehicle detoxification systems for elimination through the liver into the bile and gut, through the kidneys into the urine, through the skin into a sweat, through the lungs into the exhaled air, or directly down the gut. Meanwhile, as extraneous xenobiotic chemicals dwell circulating or stored within body vehicle cellular and tissue compartments awaiting clearance and elimination, the processing time pending xenobiotic elimination increases the prospects for producing harmful body vehicle effects.

Additionally, *all* xenobiotic substances introduced into the body vehicle especially through the gut can chemically and biologically affect gut microbial communities to impact body vehicle system function, health, and survival in ways that are only recently becoming appreciated and studied scientifically. Therefore, taking more pills and other artificially manufactured foreign chemical substances regularly into the body vehicle also introduces greater adverse health risks into the body vehicle system.

20.16 PRODUCT EXPIRATION DATE

All artificially manufactured substances chemically disintegrate and biologically decompose over time. Pharmaceutical substances made commercially for human use have a finite life-span for optimal commercial delivery and consumer utilization to produce desired product effects.

Product expiration dates estimate when significant chemical, physical, or biological deterioration or spoilage of industrially manufactured products may have occurred to reduce product effectiveness or create the potential for causing toxicities, warranting discarding of remaining or unused portions of the product.

Packaged pharmaceutical product ingredients may chemically react with air or any of the other contained product constituents comprising either the biologically active substances or the inactive components of the carrier delivery systems.

Loss of biological potency of bioactive ingredients and accumulation of toxic chemical by-products that compromise product quality and safety occur progressively during product storage through ongoing decomposition reactions that take place among unused portions of product constituents.

Product shelf life, which represents the estimated commercial life-span for acceptable product integrity and potency that produces the highest expected product activity with reliable safety, additionally may shorten unsuspectingly under nonoptimal storage conditions that accelerate product deterioration to produce toxic by-products faster.

20.17 PRODUCT CONTAMINANTS

Complete purity of artificially manufactured chemical products is an ideal goal. **Product contaminants** are undesirable substances not itemized or identified in product ingredient lists that compromise manufactured product purity, which have been inadvertently incorporated during manufacture and production to be delivered in final products for unintentional ingestion by unsuspecting consumers.

Despite stringent governmental regulatory oversight of pharmaceutical industry product manufacturing practices, numerous controlled medicinal agents are regularly recalled or made commercially unavailable due to inadvertent contamination or unacceptable production errors risking endangerment of consumer well-being and public health and safety.

Within the context of large-scale industrial operations that manufacture products supplying millions of dependent consumers, innocent and inadvertent product contamination during mass production is unavoidable and inevitable. Mechanized engineering marvels and robotic operations are designed for industries to automate the production and manufacture of enormous volumes of consumables with limited monitoring and only sparse worker oversight. Consequently, inadvertent introduction of undesirable and undetected contaminants including insects, bacterial or mold microbes, and possibly small animals and animal parts or excretory droppings, as well as other unwanted elements such as hair, metallic slivers, and plastic shavings into industrially manufactured commercial food and health products has become easier.

Microplastic particulates have been detected to contaminate water contained in plastic bottles and found within mosquito larvae and adult forms to be passed up the animal food chain. More ominously, these microplastic particulates are also being discovered in human stool. Reports have even surfaced describing chemical contamination of industrial food products such as macaroni and cheese and take-out fast foods with toxic **phthalate** chemical agents used to soften plastics, which apparently compose food wrappers and packaging materials and the conveyor belts moving food products along during the manufacturing process.

To reasonably balance the manufacture and availability of commercial food and health products with some semblance of safety regulation for consumers, industries and governmental regulatory agencies often negotiate and mutually agree upon commercial product quality guidelines.

Regulatory agencies such as the FDA establish limits designating maximum allowable content of specific detectable contaminants per category of consumable commercial product. The FDA also designates the safety of various nutritional and health supplements and chemical additives incorporated into foods and pharmaceutical agents under the separate category of generally recognized as safe (GRAS).

FDA designations for acceptable levels of contaminants in artificially manufactured food products, vitamins, and health supplements acknowledge the limitations that prevail in attempting to mass-produce pure and sanitary industrial grade consumable products, and concede the lack of understanding for potential human health consequences related to regular consumption of chemical food additives and manufacturing contaminants.

Minimally, food processing and pharmaceutical manufacturing compromises that receive the stamp-of-approval from national regulatory agencies highlight the commercial principle that industrial shows must go on to continue churning the wheels of business and economic profitability. Staffing and funding constraints logistically limit the capacity of the FDA to comprehensively survey and monitor the details of large-scale industrial manufacturing activities, and consequently, regulatory oversight only periodically assesses industry practices with announced site visits striving to enforce industry compliance with minimum acceptable standards for product quality and safety.

Given the considerable effort and enormous costs of overseeing the mass-scale manufacturing practices of more tightly regulated producers of controlled pharmaceutical substances, the operations of vitamin, herbal, and dietary health supplement industries are substantially ignored and carry on relatively unregulated and unchecked.

Despite all combined regulatory efforts to ensure the safety of commercially manufactured health and nutrition products, the potential toxicities and cumulative health risks of regularly consuming artificially mass-produced biologically active nutrient and inactive non-nutrient ingredients, chemical additives, decomposition by-products, and production and storage contaminants over many years are unknown.

20.18 POINTS TO CONSIDER BEFORE USING ARTIFICIALLY MANUFACTURED VITAMINS AND HEALTH SUPPLEMENTS

Selective circumstances not meant to be exclusive or exhaustive, whereby artificial supplementation with rescue industry products such as vitamins or herbal and dietary health supplements may beneficially complement appropriate health maintenance behaviors that naturally nourish the body vehicle include the following:

1. encountering limited availability of natural food resources necessary to adequately and appropriately supply required body vehicle vitamins and micronutrients

2. possessing religious or moral beliefs that categorically exclude the consumption of certain natural whole earth foods which exclusively provide essential micronutrients for the body vehicle system

3. having restricted access to vital natural food resources due to significant geographic, social, or political limitations such as living in a desert or icy tundra, being out at sea for prolonged periods of time, or existing deprived under oppressive or war-torn circumstances

4. suffering medical conditions which physiologically limit adequate body vehicle absorption or utilization of specific vital micronutrients that can be overcome reliably through artificial supplementation

5. experiencing documented allergies to natural foods uniquely providing particular essential micronutrients

6. requiring rapid correction of severe documented body vehicle micronutrient deficiencies causing or predisposing to well-characterized medical health disorders

7. treating distinct medical and health conditions proven scientifically to respond to aggressive supplementation with specific micronutrients

8. managing uncomplicated medically diagnosed health disorders established to improve with biologically active natural whole earth food ingredients which can be delivered more simply, reliably, conveniently, and inexpensively through artificial supplementation than through natural foods

Deliberately using artificially manufactured vitamins and dietary supplements to alter the healthy balance of an optimally functioning body vehicle system in an attempt to gain unproven or extraneous health benefits or increase survival advantages, may instead precipitate adverse health or survival consequences.

A diversified diet that supplies vital nutrients naturally directly from the manufacturer Mother Nature through crude fuel whole earth foods optimizes body vehicle health and well-being, without risking inadvertent body vehicle toxicities and detrimental health effects that may follow artificial micronutrient supplementation with commercially manufactured agents that unnecessarily deliver xenobiotic substances.

21 A STRATEGY TO LOSE EXCESS WEIGHT

Living is simple; trust the basics.

Body vehicle existence has *five fundamental requirements.* Without satisfying these five fundamental requirements, the body vehicle rapidly deteriorates and dies prematurely:

1. *air,* which supplies oxygen to run ongoing biochemical and metabolic body vehicle processes
2. *water* (H_2O), which forms the fluid medium that fills out all body vehicle cells, tissues, organs, and cavities; permits essential metabolic and biological life reactions to occur; serves to eliminate body vehicle wastes, and helps regulate body vehicle working temperatures (water is continuously lost through the urine, feces, sweat, and with every exhaled breath and requires regular replenishment)
3. *fuel,* which provides the energy substrates that power all body vehicle system functions and biological repairs and upkeep
4. *movement,* which is inherent to all visible, microscopic, and molecular kinetic actions of the living body vehicle system
5. *rest,* which permits expended body vehicle system life energies to recharge

The level and extent to which these five basic existence requirements are fulfilled determine the body vehicle life quality. For example, life quality is better breathing clean, fresh air instead of polluted air or smoke; drinking pure water as opposed to ingesting contaminated water or alcohol, soda pop, sports, or juice beverage products; eating natural whole earth foods rather than consuming processed food products; moving the body vehicle physically regularly compared to remaining sedentary and inactive, and getting plenty of rest and sleep and not running energy into the ground.

The body vehicle additionally has five basic, essential, and interdependent **maintenance needs** that when met appropriately promote body vehicle system homeostasis and proper functioning to optimize health and weight for height and maximize longevity:

1. nutrition
2. hydration
3. activity
4. rest
5. toxicity avoidance

The **Crude Fuel Monkey Food Diet** is a life strategy for fulfilling the preceding five basic maintenance categories optimally at the highest possible levels to achieve the ideal body vehicle health, wellness, and life-span as programmed into inherited body vehicle DNA genetic codes.

21.1 NUTRITION

Nutrition encompasses the entire provision of fuel energy, micronutrient, and building block atoms and molecules that maintain the body vehicle physical structure and function and allow the body vehicle to live. Natural crude fuel whole earth foods, readily available on earth dating back to the purported time of Adam and Eve in the story of the Garden of Eden in Paradise, best satisfy body vehicle nutritional needs.

The **Monkey Food Diet** embodies the entire spectrum of basic nutritional sustenance consumed naturally by the genetically related earth dwelling human relative apes, which actively forage through jungles eating plants, shrubs, fruit, animal flesh, and insects that comprise the naturally available package-free earth nutrients that are readily identifiable without requiring commercial labeling.

Humans are naturally both plant and meat eaters, as evidenced by the inherent biological design and function of the human teeth and digestive system.

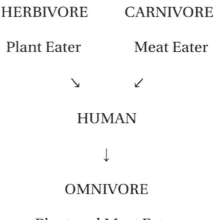

HERBIVORE   CARNIVORE

Plant Eater   Meat Eater

HUMAN

OMNIVORE

Plant and Meat Eater

Humans have adaptively evolved individually and as a species to internally process, transform, and assimilate specific indigenous earth plants, animal flesh, insects, and microorganisms that most compatibly supply critical nutrient and fuel components necessary to sustain human life on earth.

Trust what mother nature made because everything else is made for profit.

21.1.1 Crude Fuels

The name is the ingredient.

Crude fuels comprise three main categories of natural whole earth foods that optimally suit human body vehicle nutritional needs for survival. The three main crude fuel categories are plants, animal flesh and other non-plant living organisms such as insects, and direct plant or animal products.

The biological food name is the actual ingredient composing the crude fuel. Therefore, each recognizable natural crude fuel whole earth food within a nutritive category is wholly and simply the only crude fuel food ingredient.

Crude fuels utilize gut digestive capabilities more extensively and directly feed the microbiome and intestinal barrier cells situated along the entire length of the gut to promote body vehicle health maximally.

21.1.1.1 Plants

Plants are stationary nonanimal non-insect earth life-forms and their components, which substantially depend on sunlight and the process of photosynthesis to assimilate carbon dioxide (CO_2) for existence and include

1. vegetables (leafy, solid skinned, or tuber-like)
2. fruit
3. simple intact natural whole grains that entirely contain the germ, bran, and endosperm components such as delivered by whole corn, brown rice, oats, and barley
4. raw nuts
5. seeds, beans, and legumes

Consume plants fresh or cooked, whole or cut up. Diversify and combine plant intake liberally daily without concern for restricting portions, because plants have *naturally built-in portion control.*

Very few individuals can comfortably consume a whole head of cauliflower, several carrots, or several apples in one sitting which provide relatively few total calories, whereas many individuals readily eat a few donuts, several cookies or slices of pizza, or a few scoops of ice cream to consume 1,000 or more calories over a short time.

Mix, match, and cycle plant colors to broaden the nutritional value and nutrient richness delivered by ingested plants. *Chew plants thoroughly* to release vital nutrients and optimally prepare eaten plants orally for subsequent gut digestion and body vehicle utilization.

Eating the peel is part of the nutrition deal.
Eating the skin makes one thin.

Mother Nature delivers crude fuel, whole earth foods in natural skin wrappers without writing to influence decisions to purchase and consume the foods or to explain how food contents are altered to compromise nutritional value. Natural plant skins are without deceptive, explanatory, misleading, persuasive, appealing, provocative, inviting, or tempting writing to capture consumer attention and entice product purchase. Skins especially make crude fuel foods slow-later fuels.

Natural whole foods with edible skins slow gut nutrient processing to better pace and coordinate digestive activities with nutrient absorption, blood distribution, and cellular delivery to meet body vehicle energy and nutrient demands more efficiently and reduce nutrient surpluses requiring storage. Edible fruit and vegetable skins contain vitamins and other essential micronutrients and fibers that strategically feed both the body vehicle and gut microbiota. Nonedible fruit skins that are biologically indigestible by the body vehicle and require removal before plants are eaten include those wrapping bananas, melons, coconuts, avocados, and pineapples.

Diversified plant food diets ensure the best provision of essential life-sustaining nutrients and fuels necessary for body vehicle function and survival and promote diversification and richness of gut microbial floras to support healthier body vehicle existences.

21.1.1.2 Animal Flesh and Other Non-Plant Organisms

Animal flesh and other non-plant organisms comprise the fresh, whole or *recognizable* parts of *single* animals or insects decontaminated (cooked, grilled, fried, baked, etc.) for human consumption, for example, poultry, seafood, fish, beef, lamb, pork, eggs, insects. This animal and organism category excludes food products created by grinding up and combining parts of various animals and other organisms to make **community meats,** such as hamburger, sausages, and other ground-up and mixed animal flesh components.

Additionally, commercial food industries are progressively contaminating animals deliberately with artificial growth hormones, antibiotics, and other toxins to fatten up and grow animals quickly artificially, since increased animal size, weight, and quantity yield higher sales prices and industry profits. Consequently, free-range, grass-fed, wild caught, and hormone- and antibiotic-free varieties of fresh, single-source animal flesh organisms may be less contaminated for humans to consume.

Many food contaminants introduced through industry practices or environmental sources are oil soluble and preferentially store and concentrate within the fat-containing portions of foods, especially the suet or visible fat of red meats or the condensed fat and fatty skins of poultry and other birds. Trimming away visible fat and removing skins before eating animal flesh reduces dietary fat consumption and delivery of contaminants harbored in the fat.

21.1.1.3 Direct Animal, Plant, and Insect Products

Direct animal, plant, and insect products include fresh eggs, honey, milk, pure maple syrup, and water from inside of coconuts, with special consideration given to simple yogurt, kefir, and aged fermented hard cheeses that supply friendly microorganisms to the body vehicle and have been important nutrient sources for humans available through the millennia. Any direct products purchased commercially likewise should be free of hormones and antibiotics especially if originating from large-scale commercial dairy farms or industry suppliers.

21.1.2 Whole Seed Foods

The **Crude Fuel Monkey Food Diet** incorporates **whole "seed" foods** or their direct unadulterated unaltered products for body vehicle nutritional sustenance. Whole seed foods are the fully intact or segmental portions of natural earth life-forms capable of **replication,** which contain basic life-sustaining building block components packaged proportionately within biologically correct nutrient delivery systems.

Natural crude fuel, whole seed foods include living **vegetation,** such as trees, shrubs, bushes, and plants, and their component fruits and **creatures** dwelling within earth skies, waters, and lands. Eggs; beans; legumes; nuts; various edible plant seeds; genuine whole grains such as corn, oats, and barley; vegetables; fruits; animals, and insects are all biological templates theoretically possessing seed like capabilities to regenerate like-in-kind whole organisms.

Industry processing tears apart whole seed foods to radically disrupt the natural balance and composition of whole seed components and deliver separated, individual ingredients to predominantly satisfy economically driven commercial industry purposes.

The **Crude Fuel Monkey Food Diet** *excludes* processed and refined commercial food and beverage products of *indulgence, entertainment, and convenience* and any *co-conspirator taste enhancers,* which are manufactured deliberately employing taste pornography standards to arouse primal craves and promote uncontrollable devouring of foods well beyond body vehicle nutritional requirements. The crude fuel diet relies on nutritional morality to guide body vehicle fueling, with adherence to a proper nutritional code of conduct that abstains from making calorically equivalent exchanges between natural crude fuel whole earth foods and processed and refined food and beverage products during routine body vehicle maintenance fueling.

A healthy nutritional routine separates body vehicle maintenance fueling from periodic transgressions into taste pornography feeding episodes relegated to infrequent engagements such as parties, celebrations, holiday events, and special occasions, which are minimized to allow ample body vehicle metabolic recovery between unhealthy dietary digressions from otherwise healthy body vehicle fueling.

Processed food products of indulgence, entertainment, and convenience, and co-conspirator taste enhancers to be avoided during routine daily maintenance fueling include mayonnaise, ketchup, barbecue sauce, salad dressings, jellies/jams/preserves, butter/margarine, syrups, sauces, sour cream, peanut butter, French fries, pasta, white rice, white flour baked goods, ice cream, cured lunch meats and other community animal flesh products, such as hot dogs, hamburgers, and sausages that combine various flesh parts from numerous animals with artificial fillers, stabilizers, or taste enhancers.

Processed food products have made-up names and variously made-up ingredients to deliver unbalanced nutrients with additives that require protective detoxification and elimination from the body vehicle system after consumption.

21.1.3 Fueling Tips

1. Eat breakfast daily to "break" the night "fast" and nutritionally kick-start the body vehicle system engine upon awakening in the morning after a long night sleep.

First fuel the body vehicle, then drive it.

Skipping meals, especially breakfast, drives the body vehicle system into a starved mode to trigger compensatory survival fight or flight hormonal stress responses that release adrenaline and cortisol. Excessive hunger stress may precipitate adverse health consequences such as heart attacks and strokes, and predisposes to obesity by reducing metabolic fuel energy burn to lean starvation mode while intensifying craves for eating and reducing the willpower to avoid consuming pleasure and runaway escape addictification food products.

2. Fuel regularly throughout the day with slow-later delivery crude fuels to keep the gut temporary fuel holding tank filled with gradually digesting nutrients that satiate feeding drives correctly and provide continuous availability of fuel energy to smoothly power the body vehicle engine without associated metabolic energy swings often caused by eating fast-now fuels.

3. Sit down while eating. A complex behavioral connection operates between the functioning brain and the sitting butt that helps regulate eating. Sitting while eating reduces stress, allowing the body vehicle to relax and provide an opportunity for the brain to focus on food qualities communicated by mouth and gut sensors that deliver critical nutritional information helping direct eating behaviors.

4. Create convenience and facility to eat and fuel the body vehicle correctly. Plan meals and have healthy natural crude fuel whole earth foods readily available to eat and prepare for meals. Keep food recipes basic and simple incorporating easy to prepare and serve natural crude fuel whole earth food ingredients.

Make processed and refined commercial food products unavailable and inconvenient to obtain and eat and recognize that unhealthy food products that are not purchased are unavailable for inopportune consumption.

Industry peddles convenience, pleasure, and excess. Consequently, avoid buying, storing, and consuming processed and refined food and beverage products of indulgence, entertainment, and convenience, which predispose to unwanted weight gain and poor health that increase lifetime costs.

5. Avoid being distracted while eating. Strive for mindful eating. Shut off the TV, turn off electronic media devices such as the computer, get off the phone, stop texting, and put down that exciting novel or newspaper story during meal time to pay attention directly to food qualities and the eating process. Attentive eating with a direct focus on the natural appearance, smell, taste, and texture qualities of the crude fuels being ingested, communicates sensory information involving eating to the brain to register satiety and guide proper nutritional behaviors more effectively.

6. Explore the herb and spice drawer and recognize that salt is _not_ a spice. Avoid premixed commercial "seasonings" laced with preservatives and salt and other additives that artificially enhance food flavor qualities. Natural herbs and spices provide the body vehicle with an authentic taste experience. Common nutritionally healthy natural herbs and spices are anise, basil, bay leaf, caper, caraway, cayenne, chili pepper, cilantro, cinnamon, coriander, curry, dill, fennel, garlic, ginger, horseradish, jasmine, lemon, licorice, lime, marjoram, mint, mustard, nutmeg, oregano, parsley, white and black pepper, rosemary, saffron, sage, tarragon, thyme, turmeric, and vanilla.

7. Be aware of industrial adulteration and possible contamination of foods. _Soapy wash_ fruit and vegetable skins whenever possible during food preparation to remove any insects and nonvisible pesticide, herbicide, and fertilizer residues or other contaminants from food skins before cooking or ingesting foods. Avoid consuming any packaged foods labeled with ingredient lists that name chemical substances or which have descriptive modifiers or intensifiers preceding natural crude fuel whole earth food names. Avoid eating foods that appear, smell, or taste spoiled, stale, or rotten. Avoid consuming artificially manufactured food products cleverly masked by combining two or more crude fuel names, such as "almond milk."

21.2 HYDRATION

21.2.1 Hydro Pertains to Water (H₂O)

Water is a universal solvent capable of dissolving just about anything. Water composes approximately 50%–60% of adult and 65%–75% of child body vehicle volumes and is the primary medium in which body vehicle life reactions take place. Water fills and shapes body vehicle cells, tissues, organs, and certain body vehicle cavities, tubes, and vessels, and is essential for gut digestive processes, cellular fuel burning, blood circulation, fecal and urinary waste elimination, body vehicle temperature control, and ongoing life-sustaining cellular and biochemical operations to occur. Without water, body vehicle cells could not generate energy power to remain viable and would quickly become poisoned with accumulated waste products.

Water is lost continuously from the body vehicle through the skin during sweat evaporation, from the lungs with each breath, in the urine during urination, and through the feces with bowel movements, and needs to be replenished regularly daily to maintain proper body vehicle function and homeostasis. **Hydration** means to resupply the body vehicle with adequate water to preserve the appropriate balance and working concentrations of body vehicle chemical and biologic elements to permit cellular biochemical and physical processes to occur and maintain optimal body vehicle operations.

21.2.1.1 Hydration for Power Generation: Car Battery Analogy

Body vehicle cells require water to run biochemical reactions to generate energy, similarly to how water filled car batteries require water to create electrochemical currents between battery cells to produce power. When body vehicle water levels are low, body vehicle energy generation and power levels reduce.

21.2.1.2 Hydration for Waste Elimination: Toilet Analogy

Water is required to flush and eliminate toxins and wastes out from the body vehicle through urine and feces, similarly to how toilet bowls use water to flush and rid wastes out to the sewer. Low body vehicle water levels compromise body vehicle waste and toxin elimination to enable body vehicle toxins to build up and concentrate predisposing to body vehicle system poisoning.

21.2.2 Rehydration Refers to Replenishment of Body Vehicle Water Losses

Pure H_2O water is the best water.

Rehydration with pure water reestablishes the correct balance of water and non-water molecules to allow body vehicle chemical and metabolic biological reactions to proceed as intended. Body vehicle kidneys need to minimally produce approximately 0.5 milliliters (ml) of urine per kilogram (kg) of body vehicle weight per hour (h) (0.5 ml/kg/h) to filter and excrete toxic body vehicle wastes adequately.

For healthy average-sized 70 kg (154 lb.) humans, minimal water losses through urine equal approximately 35 ml per hour or 840 ml per day (3.5 cups/d). Average normal body vehicle water losses daily through stool are approximately 200 ml (5/6 cup).

Minimal body vehicle water losses through sweat evaporating to cool most humans are approximately 100 ml per day in temperate climates but can increase to several liters per day in hot climates. Daily body vehicle water losses through breathing in most unstressed adults taking 12–20 regular breaths per minute are estimated to approximate 400 ml. Therefore, the estimated minimum daily body vehicle water requirements to replace obligatory water losses for healthy unstressed 70 kg average-sized adults living in temperate environments and engaged in nonstrenuous activities equal 840 ml (urine) + 200 ml (stool) + 100 ml (sweat) + 400 ml (breath) = 1,540 ml (6.5 cups) per day or *approximately 22 ml per kg of body vehicle weight.*

For convenience and simplicity, these minimum daily body vehicle water needs for unstressed healthy adults performing nonstrenuous activities in a temperate environment can be rounded up to equal *one ounce (≈30 ml) of water for every kilogram (2.2 lbs.) of ideal body vehicle weight for height.* Consequently, approximate daily water requirements for healthy unstressed 70 kg (154 lbs.) adult humans breathing normally in comfortable room temperatures are 2,100 ml ≈ 9 cups (70 kg × 30 ml), while 100 kg (220 lbs.) humans need 3,000 ml ≈ 12.5 cups of water daily, and 50 kg (110 lbs.) humans require only approximately 1,500 ml ≈ 6.5 cups of water daily provided from all water sources.

Various factors affecting actual daily water requirements include ambient temperature; age; activity level; body vehicle temperature; illnesses, especially involving disorders that increase water losses through excessive sweating, urination, stooling, or rapid breathing; or the presence of heart, kidney, and liver conditions requiring water restriction.

Warmer ambient temperatures, vigorous physical activity, or having a fever, diarrhea, excessive urination, or profuse perspiration translates to greater daily body vehicle water requirements to compensate for increased water losses. Body vehicles that function normally readily excrete any limited excesses of body vehicle water intake through urine to maintain the appropriate body vehicle water balance. Advanced heart, kidney, and liver illness conditions reduce the body vehicle capacity to excrete water and require restriction of water intake to avoid "water logging" or drowning the body vehicle with excessively retained water.

The caloric content and chemical, mineral, and salt composition of commercially processed food and beverage products markedly impact body vehicle water balance, disposition, and requirements. Processed and refined commercial foods and beverages rapidly supply large quantities of concentrated sugars, fats, salts, minerals, and chemical additives into the body vehicle to saturate and flood body vehicle cellular water compartments with non-water atoms and molecules.

Cellular water imbalances having an increased ratio of non-water elements to water, disrupt body vehicle water equilibriums, and potently trigger biochemical and behavioral responses that increase water intake and drive more water into tissues and cells to reestablish the normal cellular homeostatic balances between the concentrations of water and non-water elements.

Commercial beverages sold as "naturally" or artificially flavored, sweetened, or taste enhanced, chemically alter natural body vehicle thirst, fluid gauging, and water satiety experiences to disturb accurate signaling of brain domains responsible for maintaining proper body vehicle rehydration efforts and water balances.

Rehydration beverages formulated with a fixed set of proprietary ingredients and additives, often comprised of secret combinations of various salts, minerals, sugars, vitamins, preservatives, artificial sweeteners, and taste enhancers, risk upsetting homeostatic salt and water balances of the body vehicle system.

Rehydration beverages deliver the same composition and amount of proprietary ingredients per recommended serving size to all, regardless of body vehicle size, existing circumstances requiring rehydration, the presence of underlying health conditions, and actual individual rehydration needs.

Examples of commercial industry beverages commonly promoted for body vehicle "rehydration" purposes that disrupt body vehicle water balances and derail efforts to regain homeostatic water equilibriums include sports "hydrating" drinks, soda pop beverages, juices, refreshment fruit drinks, alcohol products, and blender-made liquids such as smoothies.

21.2.3 Hydration Tips

1. The best rehydration liquid is pure H_2O water.
2. Normal, healthy adults under most circumstances minimally require approximately one ounce ($\approx$30 ml) of water for every 2.2 lbs. (1 kg) of ideal body vehicle weight for height daily to replace obligate body vehicle water losses.
3. Adequate water intake in healthy adults establishes steady urination throughout the day producing less concentrated lighter yellow colored urine.
4. Delaying copious hydration to replenish body vehicle water stores 15 minutes or longer before meals or 1–2 hours following meals avoids interfering with food digestion in the stomach.

Excessive ingestion of fluids during meals may dilute stomach acid and decrease the activity of stomach enzymes to reduce food digestion by the stomach, and may prematurely flush digesting stomach contents out into the small intestine before the stomach completes digestion, which generally requires approximately 1.5–2.5 hours in normal healthy adults following ingestion of a full-sized meal.

Ideally, ingest liquids during meals to orally moisten food and facilitate chewing, oral digestion, and swallowing, and defer full rehydration efforts with larger volumes of fluids to before and after meals as noted above.

21.2.4 Thirst

Thirst is a primal biological urge to drink water (H_2O) to replace body vehicle water losses, which under normal health circumstances is an excellent driving force that reliably guides body vehicle water replacement. Thirst is a survival drive that ensures proper replenishment of body vehicle water stores essential for body vehicle temperature regulation, waste elimination, and completion of cellular biological reactions.

Unsatisfied thirst may be confused with hunger and lead to unnecessary eating to disrupt body vehicle water balances further. Therefore, drinking water initially when experiencing hunger may extinguish mistaken urges to eat and fuel the body vehicle unnecessarily.

Commercial beverage industries attempt to usurp the natural biological instinctual urge to replenish lost body vehicle water appropriately and push their exclusively formulated commercial beverage products into consumers with every available opportunity. Sugar, salt, mineral, electrolyte, and artificial flavoring ingredients are cheaply mixed into water to create proprietary beverage products that leverage huge commercial profits when consumed on a mass scale.

Industry has successfully managed to confuse consumers concerning proper body vehicle rehydration needs and exploits human thirst drives to compel copious ingestion of cheaply made and expensively sold commercial industry beverages. Alcohol, concentrated sugars, salts, and other artificial chemical substances can strategically interfere with thirst satiety to promote more thirst and increase consumption of industrially created commercial beverages.

Rather than purely satisfy body vehicle water requirements, commercial beverages also may deliver toxic alcohol, unhealthy artificial preservatives and taste-enhancing substances, and excessive amounts of sugar, salt, minerals, and vitamins beyond body vehicle biological needs and handling capacities to profit commercial beverage industries at the expense of consumer health.

Many marketing strategies and advertising campaigns especially ride human thirst drives and water rehydration efforts to induce consumers to drink their proprietary commercial beverages.

21.2.5 Balance

Immediate body vehicle rehydration with pure water when thirsty restores water balances essential for cellular metabolic and biochemical reactions to proceed correctly and reduces vulnerability for survival drives to succumb to drinking unhealthy, artificially formulated rehydration beverages that perpetuate thirst and may additionally provoke unnecessary eating.

Drinking pure H_2O water and eating crude fuel whole earth foods that are already substantially composed of water help to naturally maintain appropriate body vehicle nutrient, fuel, and water balances necessary for body vehicle homeostasis and optimal function.

When body vehicle water, salt, and nutrient levels are unbalanced, programmed survival drives trigger foraging behaviors and stimulate craves that seek to correct imbalances and restore equilibrium through additional consumption of foods and beverages.

21.2.6 Dr. Zahrebelski's Two Minimum Daily Goal Strategy

Applicable to most average-sized healthy adults eating three regular-sized meals daily:

1. Minimally drink two 12-ounce containers of water *between each meal* (breakfast–2–lunch–2–dinner–2–breakfast) *daily.*
2. Minimally eat two servings of fresh fruit *daily.*
3. Minimally eat two servings of fresh vegetables *daily.*
4. Minimally eat two 2-ounce servings of natural real whole grains (such as brown rice, corn, steel cut oats, quinoa, barley, freekeh) *daily.*
5. Minimally eat two 4-ounce servings of natural real "protein" (from egg, nut, bean, or lean decontaminated fresh animal flesh sources) *daily.*
6. Minimally eat two servings of dairy foods supplying calcium (such as milk, yogurt, or aged, fermented hard cheeses) *daily.*
7. Avoid entertainment, indulgence, and convenience food and beverage products *daily* too.

21.3 ACTIVITY

21.3.1 Human Life Depends on Movement

Technologies that artificially mechanize routine body vehicle activities for human convenience and to increase the time available for disposal exact a physical toll on humanity. Too often, instead of using the body vehicle directly to perform routine physical activities or driving the body vehicle as a primary mode of transportation, technology substitutes as the body vehicle physical work, activity, and transportation surrogate to tax environmental resources and cost the human system physically and financially.

Body vehicle movement and activity are free.

There are no monetary charges or financial costs to move a normally working body vehicle or any of its physical parts. Arms and legs attached to the torso of the body vehicle are there to move and mobilize the body vehicle freely anytime without monetary fees, membership dues, or financial strings attached.

Body vehicle movement and activity provide innumerable health benefits and an immeasurable sense of well-being. Creating unnecessary requirements, impediments, or restrictions to move the body vehicle surrenders the freely available life benefits that body vehicle movement provides.

21.3.2 All Aspects of Living Involve Kinetic Activity

To be alive means to be moving.
Death brings stillness.

All aspects of human biological existence depend on physical, microscopic, and molecular kinetic actions, including

1. seeking, acquiring, and ingesting crude fuel nutrients
2. digesting ingested foods with gut secretions, enzymes, and intestinal microbes to biochemically process crude fuels for blood absorption or to nourish gastrointestinal tract lining cells
3. absorbing, circulating, and distributing micronutrients through the blood for delivery to feed body vehicle cells and tissues
4. metabolizing nutrients and fuel substrates biochemically for cellular utilization
5. detoxifying ingested toxins and metabolically generated waste products
6. purifying the body vehicle system by filtering, eliminating, and excreting ingested or metabolically produced toxins through the gut out into stool, the liver into bile and feces, kidneys into the urine, lungs into the breath, and skin into a sweat for removal from the body vehicle
7. activating the immune system of defense cells guarding body vehicle tissues against infection and cancer
8. breathing and maintaining an appropriate body vehicle heartbeat, temperature, and blood pressure

In death, when the life force that binds together and animates the living and moving body vehicle system dissipates and is lost, coordinated and purposefully organized body vehicle actions cease, and the body vehicle disintegrates into individual atoms and molecules that disperse and scatter back into the universe for recycling.

21.3.3 The Use It or Lose It Principle Governs Body Vehicle Energy Conservation

Physical activity functions as the *gauge* to inventory the utilization and productivity of individual body vehicle flesh components. The intact body vehicle is analogous to a corporation comprised of many departments and franchises.

Analogous to business corporations, whereby unproductive or inactive departments or system franchises are pared down or eliminated to conserve valuable corporate resources, the **body vehicle corporation** reduces metabolic "funding" to less active or inactive body vehicle components to save energy and channel energy resources to more active body vehicle system elements.

Active body vehicle system components demand and receive greater metabolic funding and energy distributions and recalibrate through plasticity mechanisms to function more efficiently and at higher levels. For example, walking and running increase blood flow to the heart, lungs, working muscles, and the brain to deliver more oxygen and nutrients to supply the demands of greater body vehicle activity and movement.

As walking and running continue regularly over time, the work capacity, endurance, and energy efficiency of the heart, lungs, and working muscles progressively grow to accommodate higher physical demands better.

Regular exercise and physical activity keep the brain active and mind working sharper to ward off the loss of brain function and mental decline known as dementia that can occur with aging. Similarly, regular piano practice increases finger speed and develops musical aptitude to improve manual dexterity and finger fine motor skills to augment piano playing capabilities. Sedentary routines that involve sitting on the butt all day long promote butt enlargement, with more fat deposited to cushion the seat for comfortable sitting. Additionally, excessive sitting leads to gradual atrophy of inactive body vehicle components, including muscles and brain muscle circuits involved with movement, as the body vehicle redirects valuable body vehicle energy resources to fund more active components demanding proportionately higher levels of metabolic support.

Sitting for prolonged periods of time regularly daily has even been scientifically associated with shortening of the human life-span. Therefore, while the butt grows to make sitting more comfortable, muscles normally used to move and mobilize the body vehicle shrink and wither, brain function deteriorates, and body vehicle life-span decreases.

21.3.4 Easier to Maintain than Regain Movement

Muscles that require high metabolic upkeep decondition rapidly and lose size, strength, and endurance quickly when inactive and unstimulated for significant periods of time as evidenced with unfortunately bedridden or temporarily comatose individuals, who develop incapacitating muscle weakness compromising the ability to walk or move limbs sometimes following only a few days of complete inactivity.

Severely deconditioned muscles require intensive physical therapy routines to stimulate brain muscle activity circuits, rebuild muscle endurance and strength, and reactivate movement capabilities to regain physical functioning. Unused body vehicle muscles that lose function demand proportionately more time and labor to reawaken and reprogram dormant physical capabilities, whereas continuously working muscles require less effort and energy to maintain functional capabilities at ongoing levels of physical activity.

21.3.5 Levels of Body Vehicle Physical Activity and Energy Expenditures

For simplicity, body vehicle physical activities can be conveniently grouped into three main categories being **coma, routine movement,** and **exercise,** with each category determining a certain level of body vehicle energy expenditure.

21.3.5.1 Coma

Coma energy expenditure is the minimum level of caloric energy burn essential to sustain body vehicle existence in an idle state below which the body vehicle system permanently shuts down all life functions and dies. The coma state consists of only basic electrical brain activity and limited physical functioning of vital body vehicle organs to preserve body vehicle life with stable vital signs and without any voluntary physical activity or movement.

Coma caloric energy burn can be estimated scientifically by measuring the body vehicle resting **basal metabolic rate (BMR)** of energy consumption under restrictive circumstances. The BMR is essentially the lowest obligatory caloric fuel energy burn required to keep the body vehicle alive in the absence of illness; resting quietly without any voluntary physical movements; while fasting with an empty gut; and having stable vital signs with appropriate body temperature, blood pressure, and pulse off life support. The basal metabolic rate can be calculated for various male and female heights, weights, and ages using the **Harris-Benedict Equation.** The Harris-Benedict Equation estimates routine daily resting energy expenditures to range approximately between 15–30 calories per kilogram (2.2 lbs.) of body vehicle weight, with higher caloric energy expenditures per weight for males than for females, for younger teenagers than for aged adults, and for leaner and more muscular individuals than for obese individuals.

Coma caloric energy burn constitutes the majority (up to 75%) of daily fuel energy expenditures for minimally active sedentary physical routines. *Therefore, inactive individuals mainly exist burning caloric energy in a coma state.*

21.3.5.2 Routine Movement

Routine movement energy expenditures comprise the *bonus* caloric energy burned while performing occupational or leisure activities with physical actions not deliberately intended to target specific muscles to improve muscle strength, speed, endurance, tone, or coordination, and include diverse activities such as fidgeting, accomplishing schoolwork, performing work duties, executing chores, running errands, and engaging in non-exercise-related hobbies.

Routine movement energy expenditures may easily amount to an additional 100–200 calories or more burned per hour for more physically active routines, which quickly add up to substantial quantities when specific activities continue for hours at a time.

Mentally challenging or physically demanding routines that involve intense intellectual or strenuous physical work consume larger magnitudes of caloric fuel energies that may proportionately amount to multiples of coma fuel energy burn.

21.3.5.3 Exercise

Exercise energy expenditures constitute the caloric fuel energy burned to execute and sustain physical routines specifically intended to enhance the orthopedic functioning of muscular and structural locomotive body vehicle components.

Exercise purposely targets individual muscles or muscle groups to build muscle speed, strength, endurance, tone, and coordination to improve body vehicle physical stability, mobility, and efficiency of movement, and enhance general appearance.

Regular exercise leads to numerous body vehicle physiologic adaptations. Exercise increases muscle size and contractile force to augment muscle strength, speed, endurance, and work capacity and strengthens bones, ligaments, tendons, and joints. Additionally, blood capillaries expand to deliver higher blood flow to physically working muscles and tissues, and the numbers of muscle cell mito-chondrial energy-generating powerhouses increase to meet the added energy demands of working muscles. Exercise also loosens built-up muscle tension and reduces accumulated mental stress which develop following long days performing physically demanding and mentally taxing routines.

Humans commonly misunderstand the term exercise to indicate unpleasant, tedious, painful, inconvenient, or expensive physical activities. Industry exploits misunderstandings and misperceptions concerning exercise to steer consumers into commercial behaviors that generate industry revenues such as purchasing memberships to "health" clubs charging extravagant facility fees for club usage;

hiring personal trainers to motivate and oversee individuals performing physical activities, and buying expensive exercise equipment to achieve body vehicle fitness.

The meaning and significance of exercise become clearer by substituting alternative, less ambiguous eight-letter words such as **movement, activity,** or **mobility** for exercise.

> *Movement and activity maintain mobility and increase muscular*
> *strength, function, and physical capacity.*
> *(These are all alternative eight-letter words for exercise except for*
> *and.)*

Exercise takes the body vehicle for a test drive or component check by engaging muscle, bone, joint, and brain circuits in physical actions that assess and improve the physical performance of locomotive body vehicle parts. An analogy that compares the directives of a taxi driver delivering a ride with the interests of a prospective new car buyer taking a vehicle on a test drive lends some perspective for the differences between body vehicle work and exercise routines.

The focus of the taxi driver navigating through traffic is analogous to how most individuals execute occupational or home activity routines. Taxi drivers concentrate on traffic signals, other cars and drivers, road conditions, travel routes, and travel times, which are all extraneous factors permitting the taxi to cut through traffic and are unrelated to qualities or characteristics of the driven vehicle. Meanwhile, prospective car buyer objectives are more like those of individuals engaging in exercise routines. Potential car buyers on a test drive focus internally on vehicle characteristics, including the performance, ride comfort, and function of vehicle components, analogously to how exercising individuals direct attention toward actively moving body vehicle parts.

Body vehicle movements during exercise provide feedback to the brain for further consideration concerning ongoing physical activities and body vehicle movement. Therefore, exercise deliberately engages the body vehicle in sufficient levels of physical activity specifically to improve the movement, mobility, and physical performance characteristics of the body vehicle.

Thoughtful exercise routines promote fitness, health, longevity, and a greater sense of well-being, and help protect against falls and other preventable physical injuries to increase personal safety. Physical fitness increases life-span. Ultimately, exercise engages the body vehicle in deliberate physical actions to achieve more powerful and fluid movement using less effort to allow more efficient accomplishment of physical tasks.

The main physical activity elements to integrate and maximize during exercise to optimize body vehicle movement are summarized in the acronym **FAMS-Triple B,** or "flexibility, agility, mobility, speed, and base (stability), balance, and brawn (strength)." Activity and movement keep body vehicle muscles stimulated, working, and fit. Fit working muscles pulling on bones strengthen connecting tendons, ligaments, and bones to improve body vehicle mobility and stability. More effective mobility increases available physical options to burn off excess storage fuel energy or fatness. Working muscles help prevent excessive weight gain by burning fuel energies at higher metabolic rates than nonworking muscles. Exercise also benefits behavioral health status and mental well-being by activating muscle brain nerve circuits that stimulate the release of natural pleasure-inducing brain chemicals called **endorphins,** which can improve or prevent health conditions such as depression and anxiety that predispose to overeating and unwanted weight gain. Additionally, exercise promotes mixing and a greater diversity of the intestinal microbiota to provide further body vehicle health benefits and survival advantages.

Society suffers in various ways when individuals sell out and surrender their motivation and personal responsibility to exercise in exchange for physical conveniences and commercial industry runaway escapes. Commercial rescue industry interventions inadequately compensate for the preventable health consequences that result from a lack of exercise.

Exercise strengthens bones, improves balance, and reduces risks for falls and fractures while delivering countless other health benefits to exercising individuals. On the other hand, osteoporosis medicines unpredictably benefit a minute fraction of individuals taking these chemical interventions for prolonged periods of time at great expense, and with risks of developing adverse drug reactions.

Scientific studies estimate that dozens of postmenopausal women require treatment with osteoporosis medications for several years to prevent one hip fracture for the treated group. Consider the significantly reduced personal and societal costs that these same women potentially can achieve in preventing hip and other fractures and increasing health benefits by participating in regular exercise routines for the same several year period. Exercise not only provides direct health benefits to participating women but also eliminates the need for expensive osteoporosis medications with their associated risks to cause adverse drug side effects.

Societal reliance on medications and other high-priced commercial rescue industry services to reduce the health fallout resulting from the simple failure to carry out basic maintenance exercise dramatically increases health care costs for all, unfortunately, to financially benefit only the industries that profit from the surrender of personal responsibilities to physically move.

21.3.6 Fitness Is about Exercise Whereas Fatness Is about Fueling

Frequently, exercise consumes the lowest proportion of daily fuel energy calories burned, but substantially enhances body vehicle fitness, health, mental well-being, and the odds of survival with appropriate exercise regimens. Physical activities and exercise performed at higher intensity levels and for longer durations provide even greater levels of fitness, health, and survival benefits, and burn more calories.

When exercise regimens combine with appropriate body vehicle fueling, excess body vehicle weight reduces faster and more effectively. Higher physical activity levels increase life expectancies. Regularly exercising and physically active adults generally live longer than non-exercising and sedentary or physically inactive adults. Exercising adults meeting the general **U.S. Department of Health and Human Services (HHS)** physical activity guidelines can potentially add a few extra years to their life expectancy.

Caloric usage during exercise can equal 200 calories burned per hour for lower levels of physical activity such as slow walking and rises to 1,200 or more calories burned hourly for vigorous or strenuous activities involving boxing, martial arts, basketball, soccer, or intense aerobic workouts. To burn off fuel energy calories contained in commonly ingested portions of processed food products such as one cheeseburger with French fries, two donuts, or one bagel with cream cheese (all containing approximately 700 calories) may require a few hours of exercise with lower intensity physical routines. Therefore, overindulging with calorie-rich fast-now fuels with the intention of burning off excess calories through exercise, quickly becomes a losing enterprise that instead leads to progressive fatness for most sporadically active individuals engaging in lower levels of daily physical activity.

On a positive note, heavier individuals burn proportionately more calories per hour while exercising than lighter individuals performing the same intensity and types of exercise routines, which should incentivize overweight individuals to mobilize, increase activity levels, and regularly partake in scheduled exercise routines.

21.3.7 Physical Activity Intensity and Duration

The maximum human heart rate (HR) equals 220 minus age:
Maximum HR (heartbeats per minute) = 220 − Age

For example, the estimated maximum heart rate for a 20-year-old human is 200 heartbeats per minute. **Moderate-intensity physical activity** achieves 50%–70% of maximum heart rate for age. **Vigorous-intensity physical activity** achieves 70%–85% of maximum heart rate for age. *HHS minimal activity guidelines for generally fit adults aged 18–64 years and older who have no limiting health conditions* are as follows:

> At least 150 minutes (2 hours and 30 minutes) weekly of moderate-intensity aerobic activity combined with at least two days per week of muscle-strengthening activities working all major muscle groups (legs, hips, back, abdomen, chest, shoulders, and arms);

or

75 minutes (1 hour and 15 minutes) weekly of vigorous-intensity aerobic activity combined with at least two days per week of muscle-strengthening activities working all major muscle groups (legs, hips, back, abdomen, chest, shoulders, and arms);

or

Some equivalent mix of moderate and vigorous-intensity aerobic activity weekly combined with the same two days per week minimum of muscle-strengthening activities.

Total weekly activity times can be broken up into intervals as short as 10 minutes that can be spread out over the entire week as convenient to achieve the same health and survival benefits.

For safety, individuals who are pregnant, aged, sedentary, or suffering from an orthopedic, neurologic, heart, lung, or any other significant health impairment including obesity, hypertension, and diabetes require careful medical assessment of physical fitness and exercise tolerance by a physician to receive medical clearance before initiating or engaging in any strenuous fitness or exercise regimens.[10]

21.3.8 Avoid Overfueling to Remain Active and Alert

Overfueling with fast-now fuels that absorb quickly from the gut into the blood to trigger compensatory body vehicle mechanisms to rapidly clear excessive calories from blood, creates metabolic stresses that drive the body vehicle system into a state replete with tiredness, sleepiness, and lower motivation to move, commonly experienced following overindulgent eating at holiday meals.

The reduced energy experienced following the intake of excessive energy calories can be considered an **overfueling hangover,** analogous to the toxic feeling experienced following excessive alcohol intake. Relative hunger activates body vehicle system survival drives to seek fuel energy, which stimulates the body to move, and increases alertness and brain activity sometimes to the point of irritability when hunger drives are substantial and not readily satisfied.

---

10. HHS recommendations for appropriate levels and durations of physical activity for various ages are available for review at https://www.hhs.gov/fitness/be-active/physical-activity-guidelines-for-americans/index.html.

21.3.9 **Activity Tips**

1. *Be continuously active* throughout each day.
2. *Move* as many parts of the body vehicle as often as possible daily.
3. *Mobilize* physically under natural body vehicle power to move from place to place with every available opportunity.
4. *Take the opportunity to physically get in touch and inventory working body vehicle parts daily* through yoga, calisthenics, or directed muscle stretching or massage to assess the orthopedic integrity of physically working parts, stimulate connecting circuits between working parts and the brain, and increase working part physical performance.
5. *Work* joints and muscle groups symmetrically on both sides of the body vehicle to balance strength, expand the range of motion, and promote stability in movement and mobility. Especially with aging, regular movement of all joints prevents inflammatory arthritic responses that develop from daily wear and tear to freeze up and fuse joints resulting in a restricted joint range of motion or permanent joint immobility.
6. *Add resistance* to physical movements to increase muscle strength by using free weights or elastic rubber bands, or by employing isometric exercises at least two days per week, targeting the major muscle groups of the legs, hips, back, abdomen, chest, shoulders, and arms.
7. *Keep activities safe* by being mindfully attentive to the sensory feedback delivered from moving muscles, bones, and joints, which may signal developing tiredness, fatigue, soreness, pain, or limitation in range of motion requiring adjustment or cessation of activities; and balance the intensity of physical activity to guard against overworking and injuring body vehicle parts. Body vehicle maintenance care demands reasonable levels of regular physical activity balanced safely between insufficient and excessive activity to prevent neglect disrepair and wear and tear injuries requiring repair.
8. *Breathe* rhythmically, continuously, and deeply during exercises to promote blood flow through the heart and into the lungs for oxygenation, and to relax tense muscles to facilitate circulation of oxygenated blood through working muscles and into cells.
9. *Focus* attention on working body vehicle orthopedic parts possibly by closing the eyes to reduce external distractions that divert attention and concentration away from the physical activities being performed.
10. *Overcome perceived limitations to daily movement and exercise.*

Healthy living requires prioritizing to invest personal time and energy to complete basic body vehicle maintenance activities regularly. Make exercise a priority scheduled into daily routines. Move all body vehicle orthopedic parts daily without excuses. When physical impairments limit the ability to exercise vertically or while standing, then exercise while seated or lying down. Lean on a wall for support during exercise to provide stability and a measure of safety when the balance is impaired. Similarly, when gait is unstable or physical limitations prevent walking or running, then more stationary exercises with yoga, isometrics, or using light weights and resistance bands can serve physical activity needs adequately. When outside weather is inclement, then exercise indoors.

Body vehicle movement and physical activity are naturally programmed into the body vehicle system and have been continuously carried out throughout the lifetime of humanity, without the need for "expert" advice, assistance, or training, and certainly without requiring special equipment or dedicated "health and fitness" facilities. Regular body vehicle activity and exercise produce a sense of personal accomplishment and stimulate brain release of natural pleasure-inducing endorphin chemicals, and most importantly enhance health and survival benefits to individuals and society.

From a practical standpoint, since humans expend a great deal of time and energy standing and mobilizing the body vehicle from place to place by walking or running, footwear is a crucial determinant that ensures the capability to carry out vital body vehicle locomotive activities comfortably and in a healthy manner.

Footwear provides foot protection and helps support the foot to allow comfortable standing and appropriate gait stability during mobilization. Foot friction generated during standing, walking, or running, and moisture from foot sweat and environmental elements deteriorate and wear out footwear, resulting in uneven distribution of forces on the feet, lower extremities, and back that can create orthopedic problems and fatigue muscles used for standing and ambulation. Consequently, when footwear shows the uneven wear of soles or loses foot support, and leads to pain, discomfort, or tiredness of the lower extremities or back when worn, then the footwear needs to be retired.

An additional measure by which to gauge whether to retire footwear is when walking barefoot feels substantially more comfortable compared to walking while wearing the footwear.

21.4 REST OR R&R

Perpetual motion machines that can work indefinitely without requiring additional energy inputs or having to recharge are currently nonexistent within the known universe.

The human body vehicle is not a perpetual motion machine.

21.4.1 **Rest Is the Body Vehicle R&R**

Rest will

1. Recharge and Restore depleted energy
2. Rebuild and Replace worn-out cells and cellular components
3. Repair and Regenerate deteriorated and injured tissues
4. Reboot body vehicle systems and Reprogram body vehicle operations

Rest embodies all body vehicle actions, activities, and behaviors necessary for targeted or generalized body vehicle cellular and tissue **housekeeping, regeneration,** and **recovery.** Body vehicle performance characteristics decline following vigorous or prolonged body vehicle use or stresses. Restful relaxation provides biological time for the body vehicle to refill and assimilate depleted nutrients and energy stores, patch physical and chemical wear and tear, rebuild cellular structures and constituents or degrade and replace senescent, worn-out, or malfunctioning cells.

During rest, worn-out and damaged cells and cellular components are removed, renovated, or replaced, and cellular programs are updated to maintain smooth and efficient biochemical and physiologic operations sustaining body vehicle life.

21.4.2 **Tiredness**

Tiredness is the feeling of possessing insufficient body vehicle energy to adequately meet the demands of ongoing or planned life activities, meaning that energy level is shorter than the day is long. Fighting tiredness increases stress and arouses survival fight or flight hormonal stress responses to compensate for insufficient time devoted to rest, further compromising body vehicle integrity while predisposing to stress eating and promoting body vehicle fat storage that can lead to obesity.

Excessive tiredness also facilitates the activation of any surreptitiously implanted behavioral programs that engage uncontrollable feeding impulses and craves. Tiredness reduces resolve and lowers thresholds for triggers that promote unnecessary mindless eating predisposing to unwanted weight gain. Tiredness increases distractibility and impairs focus, concentration, and attention span to increase the probability of making poor nutritional decisions. Consequently, tiredness predisposes to unwanted weight gain in many ways.

Rest relieves tiredness to decrease stress and stress hormone release, reduce fat storage and the likelihood of stress feeding, and increase self-control and resolve to improve nutritional decision-making and suppress unnecessary mindless eating. Therefore, rest is essential for appropriate weight management.

21.4.3 Sleep

Sleep is pure biological self-time that provides the body vehicle with a dedicated opportunity for physical, mental, and emotional renewal to optimize daily existence. Environmental, social, and occupational rhythms and cues program body vehicle clocks and timers to establish regular sleep-wake cycles, which adjust to feeding schedules, work cycles, and daylight nighttime exposures.

During conscious wakefulness, brains activate entirely to run with full faculties that subconsciously process and actively respond to sensory arousal and other information fed to the brain. **Sleep** suspends "real" consciousness with dream animation. During sleep, much of the usual working brain activity present with wakefulness shuts down, and the subconscious takes over to create pictorial stories that play scenarios of daily existence called dreams that are watched passively with imagined involvement.

The abstract dream forum enhancing sleep allows subconscious thoughts or life circumstances to play out imaginatively to give personal meaning to daily existence and help resolve personal life issues to promote more appropriate, efficient, effective, and balanced daily living. Better nutritional decisions are easier to make with a well-rested body vehicle after a good night sleep. Sleep helps curb unnecessary mindless eating by clearing out the mental clutter of signal noise from subconscious eating programs that cloud healthy nutritional decisions. Sleep and sleep deprivation also affect gut microbial communities which may contribute to sleep-related effects on the body vehicle system. Tired individuals commonly express "they can't think straight," reaffirming the need for rest and sleep to "refresh" routinely working body vehicle programs, so that programs function purposefully at every opportunity critical for maintaining body vehicle health.

With sleep deprivation, thinking becomes distractible, laborious, less attentive, and less productive, and automatic memory retrieval crucial for the execution of healthy behaviors becomes faulty, undesirably predisposing to unhealthy consequences such as mindless or emotional eating.

Emotional imbalances negatively affect eating behaviors, and sleep helps restore emotional balance as exemplified when crabby, tired children wake up happier after restful naps.

Numerous external factors and extenuating circumstances adversely impact the restorative quality of sleep. Viewing screens of **light-emitting diode (LED)** devices such as televisions, laptop and desktop computers, tablets, and cell phones delays sleep onset, reduces sleep quality, and increases morning tiredness upon awakening. The experience of physical pain; underlying behavioral and physical health conditions; use of alcohol products, tobacco, caffeine, and chemical recreational substances of abuse; and pharmaceutical treatments for physical pain and nerve, muscle, or behavioral health disorders can diminish sleep quality.

Sleep deprivation causes physical tiredness and impairs mental functioning to increase body vehicle stress and reduce motivation for physical activity, predisposing to inactivity and unnecessary stress eating that combine to increase risks for unwanted weight gain and development of obesity.

Physical or mental overstimulation that produces muscle tension with physical discomfort or excessive brain activity with racing thoughts and emotional distress can stimulate the release of adrenaline that maintains wakefulness and alertness to interfere with sleep onset and maintenance.

Monotony can provide a welcomed means to promote sleep, as evidenced when monotonous circumstances such as listening to dull long-winded lectures or speeches or driving down long unvarying stretches of road induce drowsiness. Monotony can be intentionally brought on at bedtime to precipitate sleep by shutting off all stimulating light-emitting electronic media devices and engaging in a regular bedtime routine—techniques often applied successfully to put children to sleep.

Reading traditional print in publications such as books or magazines may help suppress extraneous brain activity and lead to relaxation to bring on sleep. Bedtime routines incorporating gentle muscle stretching or yoga exercises with slow, rhythmic breathing can help relax built-up muscle tension and dial down overactive thoughts accumulated throughout a busy day. Spiritual prayer and meditation have long been used throughout the ages as bedtime routines to induce relaxation and sleep onset hypnotically.

Regularly scheduled **bedtime routines** serve as **programmed transition periods** that smoothly channel body vehicle wakefulness into sleep. Functional MRI scans of the brain demonstrate that the pervasive electrochemical activity present throughout the brain during wakefulness powers down to involve much smaller and limited brain areas during sleep, making abrupt transitions between wakefulness and sleep unlikely to be easily accomplished under normal circumstances.

A useful technique that directs brain activity hypnotically into a state of monotony to induce sleep involves taking a few slow deep cleansing breaths and then silently counting numbers slowly backward from 100 with eyes closed, while mentally drawing numbers being counted and refocusing any wandering thoughts back onto counting numbers.

Eventually, mental verbalizations and visualizations gradually drift wakefulness into a hypnotic trance with mental imagery that ushers in dreaming and sleep onset. Several cycles of mentally visualizing numbers slowly counted backward from 100 may be necessary to clear away any circulating body vehicle adrenaline maintaining wakefulness.

When anxiety or stress prevents sleep onset and causes awareness of heartbeats with pounding in the chest, synchronizing silently counted numbers with the experienced heartbeats may help establish a monotonous rhythm to induce sleep.

The amount of sleep that appears to generally suffice to rest and rejuvenate many adult individuals under most circumstances ranges between 6–8 hours per night. The body vehicle requires more rest and sleep to recover and reenergize when experiencing higher levels of stress and physical wear and tear. Individual sleep requirements are determined better by gauging the amount of sleep necessary to feel refreshed and energetic upon spontaneously awakening without an alarm clock in the morning after going to sleep unstressed at a reasonable bedtime. Therefore, sleep is vital for maintaining body vehicle health, mental brain function, emotional balance, and proper weight.

In busy, modern Western societies sleep is often interrupted and cut short with alarm clocks that signal the need to start busy daily routines. Consequently, to ensure adequate sleep, setting the alarm to interrupt daily routines and indicate the need to get ready for sleep is a sensible strategy for sleep-deprived individuals unable to prioritize sleep over continuing to engage in daily routines.

21.4.4 Dreams

Dreams are pictorial stories that comprise the animation of sleep. Sleep includes a restful dream state with **rapid eye movement (REM)** as part of the full body vehicle mental and physical recovery experience.

Dreams are physiologic electrochemical discharges redistributing electron energies among higher-order brain areas charged up with energy while processing life experiences and thoughts surrounding daily living. During sleep, while voluntary physical activities shut down and the body vehicle is idly suspended in a regenerative state to recover from accumulated mental and physical wear and tear, brain executive functions substantially switch off to correct accrued energy and biochemical imbalances and clear out brain toxins accumulated during wakefulness. Energy impulses and movement of electrical energies throughout brain centers during sleep create thoughts, images, and emotions recognized as dreaming.

Dreams exemplify the "real" world of illusion, perception, and recall programmed and stored within neurochemical circuits of higher-order brain areas that discharge electrochemically to create emotional and physical brain experiences imagined as real and trigger feelings that individuals have learned to experience while awake. During dreaming, flowing electrochemical brain energies encapsulating thoughts and thought fragments bleed into each other and blend into recognizable stories uncharacteristic of the orderliness, predictability, and permanence of conscious real-world experiences.

Dreaming offers the best dry-run opportunities to act out behaviors and actions risk-free without reprisal, repercussion, or suffering from negative real-life consequences. Within dreams, dramatized human scenarios and life situations are viewed or enacted to help solve problems and resolve conflicts and dilemmas encountered during daily living.

Dreaming helps provide insight into personal existence that contributes toward maintaining a healthier emotional balance. Awakening with relief to recognize that a harrowing "real" experience was only a dream and that there are no real-life injuries, deaths, or compromises provides thought-provoking perspectives concerning real-life circumstances.

For the fortunate who have skillfully mastered the ability to identify and manipulate their dream state experience, sleep offers the opportunity to tailor dream experiences to understand the operations of the real world better or to discharge pent-up emotions and frustrations. Unfulfilled need for restful sleep and dreaming increases body vehicle disrepair, dysfunction, and stress, and bottles up emotional energies from unresolved conflicts that create emotional turmoil and adversely affect the quality of wakefulness to derail choosing healthy.

Sleep deprivation and insufficient sleep duration cut off opportunities for REM sleep with dreaming that occur in short, several minute spurts throughout sleep and get progressively longer as sleep duration increases. Restorative sleep and dreaming are essential for maintaining health and appropriate weight and provide opportunities to balance emotional energies and subconsciously resolve personal conflicts, which otherwise predispose to unhealthy behaviors including emotional and mindless eating causing unwanted weight gain.

21.4.5 Mass Media and Media "Programming"

Mass media strives to usurp human attention and wakefulness.

Ironically, media programming is used frequently as an option to fill available free time and serve as a diversion from daily routines and for resting and relaxation. Media programming fills consumer free time at a price. Media steals away moments of time available for humans to rest, exercise, and perform other healthy and creative activities to ply its trade and capitalize. Mass media and media programming are instruments that industry employs to shape consumer interests and control human behaviors.

Electronic devices are the tools used to accomplish media deeds. Technological devices convert streaming free thinking into streaming of thinking through calculating media programming applications packed with manipulative advertising and propaganda. Electronic media devices deliver mentally provocative and emotionally unsettling programming interspersed with commercial advertising to interrupt and purposely redirect spontaneous mind activity, disrupt true relaxation, and gradually drain out body vehicle physical energies.

Thinking that continually engages with media devices remains "online" to be exploited. Spending excessive time watching emotionally stimulating and psychologically disturbing media programming forfeits available opportunities for dialing down overactive thoughts, regenerative rest, and healthy physical activities and ratchets up personal stress levels to impact health adversely. Plugging into electronic media devices by tuning into handheld or planted screens bleeds restorative, creative, and productive moments out of daily routines.

Fixating daily for hours at a time onto screens that generate electronic images and sounds to stimulate body vehicle visual and auditory sensory portals artificially is far from a natural and healthy human activity. The primitive lower order brain stem contains a sensory information filtering domain to protect survival called the **reticular activating system (RAS),** which acts as an **arousal gatekeeper** or **brain alert network (BAN)** that governs wakefulness and sleep-wake transitions.

Stimulation of body vehicle sensors with new information that the brain must process and act upon or disregard activates RAS BAN to arouse higher-order brain areas to alert consciousness and induce wakefulness. Body vehicle visual and auditory sensory portals bombarded with a continuous barrage of various sights and sounds, and emotionally evocative events excite RAS BAN to activate alertness and vigilance to focus attention and seize wakefulness.

Whenever the brain receives no new sensory information for processing or interpretation, RAS BAN deactivates to allow the brain to power down and enter a sleep mode. Therefore, dull or unvarying environments lacking new, exciting, or intense stimuli to excite RAS BAN lower transmission of arousal signaling to the brain to permit true rest. Media forces powerfully exploit RAS BAN to control consumer attention and accomplish media ends. Media deliberately excites RAS BAN by presenting novelty and unusual, bizarre, disturbing, inciting, or unexpected subject matter to stimulate RAS BAN and augment brain receptiveness for commercial messaging and directives. "News" alerts flash **novel information** piquing human curiosity and interest, appealing to the imagination, inciting strong emotions or outcry, or triggering survival instincts to unlock the brain to receive shipments of media couriered informational Trojan horses that inseminate commercial directives and propaganda into brain programming.

News organizations continuously "deliver news happening now" opportunistically to feed increasing societal demands for immediate gratification and the regular delivery of information and sustain undivided audience attention. Media audiences would promptly shut down their minds and withdraw attention, and media outlets would quickly lose revenues and risk market viability if viewers and listeners were routinely subjected to "olds" or "same olds," being information that has already been extensively transmitted, circulated, considered, and is "in-the-know." Additionally, the experience or anticipation of "news" events arousing excitement surges brain dopamine to drive brain pleasure-reward behavioral loops and further reinforce "news" seeking behaviors.

The continuous stimulation of RAS BAN with electronic devices that command undivided attention toward media programming and LED screens is incompatible with and sabotages rest. Electronic media devices activate RAS BAN to interrupt and disrupt ongoing rhythms of body vehicle mental and physical functioning, and derail brain, and physical activities for channeling toward media directed purposes. Rest opportunities become sacrificed casualties when encountering mass media programming.

LED devices, such as televisions, laptop and desktop computers, tablets, and cell phones, when used before bedtime especially create a lingering effect on the brain to delay sleep onset, reduce sleep quality, and lead to morning tiredness after sleep.

Media programming broadcasts numerous offerings including news; sports, talk, opinion, reality, and variety shows; infomercials; comedy and musical performances; educational presentations; etc., ostensibly to inform, provide excitement, distract from boredom and stressful daily routines, and fill available free time.

In reality, media programming competitively vies for any moments of consumer attention to sell commercial industry products and services or propaganda, while stealing valuable lifetime otherwise available to channel toward healthier, more gratifying, and personally rewarding endeavors such as rest, creative projects, intellectual pursuits, physical activity, and direct interpersonal communication and social interactions.

Human weaknesses and basic survival needs are vulnerabilities for media and commercial entities intent on influencing consumer decisions and interests to exploit for manipulating and controlling human behaviors.

Hunger is a primal human biological drive routinely exploited to influence behavior as evidenced by the higher volume of food-related advertising broadcast during typical mealtime hours. Human pleasure and reproduction drives serve as the basis for using sex commercially to captivate consumer attention and sell industry products and services.

Mind control is also accomplished more effectively when brain processing is vulnerably receptive to repetitious suggestions and subliminal messaging such as during tiredness, exemplified when hypnotists purposely induce sleep to hypnotize subjects more easily. For example, television infomercials strategically play on human ignorance and aspirations for personal improvement and societal advantage, while also opportunely capitalizing on human tiredness and need for rest to broadcast marketing pitches repetitively when psychological resistance is lower, as occurs during late night hours when body vehicle biological rhythms prefer to shut down and sleep.

The human fascination for observing others displaying unusual quirks, talents, or characteristics under a variety of life circumstances is another media target to bait viewer and listener interest and captivate attention.

Media transmitted information which alerts humans to survival threats or a drastic upset of the status quo predictably tunes in large numbers of consumers conveniently to increase the collective level of focused attention available for commercial exploitation.

Human tragedy, conflict, violence, war, murder, or death especially involving widely known entertainment celebrities and sports stars are common themes to arouse interest on a mass scale and create greater media opportunities for disseminating commercial messages and propaganda.

Media programming that incites strong human emotions and outrage stimulates a survival fight or flight adrenaline rush, which heightens attention and recall for any coincidentally advertised commercial industry products and services.

Emotionally charged, interesting, entertaining, and purportedly informational programming that strongly increases attention also lowers wariness and defensive guard against subliminal commercial directives and propaganda covertly embedded within programming transmissions. Commercially successful media outlets are unlikely to present balanced programming to relieve tension, reassure, and allow rest, since anxiety, uncertainty, and unrest grab the attention and interest of media audiences more effectively. Balanced programming that addresses salient human issues intelligently and objectively is unlikely to raise human interest to levels that draw large enough audiences, which can translate into mass consumer spending profitable enough to entice commercial industry sponsorship of the programming.

Periodicals such as magazines, newspapers, and commercially sponsored professional journals are additional media forums that intensively compete for consumer attention and available free time, and routinely come packed with persuasive advertising from various commercial and corporate sponsors. Additionally, as highlighted during the highly contentious and divisive 2016 U.S. presidential election, unscrupulous and dishonest media entities even create **fake news,** and intentionally fabricate information to incite, outrage, mislead, and manipulate media engrossed consumers to advance the commercial, corporate, or political interests of media outlets and program sponsors.

Media productions edit human experiences into compressed highlights delivered with tightly scripted language to arouse interest, curiosity, fantasy, disgust, concern, or outrage, intentionally to fixate viewer and listener attention and lock plugged in visual and auditory sensory portals into electronic media devices.

Viewers and listeners unwarily succumb to media-induced trances naively believing they are resting, recovering from taxing daily routines, being informed, or deriving temporary respite and a quick runaway escape from daily hostilities, personal stresses, unpleasant thoughts, worries, or self-neglect. Instead, their fixated attention locks sensory portals into programming mode to trap consciousness over revenue-generating media time slots in a binding spell difficult to escape. Captivated audiences baited by enticing television, radio, and other media programming modalities become unsuspectingly trapped like penned prey to be held in place until consumed by commercial and corporate interests. Therefore, media exerts large-scale mind control by plugging humanity en masse into the electronic grid, which generates electronic illusions to flood fixated sensory portals with artificial stimulation that works to brainwash and shape the behaviors of engaged minds.

Electronic media devices and media programming are the conduits that connect corporate and commercial interests with potential customers. Media outlets generate revenues by selling advertising opportunities for the highest price to commercial and corporate industry bidders. Advertisers pay top dollar for spots on prime-time media programming forums that draw large audiences to access and maximally capture media served consumer prey.

Media outlets vie to survive and prosper within competitive markets by working all available angles to build human interest for programming broadcasts and increase audience numbers to drive up network ratings and attract paying sponsors, even if working angles requires inciting mass hysteria and creating controversies where none may exist.

News talk programs continuously spin propaganda revving emotions of partisan audiences into a frenzy. Media then packs scheduled programming with overt or subliminal advertising directives to influence audience perspectives and steer consumer behaviors according to corporate and commercial industry preferences. The immense profitability of popular media programming is acknowledged by one radio talk show host who requests to be excused for an obscene profit break when commercial advertisements must interrupt his scheduled broadcasts.

Successful media personnel who have sizable numbers of followers and attract large audiences skillfully manipulate the perceptions of viewers and listeners using illusion, deception, innuendo, and controversy to profit and serve the interests of advertising sponsors and media enterprise and outlet owners. As audiences intently view and listen to media broadcasts, commercial messages from program sponsors and advertisers bombard the visual and auditory sensory portals of the face to penetrate deeply into the recesses of a receptively logged on brain.

Human weaknesses that bring together large groups of attentive prospective consumers provide strategic openings for advertisers to make profitable commercial killings that are easier than shooting game fish in a barrel. Therefore, media intentionally creates and transmits human controversy, competition, conflict, and suffering, or presents the outrageous to draw in and captivate viewer and listener attention, and then collects advertising dollars from commercial industries similarly attracted to circumstances that congregate substantial numbers of prospective customers conveniently tuned in to receive delivered advertising messages.

Successful media transmissions that predictably draw sizable numbers of potential consumers with regularity to maximize advertising impact and profit potential are the *regularly scheduled daily or weekly series programs.* Regularly scheduled series programs are promoted and advertised heavily with enticing highlights to trigger the release of motivating dopamine and train body vehicle clocks and timers to anticipate that next fix of programming, which stimulates hedonistic pleasure-reward centers of the brain on scheduled commercial industry time.

When attention glues to media device screens, marketing strategies employ state-of-the-art psychological techniques to break through protective mental barriers and drive surreptitious "programming" messages deep into brain memory banks. Brainwashing and behavioral conditioning rely on repetitive messaging to imprint directives enduringly into executive decision-making centers of the brain.

Repeated exposures to advertisements increase consumer familiarity and comfort with advertised messages to prime acceptance for advertised products and services commercially offered later. Commercials regularly interrupting media offerings with provocative and enticing messaging are eventually swallowed hook, line, and sinker into the gullet of the brain to saturate brain processing and recall areas for ready access anytime. Advertising directives repeatedly presented during various programming moments engineered to arouse consciousness become implanted like hypnotic suggestions that await germination to control consumer behaviors on the order of industry buzzwords and cues.

Electronic connectivity disseminates marketing directives, and propaganda on a mass-scale to facilitate hypnotic suggestion, strategic influence, and instantaneous manipulation of widespread segments of humanity, as evidenced when online videos go viral in a matter of hours through social media forums, or how tweeted comments spread rapidly to followers to impact societal opinions and perspectives readily. Ultimately, media programming offerings are only tasty bait on a hook, while commercial advertisements are the real hook capturing the big game consumers having the available financial means and money to spend.

Advertised messages and words from program sponsors that "interrupt" regularly scheduled program broadcasts carry out the actual "programming" of broadcast audiences. Consequently, commercial industries use various media modalities to assimilate **Trojan horse ideas** into potential consumers through advertising to reprogram subconscious minds to serve commercial industry purposes and interests.

The strategic marketing of pharmaceutical agents through television and radio advertising provides a glimpse of how media primes individuals for commercial control. Advertisements leverage health care consumers to readily accept and follow the advice of credentialed health care providers who prescribe the pharmaceutical products advertised through media outlets.

Advertisers encourage consumers with health conditions commercially targeted for industry treatments to consult their "providers" concerning the advertised therapies. Meanwhile, product detail personnel from drug companies visit "provider" practices to promote advertised therapies and leave product samples and purchase discount coupons. Subsequently, when consumers suffering health problems targeted by advertisers ask "providers" about trying advertised treatments, "providers" are more prone to accommodate health care consumer requests and prescribe the promoted treatments to consumers primed to accept prescriptions for advertised treatments without objection.

A classic forum to profitably advertise pharmaceutical products are the Olympic Games, which numerous individuals sidelined by health impairments, physical ailments and limitations, and aging watch dreaming that they could or once did accomplish such marvelous physical human feats.

21.4.6 Commercial Advertising

Commercial advertising communicates what is meant to be believed, remembered, and recalled. Advertising systematically permeates the collective consciousness of individuals subliminally to establish an expansive market presence for corporate interests and commercial products and services. Even within the Garden of Eden in Paradise, Adam and Eve were deceived to desire and misled to acquire something more than everything else available in all of Paradise, which unfortunately led them into big trouble.

Marketing strategies cleverly cater to human drives for improvement, advantage, and attainment of something better or more, and create illusions portraying enticing opportunities to increase vantage, fortune, health, and command of time, or to reduce pain, suffering, stress, and the ravages of aging and poor lifestyle choices to sell commercial industry wares. Human paranoias, uncertainties, fears, and mistrust are routine targets for marketing strategies to increase commercial sales and industry profitability. Advertisers also pander to human vices such as lust, gluttony, greed, sloth, envy, vanity, and wrath, and peddle easy and convenient ways to achieve pleasure, wealth, beauty, power, retribution, or survival advantages for money to insidiously influence consumer commercial behaviors.

Commercial advertisers hire skilled actors to adroitly cloak marketing and industry intentions behind calculated smiles, mannerisms, and staged performances on carefully designed sets to entice and commercially entrap unwary consumers attentive to media programming.

Media starts to program consumers early in life, when young children are planted in front of television screens or given handheld electronic media devices during vulnerable developmental years when brain plasticity is maximal, and behaviors are most amenable to molding and conditioning.

The evil television or other electronic babysitter media devices transmit animated characters, clowns, stories, games, and "educational" material deliberately targeting and connecting with impressionable young minds, which are easily influenced, programmed, and trained for future industry control and manipulation.

Surreptitiously implanted behavioral programming is then strategically activated later under commercial settings signaling the appropriate cues to trigger the embedded mind control opportunely. Scientific reports describe increased food industry sales of sugary cereals achieved merely by aiming the direction of eye gaze of familiar media cartoon characters advertised on cereal cartons downward toward unsuspecting children walking grocery store aisles, exemplifying successful commercial programming methods used against children.

The connecting gaze of familiar media cartoon characters displayed on cereal boxes powerfully captivates the attention of media programmed young minds, prompting preferential selection for purchase of sugary cereals that contribute toward childhood obesity, which leads to adult obesity and numerous other health problems later in life.

The costs of media programming and commercial industry advertising to steer individuals into addictification behavior traps are insignificant compared to the astronomical profits earned by establishing lifelong addictification routines in consumers for advertised products.

Some media advertising and marketing techniques employed by commercial industries include

1. inviting personal, emotional, and physical attachment to commercial products and services
2. connecting human expressions or experiences such as smiles, happiness, and feelings of exhilaration with specific commercial products
3. relating desirable human qualities such as uniqueness and independence to product use
4. creating artificial scarcity for products and service offers (only a few left), and then using scare tactics to create urgency and pressure purchases (hurry, act or call now while supplies last and before time runs out) with threats that purchase delays will miss promotional opportunities (special offer applies only for a limited time or while supplies last)
5. offering seemingly inexpensive low-priced commercial opportunities that provide surprisingly enormous benefits in return (ostensibly offering "more" for "less")
6. proposing that the purchase and use of advertised wares will somehow grant personal advantages in power, privilege, uniqueness, or social acceptance
7. providing unrealistically quick fixes to complex and difficult personal, social, occupational, or financial problems for a relatively "small price to pay"
8. offering opportunities for commercial products and services ostensibly for free or purportedly with no obligation to buy simply for investing attention and trying advertised commercial offers for a short time
9. selling the idea that spending money on products or services equals saving money, whereby in reality money spent becomes immediately unavailable to buy anything else later
10. providing seductive opportunities to buy and obtain immediate gratification with no money down and deferred payback of created debt at low "affordable" interest rates
11. convincing consumers that spending money to purchase commercial products and services somehow does the world a

good deed to help others and contributes to making the world a better place to live for everyone

21.4.7 **Working for Media**

Advertisers pay millions of dollars for choice advertising spots on television and other media forums to reach and influence large numbers of viewers and listeners. Media is an influence tool used on humanity to inseminate and disseminate concepts and ideas that allow commercial and corporate interests to manipulate and control human interests.

Advertising on television and other media outlets works well to influence, manipulate, and control consumer behaviors. Scheduled programming also powerfully shapes media audience attitudes, perspectives, frames of reference, practices, norms, and commercial spending habits. The television and movie industries purposely design programming satisfying the purposes of sponsoring investors and underwriters. Therefore, media and media programming are conduits that run agendas for corporate and commercial interests. Consequently, little controversy exists as to why various media outlets earn billions of dollars yearly from advertisers that reap great financial rewards and other successes using media outlets to market and sell their commercial products and services or ideas.

In 2013, household surveys by the U.S. Bureau of Labor and Statistics ascertained that U.S. Americans on average spent at least 2 hours daily watching television or engaging in other media programming activities, while some private companies surveying Americans estimated these activities consumed on average more than 4 hours daily of individual American time.

More recent statistics estimate that many individuals plug into electronic media devices up to eight hours per day. Directing personal attention regularly for 2 hours daily into any commercially sponsored media activity undoubtedly influences commercial, social, and health choices and behaviors.

The significance and potential impact of regularly devoting personal time to engage in any activity can be appreciated better by translating overall time investments into full-time work week or college study semester units. Watching television or engaging in other media device activities for only 2 hours daily six days per week for 50 weeks out of the year amounts to committing 600 hours to view television or engage with media devices for the year (2 hr./d × 6 d/wk. × 50 wks.). Average full-time scheduled work weeks are usually 40 hours long, and full-time college study also demands approximately 40 hours per week to attend classes and complete homework studies during semesters that typically last 15 weeks. Consequently, 600 hours per year divided by 40 hour weeks equals 15 weeks of full-time work or 1 college semester of study spent instead to watch television or engage with media devices 2 hours daily 6 days per week for 50 weeks during the year.

Over a 10-year period, devoting 2 hours daily 300 days per year to watching television or engage in other media device activities totals 150 40-hour weeks of full-time work or college study (10 yrs × 15 wks/yr); equaling an astounding 3 years of full-time work (working 50 weeks with 2 weeks off for vacation per year) or 10 semesters of full-time college study lost that could have translated instead into enormous occupational or educational opportunities to enhance personal existence.

Watching television and engaging in other media device driven activities on a regular basis without earning real lifetime benefits in return carelessly disposes of valuable lifetime otherwise available for more productive and personally enriching life endeavors.

Consumer times lost plugging into television, and other media devices amount to commercial industry and corporate mind control time gained, as over a 10-year span of connecting 2 hours daily, industry snatched a whopping 3-year opportunity to work on, condition, change, manipulate, and control viewer behaviors, choices, perceptions, and expectations to create quite a resume builder for consumers to include under lifetime accomplishments.

21.4.8 Rest & Relaxation Suggestions

1. Make adequate rest a priority and regular daily routine.
2. Plan daily activities to complete personal, social, and occupational duties and responsibilities efficiently to allow ample time for restful relaxation.
3. Reduce external sources of stimulation that heighten general states of arousal and wakefulness when resting.
4. Limit access to technological communication devices while resting.
5. Turn off the TV, stop texting, and avoid using the computer, laptop, cell phone, and other electronic media devices during rest times.
6. Take a temporary sensory time-out to lower brain stimulation when feeling excessively tired, extremely stressed, or overloaded with external demands, and meditate or vegetate for a short time without distractions to reenergize and refocus thoughts.
7. Utilize short power naps in quiet surroundings whenever necessary during the day to recharge dropping energy levels.
8. Commit to a scheduled bedtime that provides adequate sleep to feel refreshed upon awakening in the morning.
9. Avoid the use of stimulating chemical substances such as tobacco, alcohol, and caffeine, which clear slowly from the blood and linger to interfere with restful sleep and reduce sleep quality, particularly when used soon before bedtime.

21.5 TOXICITY AVOIDANCE

At birth, most body vehicles come delivered with health to be preserved, protected, and maintained and not lost and regained. The body vehicle is naturally built and programmed to heal and survive. **Toxicity** consists of any detrimental force, behavior, or activity that adversely impacts the body vehicle integrity to disturb homeostasis and create unfavorable structural or functional body vehicle consequences disadvantageous to health, well-being, or survival.

Toxicity results in injury and stresses that provoke compensatory body vehicle survival and corrective repair responses to reestablish homeostasis. Avoidance of body vehicle toxicity helps preserve and defend body vehicle health. Body vehicle toxicity that leads to deterioration of health and well-being commonly develops through body vehicle **neglect, abuse,** or **incorrect care.** Neglect indicates insufficient or absent body vehicle care. Abuse means overdoing it and excessively exposing the body vehicle to good or bad things. Incorrect care involves delivering inappropriate or inadequate body vehicle care.

The body vehicle can become toxic directly by introducing toxins through the mouth, skin and skin structures, nasal passages, lungs, genitourinary organs, and rectum, or indirectly by stimulating the physical senses of sight, hearing, smell, taste, and touch to negatively affect personal thinking, perception, and behaviors.

Body vehicle toxicity often is unintentional or incidental as commonly occurs directly through ingestion of food additives and contaminants and pharmaceutical and health product inactive ingredients; contact with industry manufactured or environmental toxins, and inhalation of air pollution; or indirectly from exposure to disturbing and stressful social circumstances. Body vehicle nutrition, health, function, and survival are particularly affected by orally ingested substances including food, food additives, drugs, and herbal and dietary health substances that pass internally down the gut.

Anything that passes down the gut interacts with and becomes further chemically and biologically transformed by the digestive juices and residing gut microbial flora to exert more complex and often unanticipated and undefined biological effects on the body vehicle system. Many of the human toxicities that economically burden individuals and society result from ingesting legal commercial products sold to feed humanity, restore or enhance health, manage weight, or provide humans with tasty fun, entertainment, and a temporary escape from reality.

Processed and refined dietary sugars, fats, and proteins, and prescribed, over-the-counter, and recreational drugs and health and weight loss supplements combine to cause the bulk of costly biochemical human injuries. Any orally ingested toxins including alcohol, tobacco residues, and toxic agents contained in foods, medicines, herbal and dietary health supplements, and hygiene products such as toothpaste and mouthwash gain direct blood access through the gut to distribute extensively throughout the entire body vehicle and exert widespread system toxicities harmful to health.

Toxins delivered through the gut can sensitize intestinal and liver immune system of defense cells to prime immune responses to subsequently develop severe adverse immune reactions, upon repeat exposure to recognized toxins passing through the gut or contacting the skin and other body vehicle membranes of the nasal passages and lungs. Noxious substances delivered into the gastrointestinal tract may also unfavorably modify existing gut microbiota to precipitate further untoward health effects. Consequently, the gut is a strategic body vehicle access point for Trojan horse toxins to enter and then destroy body vehicle health from within through numerous mechanisms.

Uniquely, the mouth is a two-way street for producing body vehicle toxicity since toxicity can occur not only through what enters but also by what comes out of the mouth as experienced by agreeing to or inappropriately saying something which then leads to unintended consequences. As noted, various other protective body vehicle barrier linings such as the skin and mucous membranes of the eyes, respiratory tract, and genitourinary system also absorb chemical toxins. Air quality affects body vehicle health, and air pollution, smoke, and indoor cooking fumes have long been known to exert harmful health effects and lead to cancer in humans. Aerosolized and evaporating chemical household cleaners, sanitizers, or beauty and hygiene products scatter toxic vaporized molecules into the air that predispose toward causing body vehicle injury when inhaled. Beauty, hygiene, and medicinal products applied to skin penetrate to become absorbed and disperse throughout the body vehicle to adversely affect many other incidentally exposed body vehicle cells. Scientific communities have growing concerns for potential human toxicities related to unregulated **cosmeceuticals,** which are formulated beauty and hygiene products sold as purportedly having antiaging or health enhancing medicinal properties.

Body vehicle toxicity then occurs unsuspectingly from skin or mucous membrane contact with potential poisons delivered through polluted air, beauty and hygiene products, skin sanitizers, and household cleaners. Consumers ultimately fail to benefit if prospective scientific determinations discover that prior use of certain manufactured products including vitamins or herbal and dietary health supplements increases body vehicle risks for cancer or other illnesses. Consequently, avoidance of all unnecessary exposures to nonessential artificially manufactured chemical substances without definitively proven benefit to body vehicle function or survival is prudent to prevent unintentional or incidental toxicity, which can develop through a multitude of complex, poorly understood, unknown, or unexpected chemical and biological mechanisms.

Finally, abusive and oppressive social interactions, personal relationships, or obligations also toxify body vehicle health and well-being. Therefore, the best health and survival approach is to avoid body vehicle toxicity through direct or casual and incidental means to prevent body vehicle harm and preserve body vehicle physical and functional integrity.

It is noteworthy to acknowledge the absence of any reputable scientific studies which have conclusively determined that long-term ingestion of plain water along with a balanced diet of diversified natural crude fuel whole earth foods causes epidemic illnesses or leads to survival disadvantages in humans.

21.5.1 General Categories for Sources of Toxicities Precipitating Body Vehicle Injury and Stress

Chemical: introduced as food additives; food container substances that migrate into wrapped or contained food products; environmental, food processing, and spoilage-generated food contaminants and toxins; refined sugars, fats, and proteins in processed foods; manufactured pharmaceutical and health industry products including medicines, vitamins, and other health and dietary supplements; alcohol, nicotine and tobacco products, and recreational substances of abuse; hygiene and beauty products; sanitizing and cleaning agents; industrial wastes, and air pollution

Physical: precipitated by excessive cellular and tissue wear and tear occurring through friction, impact, or any other mechanical forces including from extreme exercise and overuse; trauma such as from falls, motor vehicle accidents, and gunshot wounds; and prolonged immobility or inactivity.

Thermal or radiation: developing through unprotected or prolonged exposure to sun, radiation energy, or extremely hot or cold temperatures.

Biological: occurring from exposure to plant, animal, or insect organisms and their components and products that incite extreme body vehicle immune reactivity or directly poison the body vehicle system; pathologic parasitic infestations and microbial infections; and adverse alterations in friendly native body vehicle microbial compositions.

Emotional: following the experience of oppression; deprivation with unmet emotional or physical needs or expectations; personal loss; negative and abusive relationships; and overwhelming personal, social, and financial demands and obligations.

Neglect: caused by inadequate attention or time devoted to appropriately maintain body vehicle upkeep or allow tissue and cellular recovery and repair to complete after injury or excessive physical use.

21.5.2 Toxicity Leads to Body Vehicle Stress and Repair Injury

Any toxic pressures that destabilize body vehicle structure or function and disturb homeostasis or lead to biological damages induce compensatory survival stress responses and corrective repairs that can independently provoke further body vehicle damages in a vicious cycle. Engaging stress responses harms the body vehicle analogously to how mobilizing the armed forces to perform war exercises in preparation for battle coincidentally damages the environment utilized for battle practice. Stress independently activates metabolic reactions that generate toxic oxygen free radicals and reactive oxygen species to compound injuries induced by initial noxious insults.

Body vehicle injuries occurring from any cause initiate corrective biological repair mechanisms that attempt to return the body vehicle system to baseline homeostasis and function. Biological repair mechanisms can, in turn, generate secondary tissue and cellular injuries, analogously to how restorative or rebuilding construction projects create messes during repair or refurbishment activities.

Compensatory survival responses redistribute body vehicle energies and compel feeding as necessary to meet the additional energy demands of cellular and tissue repairs returning the system to homeostasis, which may lead to unwanted weight gain. Injury and stress create pain and suffering that trigger runaway escape coping behaviors including emotional eating, further predisposing to unwanted weight gain. Body vehicle toxicities causing injury and stress combine with the adverse effects of compensatory behavioral and corrective repair responses to degrade body vehicle health and well-being and accelerate aging to decrease longevity and shorten life-span.

21.5.3 Emotional Stresses Activate Emotional Feeding Impulses

Emotional stresses that develop for any reason in the context of daily living independently affect body vehicle energy metabolism and feeding behaviors. The experience of emotional stress alarms the body vehicle system and triggers stress hormone release which promotes fat storage and stress eating.

Emotional stresses distract mental clarity and focus to impair personal restraint and voluntary self-control and facilitate the discharge of primal survival feeding impulses that induce mindless eating. Emotional stresses also lead to suffering requiring relief, conveniently obtained by consuming tasty commercial food products that potently deliver fleeting on-demand taste pleasures giving runaway escapes that temporarily relieve suffering. Finally, emotional stresses affect the integrity of gut membranes and the microbiome, which, in turn, impact body vehicle well-being potentially to perpetuate emotional dysfunction in a vicious cycle.

21.5.4 Brain Drain Strain and Stress of Excess

Missing a sense of life purpose to aimlessly ride the societal hamster wheel of human activity without a destination point generates stress. Lack of directional vision and decisional uncertainty in daily living provoke anxiety and promote despair. However, highly regimented and tightly scheduled personal, social, and occupational daily routines that demand excessive attention and a heavy sacrifice of personal time and energy to complete are oppressive to body vehicle biologic clocks and timers.

The need to multitask continually to navigate and keep up with busy schedules having competing obligations creates busy on-the-go lives that lack enough opportunity for plain spontaneity to enjoy moments at hand or solely to ponder.

Excessive things and thoughts with limited time clutter the mind to cause brain overload.

Biological functional limits exist for the volume of data and information that the brain can comfortably and reliably process, interpret, organize, and act upon simultaneously at any given time. Excessive personal obligations, distractions, and life minutiae requiring all-at-once informational processing clutter and overload brain computational circuits and create stress.

The limits of functional brain processing are evident when attempting to understand what five or even two people talking at once are saying. Multitasking likewise stresses body vehicle programming and executive capabilities and works poorly for optimal brain functioning. Physical and biological limitations prevent the body vehicle from being in different places and doing different things all at the same time. When running brain programs deplete memory cache and exceed functional brain capabilities to overload brain circuits, thinking slows into bottlenecks that impede the orderly flow of thoughts to hamper brain performance and creativity. Additionally, as demands and expectations grow, and time constraints increase to reduce available time, physical and mental body vehicle performance errors increase to ultimately cost body vehicle existence.

Under duress, stress, and time constraints, central brain processing may not even reach conscious awareness, and data delivered to the brain may be stored for later or ignored entirely possibly depriving the brain of valuable survival information. Subliminal messaging delivered during times of informational brain overload targets subconscious awareness mechanisms for future exploitation.

As a behavioral default, the body vehicle system strives to execute the most efficient programs that simplify and reduce work efforts to accomplish goals, and system overload may provoke unwarranted shortcuts or neglect in completing responsibilities, meeting obligations, or performing tasks of daily living. Committing inordinate valuable personal time and energy to manage multiple priorities and life details simultaneously overloads and encumbers brain function to diminish life quality, especially when experiencing the full meaning of tasks at hand becomes neglected and sacrificed.

The accumulation of too many obligations and responsibilities to complete interferes with accomplishing the truly important. Brain clutter increases vulnerability to industry misdirection, manipulation, and exploitation.

Cluttered time→ deprivation→ misery→ suffering→ vulnerability→ exploitation

Overload stress spreads throughout brain activity like an expanding seizure focus to disrupt the orderly processing and workflow of brain cells and trigger mindless automatic behaviors. Overloaded brains lose the capability to extinguish brain signal noise that sidetracks ordered thinking and deliberate actions, compromising self-control and the ability to resist unhealthful urges and addictification behaviors predisposing to obesity. Therefore, overloading and cluttering brain function reduces self-control leading to impulsivity and behaving without thinking of future consequences, allowing behaviors to be driven automatically by programmed reactions as opposed to being guided by thoughtful and deliberate responses.

The brain channels electrical activity to efficiently accomplish tasks and goals and process sensory information and thoughts to attribute meaning to life experiences. However, channeling thinking through the brain in meaningful ways requires relaxation and life balance to focus and allow the data streaming through sensory portals to reach appropriate areas of the brain to be recognized, absorbed, processed, interpreted, organized, suitably addressed, and acted upon more comfortably and deliberately to maintain a healthy existence.

21.5.5 Maxedzurvival

Industry promotes amassing more and more, faster and faster, leaving less and less personal and humanistic time.

The commercial game is to make one obtain and then sustain through the pain to retain and maintain everything at all costs.

In modern commercially industrialized and technologically driven societies, many become maximally burdened toiling to accumulate and maintain possessions and persevering to meet unrealistic personal goals, expectations, commitments, demands, and obligations. Commercial industry systems exploit basic feeding and breeding with greed human survival drives to push consumers maximally to carry out these drives to the limits of human tolerance.

Maxedzurvival is a deliberate monetary, human existence at the extremes of physical and psychological tolerance. Maxedzurvival thinly stretches available personal energies, abilities, and resources to sustain financial spending acquiring things, maintaining possessions, and paying for various services. The self-induced, commercially driven maxedzurvival existence teeters on the brink of physical and mental breakdown and financial ruin. The maxedzurvival equilibrium consists of converting lifetime energies into money to spend on things and pay for accumulating debt. In the steady state of maxedzurvival cash flow, money earned equals money spent without leaving residual capital reserves or financial surpluses for personal leisure or to cover the expenses of unexpected emergencies.

In maxedzurvival mode, carrying out tasks such as managing personal property and possessions; meeting economic demands; fulfilling financial obligations; paying debts, and attempting to keep complicated commercially driven lives economically viable control, engulf, and consume daily existences to drain valuable physical life energies and personal lifetime eventually dry. An entourage of unwelcome service fees, taxes, interest charges, insurance costs, legal and financial consulting bills, agent and advisor commission expenses, and plain old daily costs of living line up eagerly to greet and consume excessively leveraged maxedzurvival existences.

Poor health and health care debt can complicate and greatly strain a maxedzurvival existence when illness and missed debt payments lead to insurmountable obstacles with monetary expenses and economic penalties that spell personal and financial disaster.

Maxedzurvival is a choice, whereas abject poverty is a socioeconomic hardship with insufficient life resources and inferior quality of human existence. Maxedzurvival produces extreme economic time pressures and stress from the challenge of working hectic schedules crammed with exhaustive routines to keep up commercially at all costs.

Maxedzurvival routines demand efficient and flawless execution as miscalculations or mistakes can wreck marginally tenable schedules. The strain of excessive time and monetary pressures pens up emotional stresses to diminish life quality and create feelings of sadness, anger, guilt, shame, anxiety, and depression as financially driven task-time disproportionately devours dwindling lifetime.

Struggling to work harder and longer to complete jam-packed schedules deliberately committed to obtaining, retaining, and maintaining more things, sacrifices life opportunities available to satisfy basic personal needs and predisposes to unhealthy behaviors that cause health problems and unwanted weight gain.

Maxedzurvival increases vulnerability for exploitation from profiteering industries that temptingly dangle addictification runaway escapes or rescue bail-outs to relieve individual predicaments and suffering. Greedy industry feeders seeking to extract more consumer *lifetime* in less time thrive on maxedzurvival existences.

A maxedzurvival existence chooses economic captivity with materialistic imprisonment. A rational life approach that avoids maxedzurvival navigates clear from purchases that are unaffordable with disposable income, won't regularly be utilized in any meaningful way, or will be too expensive, time-consuming, or burdensome to keep or maintain.

21.5.6 Black Holes

Black holes in the universe are stars that have imploded under the enormous weight of their amassed physical matter when the radiant internal energies keeping the star shining brightly outward have run out. Formed black holes become giant energy vortexes that vacuum up and inescapably trap all surrounding physical matter and energy within their immediate universe.

Under the weight of enormous life stresses overextended lives which regularly fail to fulfill basic body vehicle maintenance and progressively accrue unmet physical and emotional needs, become vulnerable to collapse into disrepair and dependency and implode to become **human black holes.** Human black holes unsuccessfully attempt to satisfy growing unmet body vehicle needs by spending progressively more lifetime consuming ever more commercial goods that provide limited satisfaction and diminishing personal returns for the lifetime invested in acquiring the goods. Human black holes increasingly succumb to commercial addictification and rescue bail-out dependification to drain the energies and charitable resources of the family, friends, and society helping to compensate for the repercussions erupting from the human default to meet personal maintenance needs naturally. Societal individuals who are full of positive life energy available to constructively help those genuinely in need to grow and prosper form some of the foundations of thriving human communities.

Black holes are life energy siphons.

Black holes inordinately consume the physical, mental, emotional, and financial energies and time of giving individuals and society to deplete limited resources available for helping the genuinely needy deserving of help. Human black holes renege on own responsibilities to take the initiative to establish and work toward meaningful life goals that contribute toward individual and societal improvement; and instead, undeservedly live at the expense of others to profit from the kindness and generosity of charitable individuals who share personal good fortunes and energies to help, and freely take undue advantage of societal safety net services and resources available for the truly needy.

Feeding black holes drain the resources and energies of society and charitable individuals dry. Escalating societal obesity, growing human reliance for nutritional sustenance on mass-produced processed food products, and progressive human dependence on chemical and pharmaceutical industries to counteract often personally induced health problems, reflect increasing societal and human shortcomings that are perpetuated opportunistically by profiteering commercial industries.

Societal financial, economic burdens provide the revenue streams that fund corporate and commercial interests and financially drive the profiteering systems that opportunistically thrive on temporarily remediating often self-inflicted individual and societal failures and shortcomings.

Human black holes draining societal resources and life energies are multiplying under existing commercial circumstances that miserably fail to adequately meet true basic human needs required for a long, healthy, and gratifying existence.

Accumulating numbers of human black holes having increasingly unmet personal needs are amassing to implode further to form enormous **societal black holes** causing exponentially soaring societal debt, which progressively swallows up national resources and wealth to ravage meaningful human existences paying for the escalating debt that lavishly funds burgeoning commercial industry earnings.

If the worst form of poverty is debt, then increased societal, economic time pressures with growing human self-neglect, addictification, and rescue dependification are creating an enormous societal black hole, which is collapsing into a vicious vortex of personal and societal health care debt that sucks society inescapably deeper into a gigantic hole of poverty.

Unfortunately, excessive and growing human needs with the disparity of resources to fulfill those needs lay the foundation for human conflict. Recognizing personal obligations and life responsibilities, and then taking the initiative to remain healthy, do good for self and others, and accomplish personal duties well in meaningful ways deliver greater individual life benefits for all to avert the conflicts that plunge society into disaster.

21.5.7 Planetary Escape with ME-TIME or Let-Me-Be Time

A time-honored rule for successful investing is to pay oneself first.
To take ownership of the body vehicle means to commit to its care.

Human activities invest valuable lifetime that predictably returns lifetime benefits or creates liabilities imposing lifetime costs. Successful management of the body vehicle corporation requires wise lifetime investment strategies, and prioritizing health-directed personal behaviors first is prudent. Meeting necessary body vehicle health needs promptly invests body vehicle lifetime wisely. Body vehicle health maintenance requires that adequate attention, time, and energy be devoted regularly daily to perform and complete biologic and humanistic body vehicle life functions and requisites correctly.

Basic body vehicle life activities include eating, hydrating, exercising, resting, eliminating waste, thinking creatively without interruption, socializing, and responding expeditiously to body vehicle maintenance signals, alerts, and alarms. Timely completion of required body vehicle care prevents body vehicle wear and tear from accumulating and eventually deteriorating the body vehicle to run it deep into the ground. Without committing time to care for body vehicle physical and emotional needs, the time available for necessary body vehicle upkeep is easily squandered away to lose precious opportunities to prevent body vehicle health disrepair.

Unexpected body vehicle disrepairs then create vulnerabilities for costly commercial industry rescue bail-outs. Acceptance of body vehicle physical and emotional limitations and need for maintenance acknowledges the personal obligation to attend to body vehicle needs without compromise to ensure the best chances of accomplishing individual life purpose.

Baby yourself and ask, "What have I done for me lately?"

Designate yourself as your own dependent and take full charge to fulfill essential basic personal maintenance needs as one would for a dependent baby. Always place the oxygen mask on first before attending to the needs of others as airlines safety instructions advise.

MAINTENANCE TIME
EQUALS
ME-TIME
ME-TIME is self-time.

ME-TIME is a gift of time to self to seize opportunities to perform and complete body vehicle maintenance and to ponder life meaning. Spending lifetime to pay oneself with personal maintenance increases life satisfaction and stores up energies to help others.

After meeting basic body vehicle physical and emotional needs, time can be directed to self-discovery and understanding others, and particularly to organize thinking and establish reasonable life goals and plans to carry out during the available lifetime. Therefore, ME-TIME is for body vehicle physical maintenance, and to satisfy mental and emotional needs, clear mental clutter, straighten out thinking, ponder life meaning to make sense of the world, and connect to others.

ME-TIME carried out with love and respect for the body vehicle enhances personal health, productivity, growth, and life satisfaction. A pleasurable human survival drive is spending time on self-maintenance as evidenced by the existence of SPA businesses, which have thrived for millennia fulfilling this vital human need. Humans derive happiness and gratification from a job well done, and even more so when the job well done tended toward meeting basic personal needs.

ME-TIME acknowledges the human need to meet certain fundamentals of personal care. Adding intellectual pursuits and new learning to ME-TIME completes basic self-maintenance with mental development and growth. The absence of devoted ME-TIME sacrifices precious opportunities for personal enhancement.

A starting point for satisfying ME-TIME begins with recognizing and understanding the biological time and energy limitations that apply to the body vehicle and then establishing a healthy balance between meeting internal and external body vehicle demands. ME-TIME assertiveness sets boundaries to limit outside commitments to manageable levels and reject external demands that competitively interfere with fulfilling necessary personal maintenance. Knowing when to say "no thank you" toward accepting further obligations or offers that produce hectic and unwieldy life schedules reinforces the sense of personal value to defend body vehicle health.

Failure to meet mandatory body vehicle maintenance needs can lead to body vehicle breakdown and susceptibility to addictification runaway escape or rescue bail-out behaviors that eventually compromise the ability to accommodate the needs of others. Self-neglect with absent ME-TIME deteriorates the sense of self-worth to create an opportunity for addictification and rescue industries to take over and commercially own body vehicle *lifetime.*

Proper nutrition is a vital component of ME-TIME. ME-TIME requires taking control of personal nutrition. The body vehicle dynamically repairs, refurbishes, replaces, and recycles cellular and tissue components continuously. Natural crude fuel whole earth foods deliver original "factory part" ingredients directly from the manufacturer Mother Nature to maintain top quality body vehicle parts and equipment at factory-installed specifications. Learning cooking skills that emphasize simple preparation of natural crude fuel whole earth foods assures provision of the best quality nutrients to satisfy body vehicle nutritional needs at the highest level.

Cooking and food ripeness provide a head start on digestion to compensate for any existing physical limitations that compromise the capability to chew or digest raw natural crude fuel whole earth foods properly. Occasionally, specific ingredients found only in raw foods to which the body vehicle may be sensitive or intolerant may be destroyed through cooking to allow the eating of those foods after cooking. Charring, burning, caramelizing, or overcooking foods reduces vitamin and other essential nutrient content and may produce cancer-causing substances termed carcinogens within burned or overly heated food constituents. Some inconspicuous examples of "burned" (heat prepared) foods that possibly harbor heat generated toxins or carcinogens such as **acrylamides** and **furans** include grain and potato products such as cereals, French fries, and potato chips, and roasted nuts and coffee beans. Additionally, avoiding overheating cooking oils to their **smoke point** prevents producing chemical reactions within the over-heated oils that generate toxic substances, which become unsuspectingly inhaled during cooking or ingested along with prepared foods.

Spending hard-earned money prudently to buy healthy, natural, crude fuel whole earth foods and wisely devoting precious time and energy to shop for, prepare, and eat healthy natural foods yield immeasurably greater rewards than sacrificing money, time, and energy later for health care to correct health problems developing from inappropriate body vehicle fueling. The effort to plan a weekly dietary menu creates a great blueprint to budget foods to fund basic body vehicle nutritional needs appropriately. Food selection, preparation, and cooking times constitute nutritional ME-TIME deliciously dedicated to self and exclusively set aside and made available for the thoughtful selection and preparation of choice nutrients to sensibly feed and nourish the body vehicle to maintain health.

Getting in touch with the health-promoting qualities of crude, unprocessed and unrefined, natural, whole earth foods begins with their handling and selection for purchase at the grocery store and continues through their preparation, consumption, and digestion. As an aside, healthy nutritional ME-TIME also depends on maintaining appropriate hand hygiene with the careful washing of the hands during food preparation and before eating.[11] Attending to nutritional ME-TIME complements other personal health maintenance activities to increase the probability of being around, able, and available for others when needed for a long time to come.

Commercial food industries are hijacking home food preparation and cooking times selling convenience services which create consumer dependency on artificially mass-produced and industrially delivered food products often consumed by individuals with indifference. Food industries work diligently to promote commercially profitable industry trends that turn home cooking opportunities upside down, by convincing consumers to substitute tasty artificial food pleasures and nutritionally hollow commercial eating experiences for the health benefits and satisfaction otherwise provided through the preparation of nutritious meals at home. Consequently, in hurried modern industrial societies, consumers are progressively giving up eating home prepared meals to order take-out or delivery or to eat readymade foods, which are replacing nutritional ME-TIME and contributing to societal obesity and health deterioration. Children have been especially vulnerable in succumbing to the powerful influences of the fast food industry to eat food away from home. Hints of an unfolding HESC (ʃ-shaped) time plot as depicted in the following graphs also appears to represent the progressive societal choosing to preferentially spend money for and eat meals prepared away from home.[12]

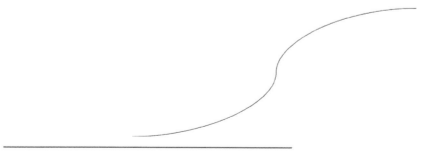

---

11. See "When & How to Wash Your Hands" at http://www.cdc.gov/.

12. https://www.ers.usda.gov/data-products/ag-and-food-statistics-charting-the-essentials/food-prices-and-spending/ https://www.bls.gov/opub/ted/2016/high-income-households-spent-half-of-their-food-budget-on-food-away-from-home-in-2015.htm https://www.ers.usda.gov/data-products/chart-gallery/gallery/chart-detail/?chartId=79201

U.S. food-away-from-home sales topped food-at-home sales in 2014.

Food-at-home and away-from-home expenditures in the United States, 1960-2014

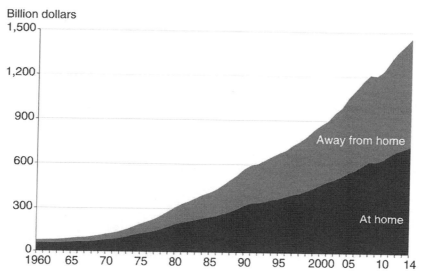

Source: USDA, Economic Research Service, Food Expenditure Series.

Percent of per capita disposable income spent on food in the United States, 1960-2014

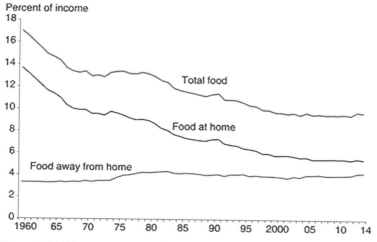

Source: USDA, Economic Research Service, Food Expenditure Series.

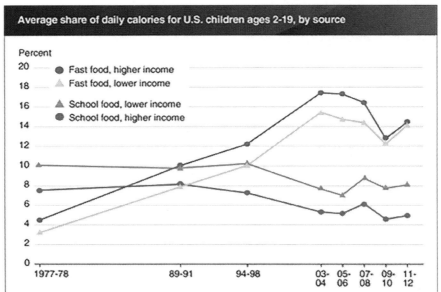

Average share of daily calories for U.S. children ages 2-19, by source

Percent

- ● Fast food, higher income
- ▲ Fast food, lower income
- ▲ School food, lower income
- ● School food, higher income

Note: Higher income (>185% of poverty) and lower income (≤ 185% of poverty).
Source: USDA, Economic Research Service using data from the USDA Nationwide Food Consumption Survey 1977-78; USDA Continuing Survey of Food Intakes by Individuals 1989-91 and 1994-98; and the National Health and Nutrition Examination Survey 2003-04, 2005-06, 2007-08, 2009-10, 2011-12.

22 DIRECTION

Where humans might be heading individually and as a group is a pertinent question undoubtedly asked repeatedly since the advent of reasoning and recognition for the concept of time. Personal life goals and the journeys chosen to reach those goals can be meaningful, gratifying, and rewarding, or burdensome, frustrating, exhausting, painful, and a constant source of anguish and personal suffering. Personal goal frustration creates stresses toxic to the body vehicle system.

LIFE GOALS, AMBITIONS, AND EXPECTATIONS
(Where one desires, sets out, or expects to be at a given point in time)

↑
↑

The divide that separates life goals, ambitions, and expectations from the perceived level of existence or state-of-being reflects the extent of life goal frustration and affects the behavioral balance and emotional, physical, and mental well-being of the body vehicle.

↑
↑

PERCEIVED LEVEL OF EXISTENCE OR STATE-OF-BEING
(Where one believes to exist at that same point in time)

Life goals, ambitions, and expectations reflect personal beliefs, dreams, and perceptions for achieving satisfaction and fulfillment of presumed individual life purpose.

Human existence is comparative.

Humans often determine their level of existence or state-of-being by comparatively appraising personal, social, and occupational accomplishments with individual capabilities and available opportunities relative to the perceived accomplishments others achieved under similar life circumstances.

The perception that a major discrepancy exists between where one is and where one expects to be at any given point in time can be a source of significant personal frustration, especially if the shortcomings in attaining own goals appear greater than the shortcomings of others having to overcome similar life challenges to reach comparable goals.

A common source of emotional frustration and unhappiness for many is the level of separation that exists between the perceived physical state of the body vehicle and the ideal body vehicle image possessed, which may be considerable when ideal body vehicle images are unrealistic or commercially devised especially concerning weight or appearance. More consequentially, the level of agreement between the actual body vehicle physical state and a truly healthy body vehicle reflects the success of individual health maintenance efforts.

Commitment and dedicated effort help to achieve realistic and sensible life goals to make daily existence healthier and more satisfying. Wisely selected life goals and intelligently conceived life course journeys permit easier goal achievement to reduce life suffering and frustration. Realistic life goals and rational personal expectations tailored to capitalize on unique individual strengths, attributes, interests, and capabilities allow far smoother and more gratifying life journeys with more certain goal attainment. Unrealistic life goals and ill-conceived life journeys with unreasonable expectations reduce opportunities for personal accomplishment and to experience the successes that contribute toward making life more fulfilling.

When necessary, setting smaller goals achieved more easily and combined stepwise to produce overall greater accomplishments and success can be an effective life strategy. Thoughtful consideration and careful planning are paramount in fashioning successful life strategies that work well. Incompletely regarded logistic, financial, and time limitations can negatively impact chosen goals or journeys to hinder goal attainment and compromise life quality.

Financial shortcomings due to poor planning, miscalculation, or setting unrealistic goals, which create insurmountable hurdles between actual *lifetime* supply and *lifetime* demands necessary to meet goal obligations, can significantly contribute to life stresses. Money matters producing financial shortcomings that limit the repayment of debt obligations are common themes of human strife and conflict. Failure to achieve life goals and the existence of formidable separations between the perceived state of being and life expectations lead to disappointment and emotional pain toxic to personal existence.

Too many loose ends accumulated by incompletely satisfying life goals create stress and increase physical and behavioral vulnerabilities for illness and commercial manipulation. Indecision to set goals and lack of motivation, commitment, and perseverance to reach goals also contribute toward stress and suffering that compromise life quality. The indecisive and weakly resolved risk being led astray by sinister forces for nefarious purposes or simply may be bypassed and abandoned by the decisive and determined who take the initiative to establish life goals and devise ways to accomplish them.

An honest reality check performed regularly to appraise the personal effort and progress toward meeting the demands of reaching goals helps reaffirm or redirect selected life journeys. Flexibility and open-mindedness to thoughtfully narrow gaps between personal expectations and the level of existence, by seizing available opportunities to redirect course journeys, adjust own behaviors, and sensibly change the mind-set to allow easier goal attainment, lowers frustration and stress levels toxic to the body vehicle.

Reasonable life journeys navigated to reach goals without excessive dependence on others or extraneous factors builds self-reliance and bolsters personal confidence to further the chances of achieving more life successes. Therefore, a successful life journey requires careful planning, commitment, hard work, perseverance, and self-control to achieve goals. The first step toward reaching set goals is to start on the planned life journey, as accomplishments occur only after getting started. Personal goals and a positive outlook provide direction for designed life journeys. Mental focus that rids the mind of irrelevant distractions and executes the life plan through appropriate action completes the life journey.

The work accomplished to achieve life goals builds appreciation for body vehicle limitations and inspires creativity and resourcefulness to operate the body vehicle intelligently to navigate successfully around obstacles encountered attaining goals. Personal gratification and fulfillment emerge from the successful completion and mastery of the challenges faced by journeying through life. Problems solved along more difficult parts of the life journey teach valuable lessons and skills available to tackle more demanding life challenges later elsewhere. Overcoming life journey difficulties creatively and constructively boosts confidence to foster a "can do" mind-set and instills a higher sense of accomplishment when life goals are reached. Milestones achieved during life journeys mark the experiences gained that can be shared to facilitate the life journeys of others.

Addictification and other human pleasure, convenience, and runaway escape peddling commercial industries that feed on human vulnerabilities profit off those pursuing life expecting immediate gratification without responsibly planning a healthy and workable life journey. Commercial industries routinely glamorize the luxuries of living the easy life, possessing expensive goods, and enjoying extravagant life amenities without addressing the need to work and sacrifice to achieve any of those luxuries. Sweepstakes, gambling, and credit industries especially hustle individuals who expect immediate rewards and gratification and easy money by beating the system, without accepting personal limitations, exercising self-control, or setting realistic life goals with reasonable life journeys.

The last-minute scramble defines the daily existence of many who depend on the very last available minute to accomplish or get anything done. Daily and long-range plans charted with ample time for completion avert the chaos of last-minute surprises and unanticipated setbacks that materialize with poor planning and inadequate time management. Poor planning creates worry and stress. Insufficient planning increases the uncertainty concerning potential outcomes of daily living to generate anxiety with suffering, which crave relief offered through runaway escape behaviors such as unnecessary eating that predisposes to unwanted weight gain.

Life plans budgeted realistically for execution with built-in contingencies and alternatives that anticipate unexpected circumstances and life events reduce anxieties to ratchet down stress and stress responses including runaway escape eating. Achievement of life goals that provide personal gratification and a sense of accomplishment requires creating rational plans to reach life goals sensibly, adjusting plans as necessary to compensate for setbacks, and persevering through difficulties to execute plans to completion. Life potential maximizes by navigating the maze of daily life choices with intelligence, forethought, and sensible planning. Luck is being in the right place at the right time. Life strategies that incorporate healthy lifestyles optimize personal capabilities for success by increasing the individual chances for taking advantage of life opportunities and realizing life goals without interruption from illness.

Healthy behaviors and lifestyle choices increase the odds that the body vehicle will continue to work properly during the journey to achieve life goals and reduce the chances of body vehicle breakdown requiring rescue bail-out and repair that derail the life course journey. Neglect of mental, emotional, physical, and spiritual body vehicle needs predisposes to body vehicle impairment that causes stress and suffering and can frustrate realization of life goals, which promote unhealthy runaway escape behaviors such as emotional eating predisposing to unwanted weight gain and obesity.

22.1 PERSONAL LIFE JOURNEY IS A WORK IN PROGRESS

Daily existence does not guarantee regular achievement of significant personal accomplishments but can be forged to be humanly meaningful and gratifying. Life journeys are passageways to discover the workings of the world and better understand self and others and one's relationship to the world, ultimately to understand individual life purpose. Life journey exploration is key to uncover individual talents and life opportunities. There are no failures in journeying through life, only unsuccessful and missed attempts at reaching personal goals, which teach valuable life lessons and provide experiences that promote self-discovery and offer prospects to redirect, redefine, and refine personal goals and traveled journey paths.

Important human qualities that lead to greater individual accomplishments along the life journey include perseverance, resiliency, resourcefulness, and flexibility. Personal improvement and growth during the life journey come from making responsible decisions and acting with the conviction and courage to own decisional outcomes and having the flexibility and resourcefulness to explore alternatives and adjust life course journeys as necessary to achieve goals successfully. Having resiliency with the capability to bounce back and persevering to continue after experiencing any setbacks are especially vital to complete life journey goals. Striving to live healthier and regularly appreciate something new about self and others satisfies deeper humanistic needs to provide contentment beyond the fleeting, superficial physical pleasures obtained using commercial industry products and services. Establishing meaningful human relationships and choosing healthy nutritional habits that nourish the life journey intelligently prevent health problems that can slow or detour life journey advances.

Projecting one's life journey beyond the immediate demands and limitations of the existing physical world propels life experiences in ways that can impact humanity constructively to benefit all. Thoughtful reflection on the toils, trials and tribulations, and events of daily existence offers greater insight into the meaning of an individual life journey and the motivations driving personal behaviors. Without reflection, personal existence easily becomes harried, disconnected, seemingly complicated, and more vulnerable to manipulation and control by external forces. Neglecting to regularly reflect on the personal life journey including choices made and reasons for choosing, can predispose one to collapse into the emotional and physical pitfalls of existence to impede life journey progress. Introspection and reflection are built-in body vehicle self-correction mind software programs that help reaffirm or redirect life course journeys.

Commercial profit industries continually vie to interrupt and distract busy lives with temporary runaway escapes and rescue bail-outs offering alcohol, tobacco products, pharmaceuticals, recreational drugs, or enticing and tasty mass-produced addictification food products loaded with sugar, fat, salt, and chemical additives, which derail healthy life journeys to trap vulnerable *lifetime* in revenue streams that feed industry profitability.

Devoting excessive lifetime engaging in media programming and riveting attention to electronic media devices slow life journey progress to reduce the potential for personal accomplishments. Enterprising corporate and commercial interests also scheme and compete to divert and steal chunks of current and future lifetime from personal life journeys by selling encumbering debt obligations represented deceptively as "credit offered for less or with no money down." Marketing campaigns run by credit industries that sell debt glamorize that acquiring debt somehow benefits the indebted. Consequently, valuable considerations concerning the life journey are whether personal efforts and time spent truly benefit self, others, or the world or principally involve hard labor to satisfy economic goals that instead predominantly benefit commercial industries. Ultimately, higher life journey personal rewards aren't about doing it faster or doing more but about doing it thoughtfully and correctly with genuine effort.

Completing a few things well gratifies more than doing many things poorly and incompletely. Mastery of completed life journey tasks rewards the commitment to travel selected course journeys. Finishing life projects generates a sense of accomplishment.

A paced, thoughtfully planned, and reflective life journey prevents living an all-consuming **maxedzurvival** that derails the life journey away from achieving meaningful and gratifying life accomplishments. Knowledge and personal experiences acquired living and saved within brain memory banks are permanently deposited lifetime, which continuously accrues intellectual interest available for transfer and application toward many alternative life endeavors.

A valuable war lesson undoubtedly learned by those unfortunate enough to have suffered the cruelty of human war conflict firsthand is that when bullets start flying and bombs start dropping, likely only three things are reasonably carried away in the mad haste to flee far away rapidly to survive. The three things immediately available upon escape are the clothes worn on the body; food filling the belly; and any knowledge, hopes, dreams, personal aspirations, human experiences, and memories stored away within brain software. The food filling the belly and clothes worn on the body are short-lived and unlikely to last much longer beyond the initial flight from terror, whereas what the brain stores endures to allow lives to rebuild anywhere anytime. The physical laws of nature limit and confine the body vehicle structure in space and time, but the human imagination and intellect are limitless and unbounded by time and space, as demonstrated through the great intellectual accomplishments of the physicist Stephen Hawking, whose disabled physical body served to house a continuously active and brilliantly productive mind. Therefore, the human intellect thinks and imaginatively conceives beyond body vehicle physical limitations to direct one's life journey strategically in infinitely creative and productive ways.

Life exists on a vast continuum. The life spectrum stretches from the infinitesimally minute to the infinitely enormous and is packed with infinite details in between to continuously offer much to see, do, appreciate, and understand. Life richness is recognized better by experiencing and learning some of the life complexities and infinite details. A fine line separates the challenge of taking advantage of living to experience, learn, and accomplish as much as possible from doing too much too often to tax brain and body vehicle capacities and produce negative life experiences. Humanity and all other enormously complex earth life-forms possessing countless individual qualities, characteristics, and behaviors populate only a microscopic speck of an infinitely large life platform.

An entire life journey encounters only a minuscule portion of a very tiny sliver of what life in the universe offers. Living in tomorrow sacrifices rich life experiences available today. The existing world provides boundless opportunities for immensely gratifying exploration and continuous discovery during the long, life journey. Journeying through life at a comfortable **speed-of-thought** pace that avoids zooming thoughtlessly with reckless abandon allows unfolding life wonders and mysteries to be noticed.

Life passes by in a virtual blur without appreciating and reflecting on life details. Successful scientific inquiry and discovery that drive human understanding, progress, and development thrive on disembarking from usual routines to explore, examine, and explain the hidden minutiae and ongoing intricacies of the apparent world. Slowing down and stopping to notice and observe the finer points in life allows for richer life outlooks that translate to more enjoyable and meaningful existences. Overly busy lives failing to notice life details desensitize to life events that continuously transpire all around. Existing without comfortably grasping life situations rapidly passing by produces frustration with overwhelming feelings of missing out and losing control leading to anxiety, depression, stress, and stress behaviors. A fast-paced existence solely focused on reaching and maintaining economic goals risks missing opportunities to recognize all the little things that make human lives more meaningful, unique, and remarkable. Learning to dawdle like a child and take time to get **in the moment** to ponder experiences in the **here-and-now** instills meaning into otherwise seemingly chaotic physical realities.

Life journeys are made more meaningful by disembarking from the crazed ride on the hamster wheel of overscheduled daily routines. Healthy life journeys open new horizons of experience that present innumerable opportunities for healthy fun. One of the many scourges of modernizing human civilizations is the derailment of spontaneous and focused thinking with constant distractions and interruptions, especially through electronic media devices. Deliberate derailment of human thinking is a mechanism to manipulate human thought.

Being in the moment seizes the opportunity to fully appreciate the life moment at hand, without permitting outside forces to spellbind and engross attention in moments artificially created for external control. Time-honored tools employed through the ages to interrupt the blind fury of frenzied daily routines and enable thoughtful reflection on the moment at hand include meditation, yoga, and spiritual prayer.

Whereas life offers richness and infinite diversity, industry delivers sameness with unwavering monotony. One-of-a-kind terminology is absent within the lexicon of industry mass production. Uniqueness and industry mass production are inherently mutually exclusive concepts. Richness, diversity, and detail evident in natural earth products are distinctly missing from mass-produced industry duplicates.

Mass production delivers sameness with precision, ensuring that manufactured products predictably elicit expected pleasures on consumer demand. Industry skillfully concocts original industrial formulations and recipes to trigger conditioned consumer behaviors driving commercial industry profits reproducibly. Carefully orchestrated marketing strategies then choreograph convincing sales pitches to highlight designer product qualities that meet consumer expectations with unvarying consistency. Industry replicates commercial product qualities that reliably achieve desired consumer outcomes and effectively maintain control of consumer loyalty and spending. Industry rarely tampers with winning product formulations that trap consumers into predictable spending rituals to spin the wheels of fortune and release "new" or "improved" versions of commercially successful industry products to entice a fresh wave of consumers for capture.

Individuals that commit significant *lifetime* to pursue commercial benchmarks for achieving personal satisfaction sacrifice opportunities to enhance personal growth and self-discovery through real-life experiences. Human lives embracing and depending on industry ideals for happiness instead experience frustration and disappointment when industry standards are unaffordable, unavailable, or become altered to satisfy the changing demands of commercial market forces. Additionally, industry uses a limited number of ingredients to create numerous assortments of tasty, processed food products that markedly reduce the diversity, richness, and composition of the indwelling body vehicle gut microbial communities to diminish the human life experience further.

Real life offers a rich palette plentifully stocked with countless options to paint individual life experiences and situational outcomes creatively. The application of abundant real-life choices is limited only by imagination and intellectual vision. Abundance and diversity are luxuries to be cherished. Cramming a life existence full of commercial objects and experiences lacking humanistic value is akin to piling up hoarded items that will never be retrieved and appreciated again.

Physical experiences and commercial objects devoid of humanistic meaning are likely to be forgotten, left behind, or discarded at the final running of the body vehicle life program, leaving only the knowledge, insight, and memories gained connecting to others. Human conduct that constructively includes others in meaningful ways to benefit humanity ingrains deeply into brain memory banks to provide more lasting fulfillment than offered by fleeting sensory experiences or physical objects.

A life course journey that reaches intensely to appreciate and better understand some of the infinite life complexities brings more opportunities to experience a richly satisfying life. Ultimately, life journeys arrive when individuals intrinsically feel valued and summon the courage to be themselves and confidently express unique talents and individuality, without seeking approval from others or needing to satisfy commercial industry standards and ideals. Positive life journeys collectively increase human knowledge, experience, and understanding to advance humanity forward, and may one day combine to mobilize all agreeably toward common goals that altruistically benefit all humans, the world, and universe in which known life exists.

23 HUMAN CONNECTIVITY

23.1 CONNECTION

A higher humanistic drive than servicing basic physical, biological needs is the drive to connect with others to establish meaningful human relationships. Humans crave companionship and want and need to connect and belong to each other to achieve personal fulfillment. Beyond the reproductive physical binding that genetically preserves and perpetuates the existence of the human species, humans need to connect more deeply to make individual life experiences complete. Connecting with the lives of others immerses individuals in-the-mix of humanity to flow within the stream of life to create new life and advance human civilization forward. The greater the number of connections with others, the deeper the immersion into the cohesive life force binding all humanity together.

The explosive commercial growth of social media engines and internet dating sites affirms the intense need humans possess to connect with each other. Whereas procreation is a primal, instinctual biological drive programmed into all physically reproducing life-forms to perpetuate species existence, the human connection is a force driving humanity to bond and integrate existentially. "Please," "thank you," "excuse me," and "I'm sorry" are four simple human expressions that acknowledge the interconnectedness of human existence and the intimate intertwining of individual behaviors that reciprocally impact interacting lives. These four expressions convey the understanding that individual life journeys occasionally disagreeably insinuate into and impose upon the life journeys of others, and especially reinforce the value and need for all to connect thoughtfully and take advantage of available opportunities to coexist peaceably and achieve individual life goals amicably.

Human existence already involves and depends on innumerable life connections with trillions of earth life-forms including other humans, animals, plants, insects, and microorganisms, all living within a vast, complex, integrated, and interdependent biological and ecological life system. The human connection is about higher-order symbiosis with interdependent coexistence and sharing of human lives to create opportunities for emotional, intellectual, and spiritual growth and development for involved individuals living together within the human life system. The ability of humans to connect beyond their immediate physical presence may exist for all animal species and possibly even across earth life-forms as minimally evidenced by the unique relationships that develop between humans and beloved their pets.

Within the known universe, there exists a fascinating scientifically unexplained physical connectivity phenomenon known as **quantum entanglements.** Quantum entanglements involve the paring of behaviors between energy particles separated by great distances so that any forces exerted on one of the paired energy particles are also expressed in kind or oppositely on the other particle separated by a considerable distance. The mystery is that the medium transmitting and synchronizing the behaviors between the separated particles is entirely unknown.

An understanding of quantum entanglements might someday unravel the deep mysteries of how humans connect on deeper levels with each other. If an alien life-form from another planet or galaxy attacked the earth, would humanity unify to ward off the alien threat or divide up and attempt to enlist the help of the animal or plant kingdoms to survive the attack? The seemingly obvious answer is that humans would overcome all relatively petty differences and band together to accomplish a common and worthwhile goal of protecting and perpetuating its own existence. Consequently, humans are driven to join and work together toward mutual goals through a multitude of inherent similarities and shared interests.

Humans are delivered naturally equipped with all the necessary tools and capabilities to establish invaluable integral connections with each other on various levels. Humans connect by interacting and sharing personal interests and life experiences. Human interactions can be intimate, peripheral, or incidental.

Intimate interactions directly intertwine human lives to pervasively affect the daily routines and living of involved individuals, while peripheral interactions affect individuals more casually to various extents depending on the level of overlap in individual routines and accompanying reciprocal fulfillment of personal needs. Incidental interactions affect individuals indirectly to the extent that individual choices may impact other lives sharing similar interests or goals, such as occurs by voting a certain way in elections or purchasing commercial items to impact item price or availability.

The extent to which encountering human life forces interact, mix, and blend determines the closeness, strength, and significance of the resultant human connectedness, with intimate encounters binding individuals more powerfully and cohesively than peripheral or incidental encounters. The quality of human life force interactions can be positive and constructive to mutually enhance interacting human existences or negative and destructive to diminish the health, safety, or well-being of interacting individuals, with the underlying motives that individuals possess to interact with others driving the consequences of life force interactions.

True human connections extend beyond parallel cohabitation, random coexistence, or brief encounters between nearby individuals that incidentally and indifferently intersect life paths, as analogously represented by live-wire coaxial electrical cables that lie side by side or over each other without ever connecting electrically. The human connection involves a reciprocal embracement that extends out and shares personal selves and human assets that become unified and protected as one. Connecting with others promotes a cohesive and mutually beneficial symbiotic existence on earth that positively contributes to advance life forward for all connected. Connecting on a human level requires taking responsibility to appropriately care for self and avoid self-neglect, while accepting responsibility to look after others and avert taking advantage of or victimizing the vulnerable for personal gain or profit as routinely carried out by commercial interests and oppressive systems of human control.

Individuals connecting through family, friendship, camaraderie, community, and country acquire vested interests inherently preserved by safeguarding everyone connected. Human connectivity achieves greater strength in numbers. The most basic level of human connection begins with ties between parents and children within nuclear family units.

Nuclear family connections evolve further when children grow up and have their own children, transforming original parents into grandparents and creating cousins, aunts, uncles, and so on. Family units are the fundamental elements composing the very fiber and substance of human societal connections that allow humanity to grow, thrive, and evolve productively. The intensity and strength of network connections among family members and between families determine the strength and stability of communal societal frameworks.

Stronger family bonds make for stronger and more cohesive societal ties and societies. The human connection is the unifying force linking humanity on deeper levels that allows humans to identify intimately with each other, separately from the ability to recognize similarities in physical features and characteristics or styles in navigating daily life challenges and complexities. Unique styles of human existence emerge and are cultivated in response to external environmental and social pressures and internal biological needs for survival.

Apparent human differences in cultural ethnicities, nationalities, political and religious affiliations, financial status, educational levels, skin color, and gender alternatively serve as convenient labels that purposely categorize and group humanity to facilitate and allow for commercial and various other forms of systemic control and domination. Labels that create divisions and appeal to commonalities among humans are especially manipulated by industry to influence human behaviors and choices. Industry uses media to emphasize artificial labels that appeal to their audiences to create an us against them mentality to steer audience perceptions and interests. Additionally, human labels become convenient economic tags of opportunity for industry to exploit and correspondingly match to industry products and services sold on commercial markets.

In contrast, real human connections require sharing of meaningful personal experiences to establish common ground and procure recognition for the commonality of basic human existence and needs, despite apparent social and economic disparities artificially created by the self-serving interests of profit industries to motivate, pressure, and drive human behaviors commercially.

Genuine human connections established among family members, teachers, schoolmates, neighbors, workers, countrymen, and organization and club members unify life journeys and tie humanity together to move in step and increase empathy and understanding among all involved. Whereas the body vehicle structure is physically confined to occupy a defined space in time, the human life force transcends physical boundaries to connect humanity across time and space. The human life force exists without the boundary limitations restricting the physical body vehicle, as evidenced when the hopes, dreams, imagination, and creativity of humanity become realized when human progress finally catches up to human potential.

Reciprocated true love with the willingness of individuals to sacrifice their physical selves entirely for another may well be the closest human experience that breaches human physical boundaries to most completely connect and blend individual human existences. Appreciation of a smile or a warm human embrace that melts two individuals into each other's realm of existence fleetingly taps into that powerful life force connecting humans. Human premonitions, family and country ties, close friendships, mother-baby bonding, sixth sense, social movements, group celebratory behaviors, and mourning of human loss, all involve that special ethereal quality that binds humanity together. Connecting individuals spiritually reenergize their body vehicle life forces.

Throughout the ages, religious worship has categorically acknowledged the existence of some connecting force or entity to which all individuals belong and are collectively bound, and which offers some opportunity for renewal of body vehicle life force energies. Having positive human relationships and sharing life with others under a variety of circumstances create supportive human networks that enhance individual life experiences and perspective, augment personal and social growth, and reaffirm the importance of collective social behaviors leading to more fulfilling and meaningful lives for all connected. Being surrounded by positive like-minded individuals who enjoy taking on the challenges of daily living and look forward toward collectively solving life problems ensures smoother, more gratifying, and accompanied personal life journeys.

Human connections, then, nourish survival during the long individual life journeys. Making every day meaningful by striving daily to connect and make positive contributions to life through others builds a better world for everyone. Societal celebrations and social rituals represent humanity attempts to connect by uniting individuals to share collectively in positive communal experiences. Ceremonial and prayer recitals counter human isolation and differences by synchronizing the activities of many gathered participants in a combined undertaking. Societal holidays are created to interrupt the madness of day-to-day individual economic survival with designated times devoted to family and the celebration of human events that reaffirm the importance of human connection.

Institutionalized systems of human connectivity such as religions inspire members to connect through participation in periodic sacrifices of materialistic human desires and pleasures such as fasts, which allow focus on the more spiritual aspects of human existence and provide a means for individuals to temporarily break away from the primal survival programming that drives activities of the "flesh."

Collective human experiences qualitatively bind, blend, and enhance individual lives to move humanity forward in unison, and create opportunities for more meaningful and gratifying personal living. Human accomplishments and progress are substantially concerted group efforts made possible through a spirit of cooperation and the combined and integrated work of many including family, friends, peers, workers, countrymen, and societal institutions. The need for humans to connect to advance human civilization forward validates the reality that successful human existence entirely depends on human community and connection. Without the involvement of many, there would be no buildings, roads, schools, cities, countries, education, travel, entertainment, social institutions, etc., existing for everyone's use and benefit.

The costs of advancing human civilization demand sacrifice from many to reap benefits available for all. All are inherently obligated to pitch in and do their part to keep life moving positively forward for everyone. Taking responsibility to choose the appropriate nutritional behaviors and healthful lifestyles that optimize own health and prevent health disrepair lowers societal costs and improves societal health.

Better societal health reduces illnesses that derail life journeys which positively contribute to overall human accomplishments and increases the chances for humanity to progress and evolve successfully to benefit all. Therefore, human connection is about community, belonging, and sacrifice leading to greater personal fulfillment and life opportunities for all.

23.2 DISCONNECTION: THE DARK SIDE

The innate need for human connection drives much of human social behaviors and interactions. Human disconnection then deprives individuals of vital bonding nourishing the human life force and causes emotional toxicity. The absence of human connections leads to feelings of loneliness and isolation. Significant interpersonal disagreements, conflicts, confrontations, discord, and alienations particularly between closely allied individuals can cause tension, stress, anxiety, and depression capable of provoking unhealthy behaviors such as stress eating and self-neglect predisposing to obesity and illness.

People connect with food to pleasurably stimulate their physical senses as well as to temporarily relieve and escape emotional suffering from absent, disconnected, or unsatisfactory human relationships that result in unfulfilled emotional needs and feelings of loneliness and exclusion creating low self-esteem. Commercial addictification food products are designed specifically to produce immediate sensory pleasures providing runaway escapes that conveniently serve to alleviate emotional pain and suffering temporarily. Likewise, alcohol bars exist for those attempting or failing human connections, with alcohol readily lowering inhibitions to facilitate human connections or numbing away the pain when connections fail.

Effective interpersonal and conflict resolution skills allow for more natural human interactions and less stressful approaches to settle disputes, which reduces the likelihood to cause human disconnection that generates anxieties and depression predisposing to unhealthy runaway escape behaviors. Respecting personal space and setting appropriate boundaries while connecting with others make human interactions more comfortable and prevent misunderstandings leading to interpersonal conflict.

Humans living a frenzied maxedzurvival hunger for genuine connection, progressively neglected and missing in financially driven and economically time-compressed lives. In modern and technologically driven industrial societies, human connectivity is being progressively devoured and owned commercially. The inherent drive for human connection offers commercial industries enormous opportunities to charge for and profit from any moments of human connectivity.

Increasingly, commercial interests persuade busy lives to connect while spending *lifetime* doing commercial activities such as eating in restaurants, exercising in commercial health clubs, drinking alcohol or smoking tobacco in bars, watching movies or shows in theaters or on pay per view, driving around in cars burning gas, shopping for items in department store malls, and interacting electronically through phone or computer devices.

Online social dating and matching services flooding electronic media sites are financially thriving by connecting time-pressured modern lives yearning to establish meaningful human relationships to satisfy deeper humanistic personal needs, which are not fulfilled by attaining wealth, acquiring physical objects, or experiencing fleeting materialistically produced sensory pleasures. Even simple human conversations are increasingly brokered commercially by cell phone, computer, or text messaging services charging by the minute, the message, or the month.

Media electronically taps into human connectivity to profit financially by offering various commercially sponsored services that establish some form of human connection, while extracting valuable personal information from media users to benefit industry and corporate media sponsors. Media advertising clichés feature representative elements of meaningful human connectivity and then invite individuals to connect impersonally through electronic devices to profit commercial interests from the ensuing electronic human interactions. Television and other media devices connect humanity electronically to drive consumer spending that generates big commercial industry profits. **Cell phones** are now personal communicators furnishing portable electronic connectivity with human **mind control**

on-the-go serving as an electronic chain to be taken everywhere to continuously offer industry profitable opportunities to dictate human behaviors and control connectivity every step of the way.

Human actions are entirely energy driven, involving biological surges and channeling of body vehicle electron energy flows to execute and complete physical, social, and occupational routines. Healthy body vehicle electron energy flows translate to healthier human existences. Energy-dependent humans need to fuel regularly to resupply electron energies continuously spent by the brain and other body vehicle physical parts to remain alive and interact socially, and increasingly rely on operating energy consuming electronic devices to communicate and carry out personal, social, and occupational activities.

Electronic media devices stimulate brain activity through RAS BAN to rev up body vehicle energies for action. Excessive use of electronic devices expends greater degrees of body vehicle energies and produces sensory overload and stress to negatively affect how the body vehicle channels and uses its internal energies; and may further provoke adverse behaviors that interfere with regenerative rest to exhaust body vehicle energies more rapidly. Consequently, owning and operating technological devices accelerates depletion of lifetime energies.

Humans interactively link and bond individual life force energies to connect and embed within humanity. Commercial and corporate interests seize upon the opportunities that technological advancements offer to provide humans with expensive interactive conduits that payoff electronically by establishing apparent human connections immediately. Electronic devices then work to control the ensuing human connections to channel the interacting life force energies into creating immense profit opportunities for commercial and corporate interests.

The growing commercial precedence is to hook consumers through electronic coupling using technological devices. Ultimately, technology indulges and further stimulates the human need to connect for which humans progressively pay the price by increasingly interacting through electronic means.

Human interactions through electronic devices can even be divisive and isolating as illustrated when individuals gather in a group only to text with outsiders, diluting group interactions to diminish immediately available opportunities for collective human experiences, or likewise when bullies use electronic social media applications to torment their victims. Dependency on using expensive technological electronic devices that charge humanity to connect is rapidly increasing as societies progressively modernize within the electronic age. Increasingly, individuals channel personal, social, financial, and occupational activities through electronic devices to carry out the business and entertainment of daily living. Consequently, **technological electronic addictification** is now the new leash tethering humanity and human interests to the control of corporate and commercial interests.

Technological electronic addictification fosters progressive human dependification on electronic devices to execute and accomplish even the simplest matters of routine human affairs. Technology and electronic devices are rapidly becoming the framework and mainstay of modern human existences and interactions, and increasingly drive the economic profitability of commercial and corporate interests. Media programming and software applications for electronic devices are industry tools to control humanity economically, and electronic devices are the equipment permitting execution of that control. Electronic devices are even becoming highly personalized to interface exclusively with single users who alone can unlock devices through fingerprint, eye, and facial recognition features that more securely fasten individual human existences to their electronic mediums of control. Electronic addictification disrupts human existences when fixating attention onto flat LED screens takes precedence over directly interacting with others or responding attentively to real-life circumstances transpiring all around. Therefore, energy-driven electronic devices impact body vehicle electron energy flows to direct human life force energies and affect human behaviors in ways that satisfy corporate and commercial interests and generate revenue streams for industry at the expense of real live human interactions.

Electronic technology to alter brain function and treat health conditions such as depression, epilepsy, and Parkinson's disease already exists. Invasive internal and noninvasive external deep brain stimulation that electronically affects brain function is accomplished by applying electrical currents through electrodes implanted directly into the brain or placed superficially on the scalp.

Recent scientific reports demonstrated the ability of the human brain to interact directly with electronic computer chips implanted into the brain. In one study, a man permanently paralyzed from the neck down was somehow able to communicate neurologically with a computer chip implanted into his brain and instruct the chip to signal an external computer source controlling hardware attached to his paralyzed arms, permitting him through computer assistance to feed independently using his paralyzed limbs. More dramatically, in another study, three participants also paralyzed from the neck down used brain implanted, multielectrode computer interface chips to turn their thoughts to work applications on an unmodified commercial computer tablet to send emails and text messages, browse the internet, play music on a piano application, and chat with other study participants. Undoubtedly, the reverse is likely to be true with the computer chips being able to communicate with and control human brains to execute more complex computer programmed directives.

In fact, externally held technological electronic devices already interface and connect with the human brain through human visual and auditory sensory portals to feed messages and directives directly into the brain to externally exert control over human behaviors. Therefore, portable electronic media devices that signal body vehicle sensory portals to engage electronically with data processing and executive functions of the brain are quickly becoming the preferred body vehicle mind control on-the-go for industry.

AR and **virtual reality (VR)** technologies open the door to control and steer human behaviors further by immersing live human existences through interfacing technological devices into artificial worlds entirely designed by outside forces. Humanity is being progressively trained to assimilate human existence and human contact through interposed electronic screens, with entirely artificial holographic human interactions fast approaching on the horizon and likely to become the new norm consuming direct physical human contact.

New rescue industry profit opportunities are surfacing as a direct consequence of excessive electronic media device usage by individuals who remain exceedingly connected electronically. Adverse behavioral and physical health disorders such as **technology addictions** and **phantom cell phone vibration syndrome** are occurring in vulnerable and especially younger individuals, who develop an unhealthy reliance on continuous internet and media connectivity and regularly lock daily existences logged into and operating electronic media devices for many hours at a time.

The irony for media device users heavily caught up using technology and believing their devices are liberating and empowering is that the devices are really just another convenient tool for corporate and commercial interests to control humanity, and are electronic versions of the usual addictification and dependification schemes that control and manipulate human behaviors to generate industry profits.

There are apparent monetary expenses as well as less obvious human costs of substantially channeling personal human encounters and moments of human communication and connectivity through electronic means that exact a billable price to pay. Individuals and humanity ultimately pay an even higher price by progressively disconnecting from direct interpersonal human interactions and sensory physical contact.

Despite permitting greater electronic connectivity, technology diminishes actual human connectivity to foment a sense of isolation and loneliness causing suffering, which raises individual vulnerability for the lure of addictification industry runaway escape relief subsequently requiring rescue industry bail-outs. The irony of social media, email, and other electronic human connectivity messenger services is that individuals that connect spend no real time connecting physically in each other's presence to interact and communicate fully and directly by mutually engaging all available senses. Interactions through technological devices deprive human encounters of the benefits of direct human contact. Direct interpersonal connectivity during human encounters with the physical engagement of all available senses and locking of minds reaches more profound levels of human connection than afforded by electronic connectivity, and additionally provides higher satisfaction than can be achieved through impersonal electronic connections. Electronically brokered connectivity suppresses the full range and expression of human emotions and sentiments when human interactions traffic through interposed electronic communication devices.

True human feelings and personal intentions are easier to ascertain during interpersonal interactions that physically engage all available human senses directly.

Technological age connectivity that interposes electronic gadgetry between human encounters and interactions permits electronic concealment of true feelings and intentions, increasing opportunities for human deception or betrayal as revealed through the popular TV program *Catfish.*

Another developing casualty of electronically brokered human connectivity is the sacred health care interaction that exists between health care providers and recipients, as **internet health care encounters** through **telehealth or telemedicine** use **virtual doctors** to conveniently substitute for direct in-person human health care interactions and eliminate face-to-face health care that best assesses the health status and individual needs of health care recipients. Health care consumers increasingly search the internet attempting to satisfy personal health needs better, while corporate and commercial rescue industries including health care insurance companies, big pharma, hospitals, and physician groups scramble to intercept and control the growing health-driven internet, consumer traffic.

For many, food and alcohol beverages opportunely serve as surrogates that substitute for missing human connections and interactions, but unfortunately, provide only transitory comfort and temporary relief from suffering the dejection resulting from living technologically isolated lives. Alcohol beverages are frequently even given human names to produce feelings of personal accompaniment while one imbibes alone.

Humanly interactive, meaningful, and constructively productive life routines seize control of living here and now fully, and lead to gratifying experiences producing contentment beyond the transient appeasement furnished by addictification and rescue industry products, or the fleeting emotional titillation delivered by electronic connectivity. During the life journey, here-and-now experiences involving direct interpersonal contacts dynamically enrich future living. Learning from here-and-now experiences to adjust personal behaviors and lifestyles constructively to live healthily and regularly interact with others in positive ways enhances future life journey experiences.

Obesity, alcoholism, and other behavioral and physical health dysfunctions reflect some of the negative consequences of addressing here-and-now experiences counterproductively to basic body vehicle connectivity and health needs. Television and media programming that exclusively offer one-way connectivity without a real opportunity for reciprocal human engagement foment growing hunger for progressively absent direct interpersonal relations, which is compounded further by wholesale media depictions of intimate human interactions which individuals yearn to experience personally. Television and other media devices ineffectually substitute for the buddy or companion people want, need, and wish to have.

Commercially sponsored media programming and electronic device software applications instead become the deceptively untrue and manipulative friend with secret ulterior motives hired by industry as an instrument of human control. Media programming must be regarded similarly to savvy story-telling politicians, who say what moves people to get the vote but then advance other agendas following their election. Therefore, media programming transmits interesting stories attempting to connect with audience interests to captivate attention, desensitize, and disarm inhibitions and suspicions to then deliver straightforward brainwashing, economic manipulation, and mind control to sell industry wares and promote financially sponsored corporate and commercial messages.

As part of the industry scheme to desensitize and brainwash consumers for commercial purposes, media campaigns promote widespread acceptance of gratuitous human violence and murder to captivate attention, analogously to how the rescue industry promotes comfortable acceptance and reliance on using pharmaceutical products that have the potential to cause harmful health effects to maintain health artificially according to industry standards.

Popping chemicals into the body vehicle to achieve health is as unnatural as beating up and killing off humans for any reason. Additionally, depicting human violence and killing for entertainment purposes to generate industry profits is even more egregious to healthy human existence. Ultimately, channeling human connectivity through electronic media devices facilitates human control and manipulation as already appreciated long ago in 1949 when George Orwell published *1984,* which illustrated how television programming was the preferred medium to mass manipulate and control humanity.

Recently, designers of addictive social media software experienced enough personal misgivings to reconsider the brilliance and utility of their addictive creations and united to issue a warning concerning the hazards surrounding the use of social media applications, perhaps as a matter of conscience but more likely after witnessing progressively more vulnerable family members and loved ones become enticingly lured and inescapably trapped to use social media applications nonstop. Undoubtedly, meals around the old dinner table with family and friends certainly are not what they used to be before the creation of electronic media devices and software applications, as more individuals engage with their devices instead of interacting with others sitting at the table.

Fortunately, the natural solution that still exists today to break free immediately from the imposed hypnotic trances and brainwashing spells cast by television, and other electronic media devices is simply to turn the television or electronic media devices *off.*

Profit industries and systems of human control attempting to connect and sell products and services or propaganda to individuals routinely exploit the inherent need for human connectivity in various ways many of which are fundamentally similar. Counter to the behavior of electrochemical particles in nature, whereby same charges repel to separate and disperse while opposite charges attract and combine, humans driven by fear and ignorance display prejudicial tendencies and band together with those having mutual ideals and qualities against those perceived as being or thinking differently.

Economic systems of human control capitalize on human tendencies toward connection and association and divisiveness and separation by artificially creating or accentuating apparent human similarities or differences to band together or separate out individuals.

Outward physical characteristics or appearances and behavioral attributes and qualities are easier for systems of human control to target to assemble or divide individuals for system management and exploitation. Human perceptions of the existing world and behavioral attributes arising from adopted ideologies, learning, available socioeconomic opportunities, environmental influences, and family ties are vulnerable to shape manipulatively by systems of human control.

Media, commercial and legal systems, and systems of government and religion utilize similarities and differences among individuals or groups as a means of human unification, segregation, and control. Similarities of insiders and differences of outsiders are easy to identify and highlight to charge premiums for group inclusion and profit from those fitting and banding together. **Connectivity terms** such as *white, black, brown, yellow, red, Democrat, Republican, liberal, progressive, communist, socialist, Christian, Hindu, Muslim, Jew, white collar,* and *blue collar* are *labels* that conveniently brand included individuals for corralling and systemic commercial and corporate exploitation. Connectivity terms translate to *tags of economic opportunity* for corporate and commercial systems. Commercial wares are disguised to fit in and appeal to the needs, interests, and biases of labeled groups to assure higher group acceptance and increased sales since wares failing to suit group requirements are likely to be resisted and excluded from economic group consumption. The greater the similarity and homogeneity of group members concerning appearance, mannerisms, behaviors, and adopted principles and ideologies the easier to design commercial wares comprehensively matching group needs, and the more favorable the circumstances are to maneuver the group. Therefore, labels which categorically separate individuals into commercially meaningful groups conveniently round up and herd individuals for more straightforward commercial and systemic processing, similarly to how specific heads of cattle are rounded up and herded through stockyards for eventual consumption.

Since individuals are inherently programmed to follow the crowd, profit industries artificially create causes or incentives deliberately to band individuals to move together for more efficient systemic manipulation and control. Commercial selling tactics additionally play on consumer frailties and insecurities to tap into human fears, uncertainties, and feelings of isolation and exclusion to peddle industry remedies, which offer to rectify or compensate for any perceived personal faults or shortcomings. Commercial industries and systems of human control even amplify self-doubts and apprehensions surrounding human connectivity and interactions and exploit failures involving human relationships to profit at the expense of human interests.

Human misperceptions concerning personal deficiencies are opportune vulnerabilities to target with compensatory or "corrective" commercial interventions, as exemplified by the sale of weight loss aids to those believing they are overweight, and the peddling of male sexual enhancement products to men perceiving their sexual potency to be inadequate.

Commercial industries also single out individuals feeling disconnected from commercially defined and propagated societal ideals and norms, encouraging the "disenfranchised" to get-with-it and belong to the in-crowd by buying commercial industry offerings. Industry opportunely offers to fill personal voids for human connection by selling products and services that create a false sense of group belonging or that temporarily relieve suffering from isolation, and which insidiously indoctrinate industry addictification and dependification coincidentally to cost individuals their freedom.

Growing societal obesity, addictification, and rescue industry dependification reflect the perverse industry accomplishments of connecting humanity and filling basic human needs commercially, which collectively derail countless human life journeys to compound stress, suffering, and expense for all. Even more devious are the intentions of media and commercial industries to underhandedly target and penetrate the family unit to achieve corporate and commercial aims.

The family is the fundamental unit of social connectivity and is a strategic target for many commercial marketing strategies and advertising campaigns looking to infiltrate consumer spending behaviors and achieve societal, economic control. Family units create ideal access points to impact economic decision-making originating at the core of society. The economic conquest of societies begins by influencing the spending habits of individuals, who in turn change commercial behaviors of family units that integrate into society to modify societal spending more broadly, which explains why commercial interests earmark family unit good times, togetherness, fears, or safety concerns as tactical starting points for sales strategies.

Unhealthy habits and obesity frequently start and are propagated within family units. Family ideals, mind-sets, biases, traditions, values, practices, and other learned behaviors including those which are inherently harmful and counterproductive may entrench within family units to pass down many future family generations. Illness or incapacity within family units shifts family member responsibilities to impose greater obligations and stress on family members that must help and compensate for sidelined members. Unfortunate family unit predicaments are problems offering commercial opportunities for addictification and rescue industries to solve with runaway escape and rescue bail-out interventions.

Therefore, the **step-up approach** operates to control societal, economic behaviors by initially influencing the commercial attitudes and spending habits of individual family unit members, who are expected to shape monetary practices of the family unit, which, in turn, is anticipated to impact the commercial activities of the community to eventually transform societal, economic norms. The step-up approach is more tedious, difficult, unpredictable, and costly for commercial interests to incorporate.

Modern technological advancements now allow corporate and commercial interests to penetrate society thinking quicker, deeper, and with less effort using group informational messaging, which conveniently permits manipulation of large segments of humanity simultaneously through a **top-down approach** that hijacks communication activities among online communities. Social media communities created to communicate pertinent information to family, friends, and special interest groups are an ideal channel for the top-down approach to rapidly control the thoughts and behaviors of extensive collections of humanity sharing common interests.

By using electronic human connectivity, corporate and commercial interests can more easily cloak their objectives and spread commercial messages and propaganda into larger consumer bases by piggybacking advertisements onto messaging boards shared online by families and friends, and by professional groups interacting through various media applications.

The primary objective of top-down communications is to use sophisticated technologies to exert rapid mass-scale control of dependent followers essentially by creating an itch that all downstream followers reflexively scratch immediately. Consequently, increased technological connectivity offering humanity enormous potential to evolve modern human existence to benefit all humankind is being hijacked surreptitiously by commercial interests as a tool to promote human addictification and dependification electronically, and increasingly trap unwary human lifetimes to transfer life force energies to serve commercial and corporate industry self-interests.

Human connectivity is a convenient means to introduce addictification and dependification and convert the living human essence into a monetary value to profit industry. Therefore, industry interests employ human connectivity in any way possible to drive commercial hooks through vulnerable live human meat and into the purse or wallet of consumers to extract *lifetime* for industry purposes.

Possessing awareness for the predatory corporate and commercial activities that generate industry profits at the expense of individuals and society and taking the responsibility to defend personal health and connect to other humans naturally enable individual life purpose and allotted human lifetime to be completed successfully with satisfaction.

Simplified human needs protect against entrapment and control by greedy industry feeders and self-serving industry systems, which enrich their own self-interests at the cost of vulnerable individuals seeking to attain more from life than the simple fulfillment of basic human needs. Genuinely human living is simple so trust the basics, and trust what Mother Nature made because everything else is made for profit.

For a successful *human connection,*

1. think beyond individuality

2. appreciate that life is bigger than any one individual
3. connect constructively with other lives to immerse in humanity
4. get involved directly in person with other individuals and develop positive human relationships that satisfy healthy living
5. avoid toxic behaviors, relationships, and human interactions that lead to stress and an emotional brain drain

23.3 THE FINAL CONNECTION

Ingesting natural crude fuel whole earth foods that are unaltered through industry processing and refinement and unadulterated with artificial additives allows the body vehicle to directly experience the nutritional completeness connecting with the vast ecosystem encompassing body vehicle earthly existence.

The sky, water, ground, and earth trees, bushes, plants, and shrubs suitably provide humanity directly with all the necessary nutritional sustenance, which the masterfully created and perfectly equipped body vehicle capably processes and refines naturally with minimal preparation to energize and sustain human existence.

Socialization, spirituality, and advancing mutual human interests fulfill higher-order humanistic needs more than commercial industry products or services, which deliver fleeting physical sensory experiences, temporary runaway escapes, or rescue bail-outs and contribute to unhealthy behaviors and lifestyles that sacrifice precious human *lifetime* to benefit corporate and commercial interests exclusively, can ever satisfy.

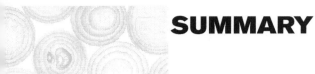

SUMMARY

Whereas life is complex,
living is simple, so trust the basics.

The story of Adam and Eve living in the Garden of Eden in Paradise exemplifies the basic tenets of healthy living and optimal body vehicle maintenance that maximize life existence. Basic body vehicle requisites for *paradise* healthy living include

1. nutritional fueling through eating unprocessed and unrefined Mother Nature–made crude fuel, whole earth plants, animals, insects, and their direct products, such as milk and honey, when hungry

2. hydration with pure water (H_2O) when thirsty

3. continuous physical movement and activity daily with every available opportunity through walking, running, climbing, swimming, stretching, etc.

4. rest and sleep for recovery and energy restoration when tired

5. the absence of clocks, economic agendas, and schedules that interrupt basic personal, mental, emotional, and spiritual activities and biological time requirements

6. the absence of chemical, biological, and emotional contaminants causing toxicity

7. human interactions carried out in person to link individuals physically and emotionally directly through the reciprocal engagement of all available senses naturally, without interposed technology or electronic devices

8. cultivation of relationships and companionship that effectively connect and harmonize individuals and allow peaceable negotiation and amicable resolution of disagreements and differences of opinion to ensure mutual happiness and contentment for all eternity

9. enjoyment of the sunshine and the outdoors regularly in natural surroundings, since human skin absorbs sunlight to produce

> vital vitamin D, and spending time away from the hustle and
> bustle of artificially constructed human surroundings provides
> a sense of health to enhance emotional well-being and lend
> greater life perspective

Healthy living is the foundation that supports the framework of biologic integrity for the body vehicle and mind. Consequently, understand and naturally meet basic body vehicle needs that maintain body vehicle physical and emotional balance to optimize personal function.

Avoid temporarily appeasing or suppressing primal, survival biological urges and impulses with behaviors and commercial industry products that produce untoward body vehicle health consequences leading to unnecessary personal expenses and suffering. Recognize the commercial market forces working to surreptitiously condition consumers through subliminal programming, attempting to control and manipulate the body vehicle mind and behaviors to generate industry profits. Realize that addictification runaway escapes are pipelines to rescue industry bail-out dependification.

Be proactive and plan healthy behaviors into daily schedules and routines. Heed and accommodate biologic time requirements necessary to carry out and complete basic body vehicle biologic functions and social activities properly. Respect body vehicle biological time and energy limitations and set boundaries for accepting or meeting any external demands or obligations that impose on body vehicle maintenance needs.

Appreciate that breathing clean air, hydrating with plain water, fueling with Mother Nature direct foods, moving physically naturally, and resting when necessary to restore energy are vital in preserving body vehicle integrity, function, and balance essential for wellness and without suitable commercial alternatives offered by addictification and rescue industries.

Avoid exposure to toxins and unnecessary chemical industry products, often introduced into the body vehicle through processed foods, hygiene products, cleaning agents, artificially manufactured health supplements, and inactive, hitch-hiker pharmaceutical ingredients that work as taxi vehicles to carry biologically active medicinal agents.

Accept and fulfill the personal obligation to maintain the health and biological balance of the body vehicle system naturally as was meant to be done, without reliance on industry products and services that predominantly satisfy profit margins for commercial industry forces. Understand that the human body vehicle is an integrated biological system that houses innumerable interdependent symbiotic microorganisms and immerses in a thriving earth ecosystem which sustains life as is known and experienced by all.

Be respectful of the earth environment in which the body vehicle lives and on which it crucially depends for existence. Establish healthy connections with other human beings. Choose meaningful life goals and journeys that positively impact and constructively improve existence for all. Take time out daily to reflect on daily life experiences to learn about self, others, and the world in which all coexist interdependently.

Thank you for your interest in wanting to live healthier and for purchasing this book, which I hope will be an investment reaping you many great, long-term, personal health rewards.

George Zahrebelski, MS, MD
Nutritional, Digestive and Liver Health Matters Institute, S.C.
https://www.nutritionaldigestiveandliverhealthmatters.institute/

Selected References and Resources

Many of the commercially sponsored references herein have excellent slideshows encapsulating the basic body vehicle health and nutritional concepts discussed in this book. The best slideshow presentations address the nutritional and health benefits that natural foods in their unprocessed and unrefined, crude fuel, whole earth food versions deliver.

When navigating through the commercially sponsored sites, take notice how advertisers work in commercial subject matter to complement featured stories, but primarily focus on the nutritional information accompanying slideshows to benefit from the valuable health-related nutritional concepts being presented.

Please visit https://www.nutritionaldigestiveandliverhealthmatters.institute/ and click on "Links" for live online access to the following listed and any new and updated reference and resource links.

1. health.com / 17 Superfoods That Fight Disease. Maryanne Gragg, March 4, 2013 https://www.health.com/health/gallery/0,,20662664,00.html#eat-your-way-healthy-1
2. health.com / The Best Foods for Every Vitamin and Mineral. Amanda Macmillan, October 8, 2015 https://www.health.com/health/gallery/0,,20660118,00.html
3. health.com / 31 Superfood Secrets for a Long and Healthy Life. Amanda Macmillan, October 1, 2014 https://www.health.com/health/gallery/0,,20610379,00.html
4. health.com / 9 Ways to Live Longer. May 22, 2013 https://www.health.com/health/gallery/0,,20366671,00.html#live-healthy-live-longer-0
5. health.com / Eating Smart for Your Whole Body. Brittani Renaud, April 3, 2013 https://www.health.com/health/gallery/0,,20307133,00.html
6. health.com / 6 Surprising Superfoods. Jennifer Matlack, June 3, 2013 https://www.health.com/health/gallery/0,,20471231,00.html
7. health.com / Want to Live to 100? Eat These Foods. Aviva Patz, October 1, 2014 https://www.health.com/health/gallery/0,,20655883,00.html
8. health.com / 15 Foods That Help You Stay Hydrated. Amanda Macmillan, June 28, 2017 https://www.health.com/health/gallery/0,,20709014,00.html
9. health.com / 7 Ways You Should Tweak Your Diet as You Age. Cynthia Sass, January 24, 2014 https://www.health.com/celebrities/7-ways-you-shoul d-tweak-your-diet-as-you-age
10. health.com / Your Nutrition Needs in Your 30s, 40s, and 50s. Joan Raymond May 5, 2014 https://www.health.com/health/article/0,,20410268,00.html
11. health.com / Best Superfoods for Weight Loss. Sarah Klein, May 29, 2017 https://www.health.com/health/gallery/0,,20475957,00.html
12. health.com / 23 Best Foods with Fiber. Anne Harding, March 1, 2015 https://www.health.com/health/gallery/0,,20553010,00.html
13. health.com / How to Buy Healthy Food without Looking at the Nutrition Label. Cynthia Sass, October 13, 2016 https://www.health.com/nutrition/nutrition-label-tips

14.   health.com / 11 Ways to Boost Your Energy with Food. Amy O'Connor, September 29, 2015 https://www.health.com/health/gallery/0,,20683067,00.html#view-all

15.   cookinglight.com / 8 Foods That Can Lower Your Cholesterol (Plus the Foods to Avoid). February 1, 2018 https://www.cookinglight.com/eating-smart/nutrition-101/cholesterol-lowering-foods

16.   health.com / Your Secret to Happiness at Every Age. Susannah Felts, November 1, 2015 https://www.health.com/health/gallery/0,,20348268,00.html

17.   health.com / Can Supplements Ease Menopause Symptoms. January 24, 2012 https://www.health.com/health/gallery/0,,20347965,00.html

18.   health.com / 12 Ways We Sabotage Our Mental Health. Amanda Gardner, November 1, 2015 https://www.health.com/health/gallery/0,,20694928,00.html

19.   health.com / 30 Foods Under 40 Calories, with Recipes. Amy O'Connor January 26, 2016 https://www.health.com/health/gallery/0,,20640804,00.html

20.   health.com / 18 Superfoods for Your Heart. Amanda Gardner, February 13, 2017 https://www.health.com/health/gallery/0,,20720182,00.html

21.   fitday.com / 8 Foods Rich in Biotin https://www.fitday.com/fitness-articles/nutrition/vitamins-minerals/8-foods-rich-in-biotin.html

22.   fitday.com / 10 Foods Rich in Selenium https://www.fitday.com/fitness-articles/nutrition/vitamins-minerals/10-foods-rich-in-selenium.html

23.   realsimple.com / 10 Organic Foods That Aren't Worth Buying. Shirley Fan https://www.realsimple.com/food-recipes/shopping-storing/food/non-organic-food

24.   realsimple.com / 10 Organic Foods That Are Worth the Money. Michele Bender https://www.realsimple.com/food-recipes/shopping-storing/more-shopping-storing/ten-organic-foods-worth-money-0

25.   realsimple.com / 11 Superfoods You Should Know About. Shirley Fan https://www.realsimple.com/food-recipes/shopping-storing/food/superfoods

26.   health.com / Eat Your Way to Health and Happiness. Nancy Rones, January 26, 2016 https://www.health.com/health/gallery/0,,20621800,00.html#shop-wisely-1

27.   health.com / America's Healthiest Superfoods for Women. Laurie Herr and Sarah Jio, October 8, 2015 http://www.health.com/health/gallery/0,,20331905,00.html

28.   health.com / 15 Best Superfoods for Fall. October 5, 2013 http://www.health.com/food/15-best-superfoods-for-fall

29.   health.com / 23 Healthiest Superfruits You Need Now. Benjamin Placket, August 1, 2012 http://www.health.com/health/gallery/0,,20606331,00.html

30.   diabetesjournals.org / Pepino MY, et al. Sucralose Affects Glycemic and Hormonal Responses to an Oral Glucose Load. Diabetes Care; 2013 Sep; 36(9): 2530–2535 https://doi.org/10.2337/dc12–2221; http://care.diabetesjournals.org/content/36/9/2530

31.   nature.com / Suez J, et al. Artificial Sweeteners Induce Glucose Intolerance by Altering the Gut Microbiota; Nature; 2014 Oct 9; 514: 181–186 https://doi:10.1038/nature13793; https://www.nature.com/articles/nature13793

32.   scientificamerican.com / How Artificial Sweeteners May Cause Us to Eat More. Bret Stetka, July 12, 2016 https://www.scientificamerican.com/article/how-artificial-sweeteners-may-cause-us-to-eat-more/

33.   theatlantic.com / This Is Your Brain on Diet Soda: How Fake Sugar Makes You Overeat. Brian Fung, June 14, 2012 https://www.theatlantic.com/health/archive/2012/06/this-is-your-brain-on-diet-soda-how-fake-sugar-makes-you-overeat/258521/

34.   scientificamerican.com / How Sugar and Fat Trick the Brain into Wanting More Food. Ferris Jabr, January 1, 2016 https://www.scientificamerican.com/article/how-sugar-and-fat-trick-the-brain-into-wanting-more-food/

35.   sciencenews.org / Diet Sodas May Confuse Brain's "Calorie Counter." Anet Raloff, June 13, 2012 https://www.sciencenews.org/article/diet-sodas-may-confus e-brains-calorie-counter

36.   thedailymeal.com / 11 Misleading Beverage Labels. Marcy Franklin, April 23, 2013 https://www.thedailymeal.com/11-misleading-beverage-labels

37.   thedailymeal.com / 8 "Healthy Drinks" That Are Actually Terrible for You. Marcy Franklin, November 13, 2012 https://www.thedailymeal.com/8-healthy-drink s-are-actually-terrible-you

38.   thedailymeal.com / 10 of the Best Nuts for Your Health Slideshow. https://www. thedailymeal.com/cook/10-best-nuts-your-health-slideshow

39.   thedailymeal.com / 10 Foods That Burn Fat. Julie Wilcox, March 19, 2014 https:// www.thedailymeal.com/10-foods-burn-fat/31914

40.   greatist.com /15 Easy Ways to Beat Anxiety Now. Giuliana Hazelwood, March 9, 2014 https://greatist.com/happiness/reduce-anxiety

41.   cookinglight.com / 12 Filling Foods. August 16, 2012 http://www.cookinglight.com/ eating-smart/nutrition-101/filling-foods

42.   health.com / 13 Comfort Foods That Burn Fat. K. Aleisha Fetters, December 23, 2013 http://www.health.com/health/gallery/0,,20735735,00.html

43.   health.com / Bone Health: Preventing Osteoporosis: 14 Surprising Facts about Healthy Bones. Alyssa Sparacino, September 16, 2013 http://www.health.com/ health/gallery/0,,20471612,00.html#-don-t-break-a-leg-0

44.   readersdigest.com / 27 Foods You Should Never Buy Again. Reader's Digest Editors https://www.rd.com/health/wellness/foods-you-should-never-buy-again/

45.   readersdigest.com / 25 Natural Energy Boosters That Just Might Change Your Life. Reader's Digest Editors https://www.rd.com/health/healthy-eating/ natural-energy-boosters/

46.   readersdigest.com / 6 Foods That Improve Your Eyesight. Diana Kelly http://www. readersdigest.ca/health/eye-health/foods-that-improve-your-eyesight/view-all/

47.   readersdigest.com / 6 Natural Cough Remedies You Can Make from Items Already in Your Kitchen. Taylor Shea https://www.rd.com/health/wellness/natural-cough-rem edies/

48.   readersdigest.com / How to Develop a Positive Attitude in 6 Easy Steps. Katie Macdonald https://www.rd.com/health/wellness/develop-positive-attitude/8/

49.   readersdigest.com / 10 Benefits of Reading: Getting Smart, Thin, Healthy and Happy. Lauren Gelman http://www.readersdigest.ca/health/healthy-living/ reading-benefits-change-life/view-all/

50.   readersdigest.com / Experts Say These Magic Words Will Change Your Life. Lauren Gelman https://www.rd.com/health/wellness/experts-magic-words-change-your-life/

51.   readersdigest.com / The 9 Best Foods to Eat to Boost Your Brain Health. Diana Kelly, Claire Nowak and Lauren Gniazdowski https://www.rd.com/health/conditions/ best-brain-food/

52.   readersdigest.com / The Best Post-Workout Snack Ideas. Diana Kelly https://www. rd.com/health/wellness/best-post-workout-snack/

53.   readersdigest.com / 7 Ways to Trick Your Taste Buds into Eating Healthier. Lauren Gelman https://www.rd.com/health/healthy-eating/trick-your-taste-bud s-eating-healthier/

54.   readersdigest.com / How to Eat More Healthy Protein without Even Trying. Diana Kelly https://www.rd.com/health/wellness/healthy-protein/

55.   readersdigest.com / 7 Ways to Eat More Omega-3 Foods That Aren't Fish. Diana Kelly https://www.rd.com/health/wellness/omega-3-foods/9/

56.   readersdigest.com / 5 Delicious Ways to Eat More Vitamin E Foods. Diana Kelly
       https://www.rd.com/health/wellness/vitamin-e-foods/
57.   readersdigest.com / Fast Food Facts: How Long Does It Take to Burn Off Your Meal?
       Perri O. Blumberg https://www.rd.com/health/healthy-eating/fast-food-facts-ho
       w-long-does-it-take-to-burn-off-your-meal/15/
58.   thedailymeal.com / Foods Americans Eat That Are Banned Around the World. Elsa
       Säätelä, October 10, 2013 https://www.thedailymeal.com/10-foods-american
       s-eat-banned-around-the-world/101013; https://www.thedailymeal.com/travel/10-f
       oods-americans-eat-are-banned-around-world-slideshow
59.   thedailymeal.com / 11 Banned Ingredients We Eat in the US. Haley Willard, July 1,
       2013 https://www.thedailymeal.com/11-banned-ingredients-we-eat-us
60.   thedailymeal.com / 7 Myths about Olive Oil. Will Budiaman, July 30, 2013 https://
       www.thedailymeal.com/7-myths-about-olive-oil
61.   cookinglight.com / Foods to Get You Fit and Beautiful. Katherine Brooking, May 27,
       2010 http://www.cookinglight.com/eating-smart/nutrition-101/beauty-foods
62.   health.com / 12 Ways We Sabotage Our Mental Health. Amanda Gardner, November
       1, 2015 http://www.health.com/health/gallery/0,,20694928,00.html
63.   health.com / 9 Foods That May Help Save Your Memory. September 21, 2017 http://
       www.health.com/health/gallery/0,,20434658,00.html
64.   health.com / New Ways to Boost Your Brain Power. Susan Hall, October 9, 2012
       http://www.health.com/health/gallery/0,,20365995,00.html
65.   health.com / Attention Sappers: 5 Reasons You Can't Concentrate. Jessica Gird-
       wain, May 12, 2010 http://www.health.com/health/gallery/0,,20307269,00.
       html#too-much-stress-0
66.   health.com / 5 Ways Your Healthy Diet Is Making You Tired. Norine
       Dworkin-McDaniel, August 26, 2013 http://www.health.com/health/
       gallery/0,,20723556,00.html
67.   health.com / 18 Superfoods for Your Heart. Amanda Gardner, February 13, 2017
       http://www.health.com/health/gallery/0,,20720182,00.html
68.   health.com / 8 Tips to Instantly Boost Your Energy. Sarah Jio, April 10, 2015 http://
       www.health.com/health/gallery/0,,20559973,00.html
69.   health.com / 12 Foods with More Vitamin C than Oranges. Christine Mattheis,
       December 30, 2013 http://www.health.com/health/gallery/0,,20745689,00.html?x-
       id=Time-calcium-090214
70.   health.com / Vitamins: What to Take, What to Skip. Amanda Gardner http://www.
       health.com/health/gallery/0%2C%2C20506267%2C00.html
71.   thedailymeal.com / What's Really in Your Fast Food? Dan Myers, November 12, 2013
       https://www.thedailymeal.com/what-s-really-your-fast-food/111213 https://www.
       thedailymeal.com/eat/what-s-really-your-fast-food-slideshow/list
72.   cookinglight.com / 20 Foods That Sound Healthy (but Aren't). Carolyn Williams,
       September 2, 2009 http://www.cookinglight.com/eating-smart/smart-choices/
       top-10-unhealthy-foods
73.   health.com / 10 Best Foods for Your Heart. October 8, 2015 http://www.health.com/
       health/gallery/0,,20307113,00.html
74.   health.com / 13 Surprising Causes of Constipation. Amanda Gardner, July 25, 2014
       http://www.health.com/health/gallery/0,,20452199,00.html
75.   thedailymeal.com / We Asked 10 Nutritionists How Much Water You Should Actu-
       ally Drink https://www.thedailymeal.com/healthy-eating/we-asked-10-nutritioni
       sts-how-much-water-you-should-actually-drink-0/slide-6; https://www.thedaily-
       meal.com/drink/how-much-water-should-you-be-drinking-slideshow

76. thedailymeal.com / 10 Foods That Promote Bone Health. Emily Jacobs, November 11, 2013 https://www.thedailymeal.com/cook/10-foods-promote-bone-health-slide-show; https://www.thedailymeal.com/10-foods-promote-bone-health/111113

77. thedailymeal.com / 5 Foods That Fight Inflammation. Elyse Cromer, November 8, 2013 https://www.thedailymeal.com/cook/5-foods-fight-inflammation-slideshow https://www.thedailymeal.com/5-foods-fight-inflammation/110813

78. health.com / 10 Reasons to Give Up Diet Soda. Mary Squillace, October 28, 2013 http://www.health.com/health/gallery/0,,20739512,00.html

79. health.com / The 25 Best Diet Tricks of All Time. February 14, 2013 http://www.health.com/health/gallery/0,,20645166,00.html

80. thedailymeal.com / 12 Superfoods You Need to Know. Emily Jacobs, June 18, 2015 https://www.thedailymeal.com/cook/12-superfoods-you-need-know-slideshow https://www.thedailymeal.com/12-superfoods-you-need-know/102113

81. health.com / 27 Mistakes Healthy People Make. Anne Harding, April 23, 2013 http://www.health.com/health/gallery/0,,20621010,00.html

82. health.com / Are You Making These Dieting Mistakes? Kate Fodor, April 27, 2012 http://www.health.com/health/gallery/0,,20584613,00.html

83. health.com / Diet Crutches: What Works, What Doesn't. Ella Quittner, May 10, 2013 http://www.health.com/health/gallery/0,,20517473,00.html

84. thedailymeal.com / 10 Foods That Are Highest in Cholesterol. Lauren Gordon, November 27, 2013 https://www.thedailymeal.com/10-foods-are-highest-cholesterol/112713

85. health.com / 14 Ways to Cut Portions without Feeling Hungry. Diana Kelly, May 13, 2015 http://www.health.com/health/gallery/0,,20769037,00.html

86. health.com / 25 Ways to Cut 500 Calories a Day. Shaun Chavis, January 23, 2014 http://www.health.com/health/gallery/0,,20454528,00.html

87. dummies.com / Seven Foods That Fight Inflammation and Belly Fat. Erin Palinski-Wade http://www.dummies.com/health/exercise/lose-belly-fat/seven-foods-that-fight-inflammation-and-belly-fat/#slide-1

88. thedailymeal.com / Fountain of Youth: 7 Anti-Aging Foods. Natalia Sloam, January 21, 2014 https://www.thedailymeal.com/fountain-youth-7-anti-aging-foods/12114

89. thedailymeal.com / 5 Ways Avocados Can Make You Prettier. Lauren Gordon, March 20, 2017 https://www.thedailymeal.com/5-ways-avocados-can-make-you-prettier/111513; https://www.thedailymeal.com/entertain/5-ways-avocados-can-make-you-prettier-slideshow

90. thedailymeal.com / 6 Kinds of Fat, and Which Foods Are Highest in Them. Dan Myers, February 21, 2014 https://www.thedailymeal.com/6-kinds-fat-and-which-foods-are-highest-them/22114

91. thedailymeal.com / The 20 Worst Things You Can Eat and Why. Dan Myers, October 14, 2015 https://www.thedailymeal.com/the-20-worst-things-you-can-eat-why/42314

92. thedailymeal.com / 10 Foods with Healthy Fats. Emily Jacobs, January 2, 2014 https://www.thedailymeal.com/10-foods-healthy-fats/1214

93. thedailymeal.com / Yogurt for Sour Cream and 7 Other Healthy Food Swaps. Emily Jacobs, Jun 5, 2014 https://www.thedailymeal.com/yogurt-sour-cream-and-7-other-healthy-food-swaps/6514

94. health.com / 14 Ways to Age in Reverse. Aviva Patz, June 25, 2014 http://www.health.com/health/gallery/0,,20825198,00.html

95. howstuffworks.com / 20 Everyday Activities and the Calories They Burn. By the editors of Publications International, LTD https://health.howstuffworks.com/well-

ness/diet-fitness/information/20-everyday-activities-and-the-calories-they-burn.
htm

96.   nutristrategy.com / Calories Burned during Exercise, Activities, Sports and Work.
http://www.nutristrategy.com/caloriesburned.htm

97.   health.harvard.edu / Calories Burned in 30 Minutes for People of Three Different
Weights https://www.health.harvard.edu/diet-and-weight-loss/calories-burned-in-
30-minutes-of-leisure-and-routine-activities

98.   en.wikipedia.org / List of Food Additives. https://en.wikipedia.org/wiki/List_of_
food_additives

99.   en.wikipedia.org / E Number. https://en.wikipedia.org/wiki/E_number

100.   thedailymeal.com / Jackfruit and 8 Other Superfoods You've Never Heard Of. Kristie
Collado, November 19, 2014 https://www.thedailymeal.com/cook/jackfruit-and-
8-other-superfoods-youve-never-heard-slideshow; https://www.thedailymeal.com/
jackfruit-and-8-other-superfoods-you-ve-never-heard

101.   thedailymeal.com / Top 5 Superfoods for a Super Mood. By Spoon University, March
9, 2014 https://www.thedailymeal.com/top-5-superfoods-super-mood

102.   thedailymeal.com / 10 Metabolism Boosting Superfoods. Lauren Gordon, June 17,
2015 https://www.thedailymeal.com/10-metabolism-boosting-superfoods/22514

103.   thedailymeal.com / Hydrate and Energize: 10 Foods for Summer Health. Emily Jacobs, May
4, 2015 https://www.thedailymeal.com/hydrate-and-energize-10-foods-summer-health;
https://www.thedailymeal.com/cook/hydrate-and-energize-10-foods-summer-health/list

104.   thedailymeal.com / 8 Foods to Beat the Heat. Emily Jacobs, June 20, 2014 https://
www.thedailymeal.com/8-foods-beat-heat/62014

105.   thedailymeal.com / 8 Summer Slim-Down Superfoods. Emily Jacobs, June 17, 2015
https://www.thedailymeal.com/8-summer-slim-down-superfoods

106.   thedailymeal.com / 12 Best and Worst Weight-Loss Programs According to
Experts. Lauren Gordon, May 13, 2014 https://www.thedailymeal.com/12-best-an
d-worst-weight-loss-programs-according-experts/51414

107.   thedailymeal.com / 10 Reasons Your Kids Are Making You Fat. Sidney Harrison, July
11, 2014 https://www.thedailymeal.com/10-reasons-your-kids-are-making-you-
fat; https://www.thedailymeal.com/entertain/10-reasons-your-kids-are-mak-
ing-you-fat-slideshow

108.   niaaa.nih.gov / Alcohol & Health. https://www.niaaa.nih.gov/alcohol-health

109.   umm.edu / Health / Medical / Altmed / Supplement / Quercetin. http://accu-
rateclinic.com/wp-content/uploads/2016/02/Quercetin-University-of-Marylan
d-Medical-Center.pdf

110.   health.harvard.edu / Listing of Vitamins. August 14, 2017 https://www.health.
harvard.edu/staying-healthy/listing of vitamins

111.   safepatientproject.org / posts / 2257-Survey Finds Close Ties between Drug Companies and Patient Groups. https://safepatientproject.org/posts/2257-survey_finds_
close_ties_between_drug_companies_and_patient_groups

112.   pogo.org / our-work / reports / 2016 / In FDA Meetings Voice of the Patient Often
Funded by Drug Companies. http://www.pogo.org/our-work/reports/2016/in-fd
a-meetings-voice-of-the-patient-often-funded-by-drug-companies.html

113.   propublica.org / blog/item / Health Advocacy Groups Take Drug Company Cash:
Often without Full Disclosures. Marian Wang, January 13, 2011 https://www.
propublica.org/article/health-advocacy-groups-take-drug-company-cashoften-w
ithout-full-disclosures

114.   nytimes.com / Health / The Selling of Attention Deficit Disorder. Alan Schwarz,
December 14, 2013 http://archive.nytimes.com/www.nytimes.com/2013/12/15/
health/the-selling-of-attention-deficit-disorder.html

115. thedailymeal.com / 11 Foods That Keep You Young. Lauren Gordon, March 3, 2015 https://www.thedailymeal.com/11-foods-keep-you-young https://www.thedaily-meal.com/entertain/11-foods-keep-you-young/list

116. en.wikipedia.org / Resin Identification Code (plastics recycling numbers) https://en.wikipedia.org/wiki/Resin_identification_code

117. nrdc.org / Natural Resources Defense Council / 4 Ways to Avoid Toxic Chemicals in Food Packaging. https://www.nrdc.org/stories/4-ways-avoi d-toxic-chemicals-food-packaging

118. thealternativedaily.com / The Final Verdict on Non-Toxic Food Containers. October 6, 2015 https://www.thealternativedaily.com/final-verdict-on-non-toxic-food-con-tainers/

119. theactivetimes.com / Surprising Reasons You're Gaining Weight. Catarina Cowden, October 23, 2014 https://www.theactivetimes.com/11-surprising-reason s-youre-gaining-weight-slideshow; https://www.theactivetimes.com/surprising-reasons-youre-gaining-weight

120. thedailymeal.com / 8 Grossest Things You Didn't Know You Were Eating. Kristie Collado, August 19, 2014 https://www.thedailymeal.com/8-grossest-things-you-did n-t-know-you-were-eating

121. fda.gov / Food / Guidance Regulation / Defect levels Handbook / The Food Defect Action Levels: Levels of Natural or Avoidable Defects in Foods That Present No Health Hazards for Humans. https://www.fda.gov/Food/GuidanceRegulation/Guid-anceDocumentsRegulatoryInformation/SanitationTransportation/ucm056174.htm

122. fda.gov / Food / Guidance Regulation / Guidance Documents Regulatory Infor-mation by Topic / Sanitation & Transportation Guidance Documents & Regulatory Information. https://www.fda.gov/Food/GuidanceRegulation/GuidanceDocu-mentsRegulatoryInformation/SanitationTransportation/default.htm

123. thedailymeal.com / 13 Carbohydrates That Can Help You Lose Weight. Sara Kay, September 25, 2014 https://www.thedailymeal.com/13-carbohydrates-ca n-help-you-lose-weight; https://www.thedailymeal.com/cook/13-carbohydrates-ca n-help-you-lose-weight/list

124. thedailymeal.com / Beware: These 7 Ingredients Aren't What You Think They Are. Kristie Collado, September 25, 2014 https://www.thedailymeal.com/beware-these-7-ingredients-arent-what-you-think-they-are; https://www.thedailymeal.com/cook/7-ingredients-arent-what-you-think-slideshow

125. health.com / Best and Worst Foods for Your Teeth. Amanda Gardner, September 18, 2016 http://www.health.com/health/gallery/0,,20687551,00.html

126. theactivetimes.com / Ways Stress Causes Weight Gain. Catarina Cowden, September 5, 2014 https://www.theactivetimes.com/8-ways-stress-making-you-gain-weight; https://www.theactivetimes.com/ways-stress-causes-weight-gain/slide-4

127. health.usnews.com / Health / Wellness / The Best Foods for Lowering Your Blood Pressure. Angela Haupt, April 1, 2014 https://health.usnews.com/health-news/health-wellness/slideshows/the-best-foods-for-lowering-your-blood-pressure

128. theactivetimes.com / Sneaky Holiday Habits That Cause Weight Gain. Katie Rosenbrock, November 6, 2014 https://www.theactivetimes.com/sneaky-holida y-habits-cause-weight-gain

129. health.com / 10 Signs Your House Is Making You Fat. Jessica Migala, January 13, 2015 http://www.health.com/health/gallery/0,,20857242,00.html

130. theactivetimes.com / Stop Drinking Pop / Reasons Soda Is Killing You. Cata-rina Cowden, October 24, 2014 https://www.theactivetimes.com/stop-drinkin g-pop-reasons-soda-killing-you

131.   grainstorm.com / What's Wrong with Modern Wheat? https://grainstorm.com/pages/modern-wheat

132.   healthline.com / Why Modern Wheat Is Worse Than Older Wheat. https://www.healthline.com/nutrition/modern-wheat-health-nightmare

133.   nejm.org / Longo, DL; Cancer Drug Discovery: Let's Get Ready for the Next Period. NEJM; 2014 Dec 4; 371(23): 2227–2228 DOI: 10.1056/NEJMe1412624 https://www.nejm.org/doi/full/10.1056/NEJMe1412624

134.   thedailymeal.com / 7 Underrated Foods for Weight Loss. Kristie Collado, March 10, 2015 https://www.thedailymeal.com/cook/7-underrated-foods-weight-loss

135.   menshealth.com / 7 Vegetables You're Not Eating: but Should Be. Cassie Shortsleeve, March 7, 2014 https://www.menshealth.com/nutrition/a19538737/vegetables-you-should-be-eating/

136.   readersdigest.com / What to Eat When You Have a Cold: 8 Healing Foods. Alyssa Jung https://www.rd.com/health/conditions/what-to-eat-when-you-have-a-cold/

137.   health.com / Superfoods That Fight Colds. Amanda Macmillan, September 8, 2015 http://www.health.com/health/gallery/0,,20631007,00.html

138.   thedailymeal.com / How Lack of Sleep Can Affect Your Diet. Fabiana Santana, March 26, 2015 https://www.thedailymeal.com/entertain/how-lack-sleep-can-affect-your-diet

139.   usatoday.com / How Sleep Loss Leads to Significant Weight Gain. Nanci Hellmich, July 20, 2014 https://www.usatoday.com/story/news/nation/2014/07/20/sleep-loss-weight-gain/7507503/

140.   thedailymeal.com / Foods and Drinks That Make You More Forgetful. Natalia Sloam, December 4, 2014 https://www.thedailymeal.com/entertain/foods-and-drinks-make-you-more-forgetful

141.   thedailymeal.com / 10 Reasons You Should Never Drink Soda. Dr. Verma, December 17, 2015 https://www.thedailymeal.com/10-reasons-you-should-never-drink-soda/21214

142.   thedailymeal.com / Surprisingly Unhealthy Drinks. Kim Cooper, November 24, 2014 https://www.thedailymeal.com/drink/surprisingly-unhealthly-drinks

143.   commonsensemedia.org / The Ugly Truth behind Pretty Pictures. Sierra Filucci, January 18, 2017 https://www.commonsensemedia.org/blog/the-ugly-truth-behind-pretty-pictures

144.   en.wikipedia.org / Mass-Energy Equivalence. https://en.wikipedia.org/wiki/Mass%E2%80%93energy_equivalence

145.   health.com / 15 Things Nobody Tells You About Losing Weight. Amanda Macmillan, February 10, 2015 http://www.health.com/health/gallery/0,,20888773,00.html

146.   health.com / Bloated All the Time? 11 Reasons Why. Esther Crain, August 28, 2015 http://www.health.com/health/gallery/0,,20872171,00.html

147.   health.com / 20 Things You Should Throw Away for Better Health. Nicole Cherie Jones, March 4, 2015 http://www.health.com/health/gallery/0,,20892663,00.html

148.   health.com / 12 Worst Habits for Your Mental Health. Carey Rossi, December 11, 2015 http://www.health.com/health/gallery/0,,20866947,00.html#hang-on-to-your-happiness-0

149.   thedailymeal.com / Supersize That? 10 Ways Fast-Food Chains Are Playing with Your Head. Dan Myers, September 30, 2016 https://www.thedailymeal.com/eat/supersize-10-mind-games-fast-food-restaurants-play-you; https://www.thedailymeal.com/eat/supersize-10-mind-games-fast-food-restaurants-play-you-0/list

150.   bls.gov / US Department of Labor / Bureau of Labor Statistics / Economic News Release / American Time Use Survey Summary. https://www.bls.gov/news.release/atus.nr0.htm

151.   nielson.com / How Smartphones Are Changing Consumers' Daily Routines around the Globe. February 24, 2014 http://www.nielsen.com/us/en/insights/news/2014/how-smartphones-are-changing-consumers-daily-routines-around-the-globe.html

152.   emarketer.com / Mobile Continues to Steal Share of US Adults' Daily Time Spent with Media. https://www.emarketer.com/Article/Mobile-Continues-Steal-Share-of-US-Adults-Daily-Time-Spent-with-Media/1010782

153.   thedailymeal.com / Foods That Could Be Weakening Your Immune System. Lauren Fusilier, December 3, 2015 https://www.thedailymeal.com/entertain/foods-could-be-weakening-your-immune-system; https://www.thedailymeal.com/cook/learn-which-foods-weaken-immune-system/list

154.   thedailymeal.com / These 10 Foods Will Help You Get a Better Night's Sleep. Kristie Collado, February 2, 2015 https://www.thedailymeal.com/cook/these-10-foods-will-help-you-get-better-nights-sleep; https://www.thedailymeal.com/cook/these-10-foods-will-help-you-get-better-nights-sleep-slideshow/list

155.   theactivetimes.com / Ageing Well: Healthy Habits That Keep You Young. Katie Rosenbrock, January 27, 2015 https://www.theactivetimes.com/aging-well-healthy-habits-keep-you-young

156.   health.com / 10 Reasons Your Belly Fat Isn't Going Away. Camille Noe Pagan, February 3, 2017 http://www.health.com/health/gallery/0,,20905682,00.html#lose-the-pudge-1

157.   theactivetimes.com / Myths about Weight Loss, and What Science Really Says. Katie Rosenbrock, March 5, 2015 https://www.theactivetimes.com/myths-about-weight-loss-and-what-science-really-says; https://www.theactivetimes.com/10-myths-about-weight-loss-and-what-science-really-says-slideshow

158.   theactivetimes.com / 10 Healthy Eating Obstacles (and How to Overcome Them). Katie Rosenbrock, February 26, 2015 https://www.theactivetimes.com/10-healthy-eating-obstacles-and-how-overcome-them

159.   thedailymeal.com / 27 Foods Doctors Won't Eat and Why. Christian Kogler, February 11, 2016 https://www.thedailymeal.com/healthy-eating/27-foods-doctors-wont-eat-and-why; https://www.thedailymeal.com/healthy-eating/27-foods-doctors-wont-eat-and-why-slideshow/list

160.   tandfonline.com / Bianconi, E, et al. An Estimation of the Number of Cells in the Human Body; Annals of Human Biology; 2013 Jul 05 online; 40(6): 463–471 https://www.tandfonline.com/doi/full/10.3109/03014460.2013.807878

161.   healthaliciousness.com / Nutrition Facts. https://www.myfooddata.com/

162.   health.harvard.edu / Top Foods to Help Protect Your Vision. August 1, 2013 https://www.health.harvard.edu/staying-healthy/top-foods-to-help-protect-your-vision

163.   health.com / 15 Eating Habits That Make You Live Longer. Dan Buettner, May 29, 2015 http://www.health.com/health/gallery/0,,20922657,00.html

164.   health.com / Want to Live to 100? Eat These Foods. Aviva Patz, October 1, 2014 http://www.health.com/health/gallery/0,,20655883,00.html

165.   health.com / Eat Your Way to Health and Happiness. Nancy Rones, January 26, 2016 http://www.health.com/health/gallery/0,,20621800,00.html

166.   onlinelibrary.wiley.com / Gross, K; Framing Persuasive Appeals: Episodic and Thematic Framing, Emotional Response, and Policy Opinion; Political Psychology 2008; 29(2): 162–192 https://doi.org/10.1111/j.1467-9221.2008.00622.x https://onlinelibrary.wiley.com/doi/abs/10.1111/j.1467-9221.2008.00622.x

167.   theactivetimes.com / 11 Habits That Cause Premature Aging. Catarina Cowden, October 8, 2015 https://www.theactivetimes.com/habits-are-making-you-age-prematurely

168.   crohnsforum.com / Emulsifiers Detergents and IBD-Crohn's Disease Forum. https://www.crohnsforum.com/showthread.php?t=46181

169.   ncbi.nlm.nih.gov / McGill SL, Smyth HDC. Disruption of the Mucus Barrier by Topically Applied Exogenous Particles; Molecular Pharmaceutics 2010; 7(6): 2280–2288 https://www.ncbi.nlm.nih.gov/pmc/articles/PMC3654807/

170.   clinicaleducation.org / Food Additives Feed the Fire via Microbiome Dysbiosis Induction. Michael Ash, April 8, 2015 https://www.clinicaleducation.org/news/food-additives-feed-the-fire-via-microbiome-dysbiosis-induction/

171.   nature.com / Bordon Y. Food Additives Feed the Fire; Nature Reviews Immunology; 2015 Apr; 15(4); 200–201 DOI: 10.1038/nri3833. Epub 2015 Mar 6 https://www.ncbi.nlm.nih.gov/pubmed/25743220 https://www.nature.com/articles/nri3833

172.   ncbi.nlm.nih.gov / Chassaing B, Gewirtz AT. Gut Microbiota, Low-Grade Inflammation, and Metabolic Syndrome; Toxicologic Pathology; 2014 Jan; 42(1): 49–53 DOI: 10.1177/0192623313508481 https://www.ncbi.nlm.nih.gov/pubmed/24285672 Epub 2013 Nov 27 http://journals.sagepub.com/doi/full/10.1177/0192623313508481

173.   lpi.oregonstate.edu / mic / Linus Pauling Institute, Oregon State University, Micronutrient Center. http://lpi.oregonstate.edu/mic

174.   theactivetimes.com / Fall Superfoods That Help with Weight Loss. October 12, 2016 https://www.theactivetimes.com/content/fall-superfoods-help-weight-loss/slide-4; https://www.theactivetimes.com/content/fall-superfoods-help-weight-loss/slide-1

175.   health.com / 17 Ways to Age-Proof Your Brain. Amanda Gardner, May 29, 2017 http://www.health.com/health/gallery/0,,20892550,00.html

176.   thedailymeal.com / 8 Reasons Why Fast Food Is Making You Sick and Tired. Dan Myers, May 15, 2015 https://www.thedailymeal.com/eat/8-reasons-why-fast-food-making-you-sick-and-tired; https://www.thedailymeal.com/eat/8-reasons-why-fast-food-making-you-sick-and-tired-0/list

177.   health.com / 10 Things You Should Never Do When You're Angry. Linda Melone, June 15, 2015 http://www.health.com/health/gallery/0,,20805851,00.html

178.   thedailymeal.com / Pay Attention! 14 Foods That Will Boost Your Concentration. Bridget Creel, September 16, 2015 https://www.thedailymeal.com/healthy-eating/pay-attention-14-foods-will-boost-your-concentration; https://www.thedailymeal.com/healthy-eating/pay-attention-14-foods-will-boost-your-concentration-0

179.   rsc.org / Education / Teachers / Resources / Chemistry for Biologists. http://www.rsc.org/Education/Teachers/Resources/cfb/

180.   thedailymeal.com / You Don't Really Need to Be Taking These Vitamins. Bridget Creel, December 14, 2015 https://www.thedailymeal.com/healthy-eating/you-don-t-really-need-be-taking-these-vitamins; https://www.thedailymeal.com/healthy-eating/you-don-t-really-need-be-taking-these-vitamins-0

181.   today.com / Series / Wired / Are Cellphones Causing Hallucinations? The Reason Why You Felt That "Phantom Buzz." Chloe Vincente, January 15, 2016 https://www.today.com/series/wired/are-cellphones-causing-hallucinations-reason-why-you-felt-phantom-buzz-t67231

182.   ncbi.nlm.nih.gov / Hartmann P. Normal Weight of the Brain in Adults in Relation to Age, Sex, Body Height and Weight; Pathologe; 1994 Jun; 15(3): 165–170 https://www.ncbi.nlm.nih.gov/pubmed/8072950

183.   en.wikipedia.org / List of Culinary Herbs and Spices. https://en.wikipedia.org/wiki/List_of_culinary_herbs_and_spices

184.   nih.gov / US Department of Health and Human Services / National Institutes of Health / Office of Dietary Supplements / Health Information / Dietary Supplement Fact Sheets. https://ods.od.nih.gov/; https://ods.od.nih.gov/factsheets/list-all/

185.   journals.plos.org / Moore SC, et al. Leisure Time Physical Activity of Moderate to Vigorous Intensity and Mortality: A Large Pooled Cohort Analysis; PLOS Medicine;

2012 Nov; 9(11): e1001335 https://doi.org/10.1371/journal.pmed.1001335; http://journals.plos.org/plosmedicine/article?id=10.1371/journal.pmed.1001335

186. ncbi.nlm.nih.gov / Woolf SH. Potential Benefits, Limitations, and Harms of Clinical Guidelines; The BMJ; 1999 Feb 20; 318(7182): 527–530 https://www.ncbi.nlm.nih.gov/pmc/articles/PMC1114973/

187. addiction.com / Technology Addiction 101. https://www.addiction.com/addiction-a-to-z/technology-addiction/technology-addiction-101/

188. ncbi.nlm.nih.gov / Brand M, et al. Prefrontal Control and Internet Addiction: A Theoretical Model and Review of Neuropsychological and Neuroimaging Findings. Frontiers in Human Neuroscience 2014 May 27; 8: 375 https://www.ncbi.nlm.nih.gov/pmc/articles/PMC4034340/

189. ers.usda.gov / Food Expenditures Data. https://www.ers.usda.gov/data-products/food-expenditures.aspx

190. khn.org / Kaiser Health News: Accountable Care Organizations Explained. https://khn.org/news/aco-accountable-care-organization-faq/

191. gastrojournal.org / Owyang C, Wu GD. The Gut Microbiome in Health and Disease; Gastroenterology 2014 May; 146(6); 1433–1436 https://doi.org/10.1053/j.gastro.2014.03.032 ; https://www.gastrojournal.org/article/S0016-5085(14)00381-3/fulltext?referrer=https%3A%2F%2Fwww.ncbi.nlm.nih.gov%2F

192. ncbi.nlm.nih.gov / Shreiner AB, et al. The Gut Microbiome in Health and in Disease; Current Opinion in Gastroenterology; 2015 Jan; 31(1): 69–75 DOI:10.1097/MOG.0000000000000139 https://www.ncbi.nlm.nih.gov/pmc/articles/PMC4290017/

193. ncbi.nlm.nih.gov / Hollister EB, et al. Compositional and Functional Features of the Gastrointestinal Microbiome and Their Effects on Human Health; Gastroenterology; 2014 May; 146(6): 1449–1458 DOI: 10.1053/j.gastro.2014.01.052 https://www.ncbi.nlm.nih.gov/pmc/articles/PMC4181834/

194. ncbi.nlm.nih.gov / Ursell LK, et al. The Intestinal Metabolome: An Intersection Between Microbiota and Host; Gastroenterology; 2014 May; 146(6): 1470–1476 DOI: 10.1053/j.gastro.2014.03.001 https://www.ncbi.nlm.nih.gov/pmc/articles/PMC4102302/

195. ncbi.nlm.nih.gov / Kamada N, Nunez G. Regulation of the Immune System by the Resident Intestinal Bacteria; Gastroenterology; 2014 May; 146(6): 1477–1488 DOI: 10.1053/j.gastro.2014.01.060 https://www.ncbi.nlm.nih.gov/pmc/articles/PMC3995843/

196. ncbi.nlm.nih.gov / Mayer EA, et al. Brain-Gut Interactions and Functional Bowel Disorders; Gastroenterology; 2014 May; 146(6): 1500–1512 DOI: 10.1053/j.gastro.2014.02.037 https://www.ncbi.nlm.nih.gov/pmc/articles/PMC4114504/

197. ncbi.nlm.nih.gov / Schnabl B, Brenner DA. Interactions between the Intestinal Microbiome and Liver Diseases; Gastroenterology; 2014 May; 146(6): 1513–1524 DOI: 10.1053/j.gastro.2014.01.020 https://www.ncbi.nlm.nih.gov/pmc/articles/PMC3996054/

198. gastrojournal.org / Nieuwdorp M, et al. Role of the Microbiome in Energy Regulation and Metabolism; Gastroenterology; 2014 May; 146(6): 1525–1533 https://www.gastrojournal.org/article/S0016-5085(14)00219-4/fulltext?referrer=https%3A%2F%2Fwww.ncbi.nlm.nih.gov%2F

199. ncbi.nlm.nih.gov / Abreu MT, Peek RM Jr. Gastrointestinal Malignancy and the Microbiome; Gastroenterology; 2014 May; 146(6): 1534–1546 DOI: 10.1053/j.gastro.2014.01.001 https://www.ncbi.nlm.nih.gov/pmc/articles/PMC3995897/

200. gastrojournal.org / Shanahan F, Quigley EMM. Manipulation of the Microbiota for the Treatment of IBS and IBD: Challenges and Controversies; Gastroenterol-

ogy: 2014 May; 146(6); 1543–1563 https://www.gastrojournal.org/article/S0016-5085(14)00141-3/fulltext?referrer=https%3A%2F%2Fwww.ncbi.nlm.nih.gov%2F

201. ncbi.nlm.nih.gov / Albenberg LG, Wu GD. Diet and the Intestinal Microbiome: Associations, Functions, and Implications for Health and Disease; Gastroenterology; 2014 May; 146(6): 1564–1572 DOI: 10.1053/j.gastro.2014.01.058 https://www.ncbi.nlm.nih.gov/pmc/articles/PMC4216184/

202. ncbi.nlm.nih.gov / Corley DA, Schuppan D. Food, the Immune System, and the Gastrointestinal Tract; Gastroenterology; 2015 May; 148(6); 1083–1086 DOI: 10.1053/j.gastro.2015.03.043 https://www.ncbi.nlm.nih.gov/pmc/articles/PMC4409565/

203. gastrojournal.org / Tilg H, Moschen AR. Food, Immunity, and the Microbiome; Gastroenterology; 2015 May; 148(6): 1107–1119 https://www.gastrojournal.org/article/S0016-5085(15)00012-8/fulltext?referrer=https%3A%2F%2Fwww.ncbi.nlm.nih.gov%2F

204. ncbi.nlm.nih.gov / Valenta R, et al. Food Allergies: The Basics; Gastroenterology; 2015 May; 148(6): 1120–1131 DOI: 10.1053/j.gastro.2015.02.006 https://www.ncbi.nlm.nih.gov/pmc/articles/PMC4414527/

205. gastrojournal.org / Tulloch AJ, et al. Neural Responses to Macronutrients: Hedonic and Homeostatic mechanisms; Gastroenterology; 2015 May; 148(6): 1205–1218 https://www.gastrojournal.org/article/S0016-5085(15)00153-5/fulltext?referrer=https%3A%2F%2Fwww.ncbi.nlm.nih.gov%2F

206. ncbi.nlm.nih.gov / Camilleri M. Peripheral Mechanisms in Appetite Regulation; Gastroenterology; 2015 May; 148(6): 1219–1233 DOI: 10.1053/j.gastro.2014.09.016 https://www.ncbi.nlm.nih.gov/pmc/articles/PMC4369188/

207. ncbi.nlm.nih.gov / Abnet CC, et al. Diet and Upper Gastrointestinal Malignancies; Gastroenterology; 2015 May; 148(6): 1234–1243 DOI: 10.1053/j.gastro.2015.02.007 https://www.ncbi.nlm.nih.gov/pmc/articles/PMC4414068/

208. ncbi.nlm.nih.gov / Song M, et al. Nutrients, Foods, and Colorectal Cancer Prevention; Gastroenterology; 2015 May; 148(6): 1244–1260 DOI: 10.1053/j.gastro.2014.12.03 https://www.ncbi.nlm.nih.gov/pmc/articles/PMC4409470/

209. gastrojournal.org / Sookian S, Pirola CJ. How Safe Is Moderate Alcohol Consumption in Overweight and Obese Individuals? Gastroenterology; 2016 June; 150(8): 1698–1703 https://doi.org/10.1053/j.gastro.2016.01.002 ; https://www.gastrojournal.org/article/S0016-5085(16)00005-6/pdf

210. Eagleman D (2015). The Brain: The Story of You; 218 pp. New York. Penguin Random House LLC

211. nationalgeographic.com / Zimmer C. Secrets of the Brain; National Geographic; 2014 February; 225(2): 28–57 https://www.nationalgeographic.com/magazine/2014/02/brain/

212. cghjournal.org / Rossi S, Navarro VJ. Herbs and Liver Injury: A Clinical Perspective; Clinical Gastroenterology and Hepatology; 2014 July; 12(7): 1069–1076 https://www.cghjournal.org/article/S1542-3565(13)01094-X/pdf

213. ncbi.nlm.nih.gov / Vally H, Misso N LA. Adverse Reactions to the Sulphite Additives; Gastroenterology and Hepatology from Bed to Bench; 2012 Winter; 5(1): 16–23 https://www.ncbi.nlm.nih.gov/pmc/articles/PMC4017440/

214. ncbi.nlm.nih.gov / Benedict C, et al. Gut Microbiota and Glucometabolic Alterations in Response to Recurrent Partial Sleep Deprivation in Normal-Weight Young Individuals; Molecular Metabolism; 2016 Dec.; 5(12): 1175–1186 DOI: 10.1016/j.molmet.2016.10.003 https://www.ncbi.nlm.nih.gov/pmc/articles/PMC5123208/

215. healthysleep.med.harvard.edu / Natural Patterns of Sleep. http://healthysleep.med.harvard.edu/healthy/science/what/sleep-patterns-rem-nrem

216.   techcrunch.com / The Internet of Medicine Is Just What the Doctor Ordered. Brendan O'Brien, February 16, 2016 https://techcrunch.com/2016/02/16/the-internet-of-medicine-is-just-what-the-doctor-ordered/

217.   health.com / 13 Everyday Habits That Are Aging You. Linda Melone, May 30, 2017 http://www.health.com/health/gallery/0,,20788790,00.html

218.   health.com / 11 Fitness Foods to Help You Get in Shape Faster. Cynthia Sass, January 28, 2016 http://www.health.com/health/gallery/0,,20799877,00.html

219.   nbcnews.com / Cereal Characters Lure Kiddies with Eye Gaze: Study. April 3, 2014 https://www.nbcnews.com/business/consumer/cereal-characters-lure-kiddies-eye-gaze-study-n70826

220.   foodpsychology.cornell.edu / Cereal Box Psychology: Eyes in the Aisles: Why Is Cap'n Crunch Looking Down at My Child? https://foodpsychology.cornell.edu/discoveries/cereal-box-psychology

221.   journals.sagepub.com / Musicus A, et al. Eyes in the Aisles: Why Is Cap'n Crunch Looking Down at My Child? Environment and Behavior; 2015 Aug; 47(7): 715–733 http://journals.sagepub.com/doi/abs/10.1177/0013916514528793

222.   thedailymeal.com / 8 Reasons Skim Milk Is Unhealthier Than 2% or Whole. Jess Novak, Mar 19, 2014 https://www.thedailymeal.com/8-reasons-skim-milk-unhealthier-2-or-whole/31914; https://www.thedailymeal.com/drink/8-reasons-skim-milk-unhealthier-2-or-whole-slideshow

223.   thedailymeal.com / 9 Foods You Should Never Eat Raw. Dan Myers, January 7, 2014 https://www.thedailymeal.com/9-foods-you-should-never-eat-raw/1714; https://www.thedailymeal.com/eat/9-foods-you-should-never-eat-raw-slideshow

224.   thedailymeal.com / 10 Memory Boosting Foods. Jonathan Hirsch, March 11, 2014 https://www.thedailymeal.com/10-memory-boosting-foods/31114; https://www.thedailymeal.com/cook/10-memory-boosting-foods-slideshow

225.   thedailymeal.com / 7 Foods That Fight Stress. Jan Bruce, January 6, 2016 https://www.thedailymeal.com/7-foods-fight-stress/121313; https://www.thedailymeal.com/entertain/foods-fight-stress

226.   cookinglight.com / 10 Surprisingly Healthy Foods. Katherine Brooking, November 16, 2009 http://www.cookinglight.com/eating-smart/smart-choices/surprisingly-healthy-foods

227.   cookinglight.com / Top 8 Cholesterol Lowering Foods. February 1, 2018 http://www.cookinglight.com/eating-smart/nutrition-101/cholesterol-lowering-foods

228.   thedailymeal.com / 9 Diet "Miracles" You Might Want To Avoid. Victoria Barton, February 24, 2014 https://www.thedailymeal.com/9-diet-miracles-you-might-want-avoid/22514

229.   thedailymeal.com / The 13 Most Fattening Foods on Earth. Dan Myers, December 19, 2014 https://www.thedailymeal.com/13-most-fattening-foods-earth/2714; https://www.thedailymeal.com/eat/13-most-fattening-foods-earth

230.   today.com / Too Much Added Sugar Can Do You In. Melissa Dahl, October 14, 2016 https://www.today.com/health/too-much-added-sugar-can-do-you-2D12047404

231.   thedailymeal.com / 10 Foods for Healthy Hair. Lauren Gordon, March 6, 2017 https://www.thedailymeal.com/10-foods-healthy-hair/110713; https://www.thedailymeal.com/entertain/10-foods-healthy-hair-slideshow

232.   cookinglight.com / Foods to Boost Your Mind. August 19, 2010 http://www.cookinglight.com/eating-smart/nutrition-101/brain-foods

233.   health.com / Foods That Make You Feel Better. Norine Dworkin-McDaniel, January 12, 2015 http://www.health.com/health/gallery/0,,20752367,00.html

234.   theactivetimes.com / Better Sex, Healthier Teeth, Clearer Skin: 12 Surprise Benefits of Exercise. Jess Scanlon, June 27, 2013 https://www.theactivetimes.com/
sex-smile-skin-exercise-benefits

235.   ncbi.nlm.nih.gov / Green E, Murphy C. Altered Processing of Sweet Taste in the
Brain of Diet Soda Drinkers. Physiology & Behavior; 2012 Nov 5; 107(4): 560–567
DOI: 10.1016/j.physbeh.2012.05.006 https://www.ncbi.nlm.nih.gov/pmc/articles/
PMC3465626/

236.   ncbi.nlm.nih.gov / Swithers SE. Not So Sweet Revenge: Unanticipated Conse-
quences of High-Intensity Sweeteners; The Behavior Analyst; 2015 May; 38(1): 1–17
DOI: 10.1007/s40614-015-0028-3 https://www.ncbi.nlm.nih.gov/pmc/articles/
PMC4883499/

237.   health.com / Your Secret to Happiness at Every Age. Susannah Felts, November 1,
2015 http://www.health.com/health/gallery/0,,20348268,00.html

238.   choosingwisely.org / http://www.choosingwisely.org/

239.   ncbi.nlm.nih.gov / Nickerson KP, et al. Deregulation of Intestinal Anti-Microbial
Defense by the Dietary Additive, Maltodextrin. Gut Microbes; 2015 Jan; 6(1): 78–83
DOI: 10.1080/19490976.2015.1005477 https://www.ncbi.nlm.nih.gov/pmc/articles/
PMC4615306/

240.   ncbi.nlm.nih.gov / Dixon LJ, et al. Combinatorial Effects of Diet and Genetics on
Inflammatory Bowel Disease Pathogenesis. Inflammatory Bowel Diseases; 2015
April; 21(4): 912–922 DOI: 10.1097/MIB.0000000000000289 https://www.ncbi.nlm.
nih.gov/pmc/articles/PMC4366276/

241.   cspinet.org / Resource / Food Additives Infographic. https://cspinet.org/resource/
food-additives-infographic

242.   cspinet.org / sites / CSPI's Annual Report to Members. Make Your Food Safer!
Michael F. Jacobson, November 18, 2016 https://cspinet.org/sites/default/files/
attachment/Year%20End%20Report.pdf

243.   ncbi.nlm.nih.gov / Fishman JE, et al. Oxidative Modification of the Intestinal
Mucus Layer Is a Critical but Unrecognized Component of Trauma Hemorrhagic
Shock-Induced Gut Barrier Failure; American Journal of Physiology Gastrointestinal
and Liver Physiology; 2013 Jan 1; 304(1): G57–G63 DOI: 10.1152/ajpgi.00170.2012
https://www.ncbi.nlm.nih.gov/pmc/articles/PMC3543631/

244.   thelancet.com / Bouvard V, et al. Carcinogenicity of Consumption of Red and
Processed Meat; The Lancet Oncology; 2015 Dec; 16(16): 1599–600 DOI: https://doi.
org/10.1016/S1470-2045(15)00444-1; https://www.thelancet.com/journals/lanonc/
article/PIIS1470-2045(15)00444-1/fulltext

245.   health.com / 13 Healthy High-Fat Foods You Should Eat More. Selene Yeager, February 22, 2016 http://www.health.com/health/gallery/0,,20986165,00.html

246.   medicaleconomics.com / Alternative Payment Model Could Be Saving
Grace for Quality Improvement. July 18, 2016 http://www.medicaleco-
nomics.com/medical-economics-blog/alternative-payment-model-coul
d-be-saving-grace-quality-improvement

247.   medicaleconomics.com / MIPS: The "Death Knell" for Small Practices? Joseph Burns,
February 25, 2016 http://www.medicaleconomics.com/medical-economics-blog/
mips-death-knell-small-practices

248.   medicaleconomics.com / 4 Crucial Tips to Consider When Picking MIPS or APM.
September 22, 2015 http://www.medicaleconomics.com/health-law-policy/4-crucia
l-tips-consider-when-picking-mips-or-apm

249.   medicaleconomics.com / Top 9 MACRA Threats That Could Become Reality for Doctors, Patients. July 23, 2016 http://www.medicaleconomics.com/

modern-medicine-cases/top-9-macra-threats-could-become-reality-doctors-patients

250.   jem-journal.com / Derlet RW, et al. Corporate and Hospital Profiteering in Emergency Medicine: Problems of the Past, Present, and Future; The Journal of Emergency Medicine; 2016; 50(6): 902–909 http://dx.doi.org/10.1016/j.jemermed.2016.01.006; https://www.jem-journal.com/article/S0736-4679(16)00007-X/pdf

251.   ers.usda.gov / webdocs / publications / Let's Eat Out: Americans Weigh Taste, Convenience, and Nutrition. Hayden Stewart, Noel Blisard, and Dean Jolliffe, October 2006 https://www.ers.usda.gov/publications/pub-details/?pubid=44119; https://www.ers.usda.gov/webdocs/publications/44117/29269_eib19.pdf?v=41305

252.   ncbi.nlm.nih.gov / Cash H. et al. Internet Addiction: A Brief Summary of Research and Practice; Current Psychiatry Reviews; 2012 Nov; 8(4): 292–298 DOI: 10.2174/157340012803520513 https://www.ncbi.nlm.nih.gov/pmc/articles/PMC3480687/

253.   spiegel.de / international / zeitgeist / Spiegel Online. Smartphone Addiction; The Slot Machine in Your Pocket. Tristan Harris, July 27, 2016 http://www.spiegel.de/international/zeitgeist/smartphone-addiction-is-part-of-the-design-a-1104237.html

254.   ncbi.nlm.nih.gov / Sussman S, Moran MB. Hidden Addiction: Television; Journal of Behavioral Addictions; 2013 Sept; 2(3): 125–132 DOI: 10.1556/JBA.2.2013.008 https://www.ncbi.nlm.nih.gov/pmc/articles/PMC4114517/

255.   nbcnews.com / What Happens to Your Brain When You Binge-Watch a TV Series. Danielle Page, November 4.2017 https://www.nbcnews.com/better/health/what-happens-your-brain-when-you-binge-watch-tv-series-ncna816991

256.   ama.org / American Marketing Association / Social Media Triggers a Dopamine High. Molly Soat. Key Takeaways: WHAT? According to Recent Research, People Get a Rush of Dopamine When They Post, Share or 'Like' Something Online. SO WHAT? Customers Get a "High" from Positive Interactions with One Another, or with Brands, on Social Media. NOW WHAT? Make Branded Social Media Posts Personable, Timely and Informative to Trigger a Pleasure-Causing Dopamine Release. https://www.ama.org/publications/MarketingNews/Pages/feeding-the-addiction.aspx

257.   distractify.com / 21 Ways Advertisers Are Manipulating You and You Don't Even Know It. Jason Iannone, December 12, 2014

258.   nbcnews.com / Are You Hooked on Screens? Here's Why You Can't Look Away. Lisa Tolin, April 18, 2017 https://www.nbcnews.com/better/wellness/are-you-hooked-screens-here-s-why-you-can-t-n745801

259.   ncbi.nlm.nih.gov / Salamone JD, Correa M. The Mysterious Motivational Functions of Mesolimbic Dopamine; Neuron; 2012 Nov 8; 76(3): 470–485 DOI: 10.1016/j.neuron.2012.10.021 https://www.ncbi.nlm.nih.gov/pmc/articles/PMC4450094/

260.   stopad.io / Manipulating Maslow: How Advertising Is Hijacking Our Heads and Making Us Unhappy. Kimberly Tytyk, October 23, 2017 https://stopad.io/blog/manipulating-maslow-how-advertising-is-hijacking-our-heads-and-making-us-unhappy

261.   lifehacker.com / How Advertising Manipulates Your Choices and Spending Habits (and What to Do about It). Adam Dachis, July 25, 2011 https://lifehacker.com/5824328/how-advertising-manipulates-your-choices-and-spending-habits-and-what-to-do-about-it

262.   kirklintaylor.weebly.com / Rogerian Argument / The Power of Advertising. http://kirklintaylor.weebly.com/rogerian-argument.html

263.   fastcompany.com / 5 Psychological Tactics Marketers Use to Influence Consumer Behavior. Robert Rosenthal, July 7, 2014 https://www.fastcompany.com/3032675/5-psychological-tactics-marketers-use-to-influence-consumer-behavior

264.   contently.com / The Dangerous Power of Emotional Advertising. Carly Miller, April 14, 2016 https://contently.com/strategist/2016/04/14/dangerous-powe r-emotional-advertising/

265.   theguardian.com / Report Reveals Tricks of Pharmaceutical Trade. Sarah Boseley https://www.theguardian.com/guardianweekly/story/0,,1807960,00.html

266.   reviews.financesonline.com / The Art of Deceptive Advertising: Quick Review of False and Misleading Tricks Used in Ads. Alex Hillsberg, June 10, 2014 https:// reviews.financesonline.com/the-art-of-deceptive-advertising-reviewed/

267.   conversionXL.com / Online Manipulation: All the Ways You're Currently Being Deceived. Alex Birkett, August 11, 2017 https://conversionxl.com/blog/ online-manipulation-all-the-ways-youre-currently-being-deceived/

268.   darkpatterns.org / What Are Dark Patterns? How Do Dark Patterns Work? Types of Dark Patterns. https://darkpatterns.org/types-of-dark-pattern

269.   cancer.org / Acrylamide and Cancer Risk. https://www.cancer.org/cancer/ cancer-causes/acrylamide.html

270.   ncbi.nlm.nih.gov / Coelho M, et al. Biochemistry of Adipose Tissue: An Endocrine Organ. Archives of Medical Science; 2013 Apr 20; 9(2): 191–200 DOI: 10.5114/ aoms.2013.33181 https://www.ncbi.nlm.nih.gov/pmc/articles/PMC3648822/

271.   foodsafetymagazine.com / Acrylamide, Furan, and the FDA. https://www.foodsafet-ymagazine.com/magazine-archive1/junejuly-2007/acrylamide-furan-and-the-fda/; https://www.cdc.gov/nutritionreport/pdf/Acrylamide.pdf

272.   ua-magazine.com / Coffee's Dirty Secret: Would You Like Carcinogens with That? Elisabeth Buhl Thubron, March 26, 2015 https://www.ua-magazine.com/coffees-dirt y-secret-like-carcinogens-with-that/

273.   healthit.gov / Meaningful Use and MACRA. https://www.healthit.gov/topic/ meaningful-use-and-macra/meaningful-use-and-macra

274.   cdc.gov / Meaningful Use. https://www.cdc.gov/ehrmeaningfuluse/introduction.html

275.   ncbi.nlm.nih.gov / Cheng CW, et al. Fasting-Mimicking Diet Promotes Ngn3 Driven Beta-Cell Regeneration to Reverse Diabetes. Cell; 2017 Feb 23; 168(5): 775–788e12 DOI: 10.1016/j.cell.2017.01.040 https://www.ncbi.nlm.nih.gov/pmc/articles/ PMC5357144/

276.   pnas.org / Scholz C, et al. A Neural Model of Valuation and Information Virality; PNAS; 2017 Mar 14; 114(11): 2881–2886 https://doi.org/10.1073/pnas.1615259114 http://www.pnas.org/content/114/11/2881

277.   reuters.com / Toxic Chemicals in One-Third of Fast Food Packaging. Lisa Rapaport, February 1, 2017 https://www.reuters.com/article/us-health-fastfood-wrappers-id USKBN15G5KH

278.   pubs.acs.org / Schaider LA, et al. Fluorinated Compounds in U.S. Fast Food Pack-aging. Environmental Science & Technology Letters; 2017 Mar 14; 4(3): 105–111 https://pubs.acs.org/doi/abs/10.1021/acs.estlett.6b00435; https://pubs.acs.org/doi/ ipdf/10.1021/acs.estlett.6b00435

279.   mayoclinic.org / Red Wine and Resveratrol: Good for Your Heart? November 12, 2016 https://www.mayoclinic.org/diseases-conditions/heart-disease/in-depth/ red-wine/art-20048281

280.   forbes.com / Study Suggests People Start Drinking Alcohol for Health Bene-fits: Should We Believe It? Alice G. Walton, January 17, 2015 https://www.forbes. com/sites/alicegwalton/2015/01/17/abstain-or-enjoy-the-health-benefits-a nd-risks-of-alcohol/#1038bd68ed2e

281.   forbes.com / Is Moderate Drinking Not as "Healthy" as We Thought? Alice G. Walton, March 23, 2016 https://www.forbes.com/sites/alicegwalton/2016/03/23/ moderate-drinking-may-not-be-as-healthy-as-we-thought/#1409cb5f51cd

282.   pubs.niaaa.nih.gov / National Institute on Alcohol Abuse and Alcoholism. Bagnardi V, et al. Alcohol Consumption and the Risk of Cancer: A Meta-Analysis. Alcohol Research & Health; 2001; 25(4): 263–270 https://pubs.niaaa.nih.gov/publications/arh25–4/263–270.htm

283.   cnn.com / Bat Reportedly Found in Packaged Fresh Express Salad Mix. Steve Almasy, April 8, 2017 https://www.cnn.com/2017/04/08/health/fresh-express-salad-bat-cdc/index.html

284.   businessinsider.com / The Smartphone Is Eventually Going to Die: This Is Mark Zukerberg's Crazy Vision for What Comes Next (FB). Matt Weinberger, April 24, 2017 https://www.businessinsider.com.au/facebook-f8-mark-zuckerberg-augmented-reality-2026-2017-4

285.   businessinsider.com / Facebook's Mysterious Hardware Division Is Working on Tech to Read Brain Waves That Could Let Users Send Thoughts to Each Other. Alex Heath, January 12, 2017 https://nordic.businessinsider.com/facebooks-building-8-working-on-brain-computer-communication-platform-2017-1/

286.   ncbi.nlm.nih.gov / Ursell LK, et al. Defining the Human Microbiome. Nutrition Reviews; 2012 Aug 1; 70(suppl 1): S38–S44 DOI: 10.1111/j.1753–4887.2012.00493.x https://www.ncbi.nlm.nih.gov/pmc/articles/PMC3426293/

287.   huffingtonpost.com / Here's What Gluten Really Does to Your Food. Alison Spiegel, April 16, 2015 https://www.huffingtonpost.com/2015/04/15/gluten-in-baking_n_7073556.html

288.   bakeinfo.co.nz / Uses of Gluten-BakeInfo (Bake Industry Research Trust) http://www.bakeinfo.co.nz/Facts/Gluten/Uses-of-Gluten

289.   ncbi.nlm.nih.gov / books / Molecular Cell Biology. 4th edition

290.   en.wikipedia.org / Composition of the Human Body https://en.wikipedia.org/wiki/Composition_of_the_human_body

291.   nature.com / Cross JH, et al. Oral Iron Acutely Elevates Bacterial Growth in Human Serum. Scientific Reports 5; 2015 Nov 23; 16670 https://www.nature.com/articles/srep16670; https://www.nature.com/articles/srep16670.pdf

292.   gizmodo.com / Google Photos Provides a Friendly Reminder That Google Owns You. Alex Cranz, May 17, 2017 https://gizmodo.com/google-photos-provides-a-friendly-reminder-that-google-1795304744

293.   sacbee.com / 100 Tons of Hot Dogs Recalled after "Metal Objects" Found in the Franks. Charles Duncan, May 20, 2017 https://www.sacbee.com/news/nation-world/national/article151707787.html

294.   kvdr.com / Colorado Group Wants to Ban Sale of Cell Phones for Kids under 13. June 18, 2017 https://kdvr.com/2017/06/18/colorado-group-wants-to-ban-sale-of-cell-phones-for-kids-under-13/

295.   ncbi.nlm.nih.gov / Ryan AM, et al. Changes in Hospital Quality Associated with Hospital Value-Based Purchasing. NEJM; 2017 Jun 15; 376(24): 2358–2366 DOI: 10.1056/NEJMsa1613412 https://www.ncbi.nlm.nih.gov/pmc/articles/PMC5841552/

296.   ncbi.nlm.nih.gov / Kwa M, et al. Adverse Events Reported to the US Food and Drug Administration for Cosmetics and Personal Care Products; JAMA Internal Medicine; 2017 August 1; 177(8): 1202–1204 DOI: 10.1001/jamainternmed.2017.2762 https://www.ncbi.nlm.nih.gov/pmc/articles/PMC5818793/

297.   jamanetwork.com / Cailiff RM, et al. Cosmetics, Regulations, and the Public Health: Understanding the Safety of Medical and Other Products. JAMA Internal Medicine; 2017 August 1; 177(8): 1080–1082 DOI: 10.1001/jamainternmed.2017.2773 https://jamanetwork.com/journals/jamainternalmedicine/article-abstract/2633254

298.   en.wikipedia.org / Quantum Entanglement https://en.wikipedia.org/wiki/Quantum_entanglement

299.   ncsf.org / National Council on Strength & Fitness: Obesity and Inflammation https://www.ncsf.org/enew/articles/articles-obesityandinflammation.aspx

300.   ncbi.nlm.nih.gov / Monteiro R, Azevedo I. Chronic Inflammation in Obesity and the Metabolic Syndrome; Mediators of Inflammation; 2010 July 14; 2010(2010): 289645 DOI: 10.1155/2010/289645 https://www.ncbi.nlm.nih.gov/pmc/articles/PMC2913796/

301.   ncbi.nlm.nih.gov / Ellulu MS, et al. Obesity and Inflammation: The Linking Mechanism and the Complications; Archives of Medical Science; 2017 Jun; 13(4): 851–863 DOI: 10.5114/aoms.2016.58928 https://www.ncbi.nlm.nih.gov/pmc/articles/PMC5507106/

302.   sciencedirect.com / Castro AM, et al. Low-Grade Inflammation and Its Relation to Obesity and Chronic Degenerative Diseases; Revista Medica del Hospital general de Mexico; 2017 April–June 2017; 80(2): 101–105 https://doi.org/10.1016/j.hgmx.2016.06.011; https://www.sciencedirect.com/science/article/pii/S0185106316300737

303.   seatletimes.com / Phthalates Found in Powdered Mac-and-Cheese Mixes. Roni Caryn Rabin, July 14, 2017 https://www.seattletimes.com/nation-world/whats-in-your-childs-mac-and-cheese-toxic-chemicals-a-new-study-says/

304.   ehjournal.biomedcentral.com / Serrano SE, et al. Phthalates and Diet: A Review of the Food Monitoring and Epidemiology Data; Environmental Health; 2014 Jun 2; 13(1): 43 DOI: 10.1186/1476–069X-13–43 https://www.ncbi.nlm.nih.gov/pmc/articles/PMC4050989/

305.   latimes.com / Bush's Baked Beans Recalled because of Defective Cans. Rachel Spacek, July 24, 2017 http://www.latimes.com/business/la-fi-bushs-bean-recall-20170724-story.html

306.   bbc.com / Time, Not Material Goods, "Raises Happiness." Helen Briggs, July 25, 2017 https://www.bbc.com/news/science-environment-40703519

307.   ncbi.nlm.nih.gov / Whillans AV, et al. Buying Time Promotes Happiness. PNAS (Proceedings of the National Academy of Sciences of the United States of America); 2017 Aug 8; 114(32): 8523–8527 DOI: 10.1073/pnas.1706541114 https://www.ncbi.nlm.nih.gov/pmc/articles/PMC5559044/

308.   sciencealert.com / Widespread Loneliness Is Killing People and We Need to Start Taking This Seriously. Signe Dean, August 7, 2017 https://www.sciencealert.com/widespread-loneliness-is-killing-people-and-we-need-to-start-taking-this-seriously

309.   ncbi.nlm.nih.gov / Holt-Lunstad J, et al. Social Relationships and Mortality Risk: A Meta-analytic Review. PLOS Medicine; 2010 Jul; 7(7): e1000316 DOI: 10.1371/journal.pmed.1000316 https://www.ncbi.nlm.nih.gov/pmc/articles/PMC2910600/

310.   ncbi.nlm.nih.gov / Holt-Lunstad J, et al. Loneliness and Social Isolation as Risk Factors for Mortality: A Meta-analytic Review; Perspectives on Psychological Science; 2015 Mar; 10(2): 227–237 DOI: 10.1177/1745691614568352 https://www.ahsw.org.uk/userfiles/Research/Perspectives%20on%20Psychological%20Science-2015-Holt-Lunstad-227-37.pdf

311.   sciencealert.com / Here's Why Friendships Can Be Even More Important Than Family as We Age. Bec Crew, June 10, 2017 https://www.sciencealert.com/here-s-why-friendships-could-be-more-even-important-than-family-as-we-age

312.   onlinelibrary.wiley.com / Chopik WJ. Associations among Relational Values, Support, Health, and Well-Being across the Adult Lifespan; Personal Relationships; 2017 June; 24(2): 408–422 https://doi.org/10.1111/pere.12187; https://onlinelibrary.wiley.com/doi/full/10.1111/pere.12187; https://onlinelibrary.wiley.com/doi/epdf/10.1111/pere.12187

313. ncbi.nlm.nih.gov / Vogel SA. The Politics of Plastics: The Making and Unmaking of Bisphenol A "Safety"; American Journal of Public Health; 2009 Nov; 99(Suppl 3): s559-s566 DOI: 10.2105/AJPH.2008.159228 https://www.ncbi.nlm.nih.gov/pmc/articles/PMC2774166/

314. npr.org / Is the Secret to a Healthier Microbiome Hidden in the Hadza Diet? Michaeleen Doucleff, August 24,2017 https://www.npr.org/sections/goatsand-soda/2017/08/24/545631521/is-the-secret-to-a-healthier-microbiome-hi dden-in-the-hadza-diet

315. ncbi.nlm.nih.gov / Smits SA, et al. Seasonal Cycling in the Gut Microbiome of the Hadza Hunter-Gatherers of Tanzania; Science; 2017 Aug 25; 357(6353): 802–806 DOI: 10.1126/science.aan4834 https://www.ncbi.nlm.nih.gov/pubmed/28839072; http://science.sciencemag.org/content/357/6353/802.long

316. ncbi.nlm.nih.gov / Sozio M, Crabb DW. Alcohol and Lipid Metabolism; American Journal of Physiology, Endocrinology and Metabolism; 2008 July; 295(1): E10-E16 DOI: 10.1152/ajpendo.00011.2008 https://www.ncbi.nlm.nih.gov/pmc/articles/PMC2493591/

317. thelancet.com/ Dehghan M, et al. Associations of Fats and Carbohydrate Intake with Cardiovascular Disease and Mortality in 18 Countries from Five Continents (PURE): A Prospective Cohort Study; The Lancet; 2017 Nov 4; 390(10107): 2050–2062 DOI: 10.1016/S0140-6736(17)32252-3 https://www.thelancet.com/journals/lancet/article/PIIS0140-6736(17)32252-3/fulltext

318. circres.ahajournals.org / Giacco F, Brownlee M. Oxidative Stress and Diabetic Complications; Circulation Research; 2010 Oct 29; 107(9): 1058–1070 DOI: https://doi.org/10.1161/CIRCRESAHA.110.223545; http://circres.ahajournals.org/content/107/9/1058.long

319. ncbi.nlm.nih.gov / Matough FA, et al. The Role of Oxidative Stress and Antioxidants in Diabetic Complications; Sultan Qaboos University Medical Journal; 2012 Feb; 12(1): 5–18 https://www.ncbi.nlm.nih.gov/pmc/articles/PMC3286717/

320. nature.com / Dong X, et al. Evidence for a Limit to Human Lifespan; Nature; 2016 Oct 13; 538(7624): 257–259: Online DOI: 10.1038/nature19793 https://www.ncbi.nlm.nih.gov/pubmed/27706136; https://www.nature.com/articles/nature19793

321. npr.org / Brains Sweep Themselves Clean of Toxins during Sleep. Jon Hamilton, October 17, 2013 https://www.npr.org/sections/health-shots/2013/10/18/236211811/brains-sweep-themselves-clean-of-toxins-during-sleep

322. ncbi.nlm.nih.gov / Xie L, et al. Sleep Drives Metabolic Clearance from the Adult Brain; Science; 2013 Oct 18; 342(6156): 373–377 DOI: 10.1126/science.1241224 https://www.ncbi.nlm.nih.gov/pmc/articles/PMC3880190/

323. ncbi.nlm.nih.gov / Cirelli C, Tononi G. The Sleeping Brain; Cerebrum; 2017 May–Jun; v. 2017: cer-07-17 https://www.ncbi.nlm.nih.gov/pmc/articles/PMC5501041/

324. fda.gov / Cosmetics / "Cosmeceutical." https://www.fda.gov/cosmetics/labeling/claims/ucm127064.htm

325. almonds.com / Nutrient Comparison Chart for Tree Nuts. https://www.almonds.com/sites/default/files/content/Tree%20Nut%20Nutrient%20Comparison%20Chart%20Web%20File.pdf

326. ncbi.nlm.nih.gov / Zalvan CH, et al. A Comparison of Alkaline Water and Mediterranean Diet vs Proton Pump Inhibition for the Treatment of Laryngopharyngeal Reflux; JAMA Otolaryngology-Head & Neck Surgery; 2017 Oct; 143(100): 1023–1029 DOI:10.1001/jamaoto.2017.1454 https://jamanetwork.com/journals/jamaotolaryngology/article-abstract/2652893

327. foxnews.com / CDC: 40 Percent of Cancers Linked to Obesity, Overweight. Mary Figuers Stallings, October 4, 2017 http://www.foxnews.com/health/2017/10/04/cdc-40-percent-cancers-linked-to-obesity-overweight.html

328.   annals.org / Diaz KM, et al. Patterns of Sedentary Behavior and Mortality in U.S. Middle-Aged and Older Adults: A National Cohort Study; Annals of Internal Medicine; 2017 Oct 3; 167(7): 465–475 DOI: 10.7326/M17-0212 http://annals.org/aim/article-abstract/2653704/patterns-sedentary-behavior-mortality-u-s-middle-aged-older-adults

329.   cdc.gov / Vital Signs / Cancer and Obesity. https://www.cdc.gov/vitalsigns/obesity-cancer/index.html

330.   cdc.gov / Steele CB, et al. Vital Signs: Trends in Incidence of Cancers Associated with Overweight and Obesity: United States, 2005–2014; Morbidity and Mortality Weekly Report (MMWR); 2017 Oct 6, 2017; 66(39): 1052–1058 https://www.cdc.gov/mmwr/volumes/66/wr/mm6639e1.htm

331.   psychiatryonline.org. / Harvey SB, et al. Exercise and the Prevention of Depression: Results of the HUNT Cohort Study; American Journal of Psychiatry; 2017 Oct; 175(1): 28–36 https://doi.org/10.1176/appi.ajp.2017.16111223; https://ajp.psychiatryonline.org/doi/10.1176/appi.ajp.2017.16111223

332.   theguardian.com / "Western Society Is Chronically Sleep Deprived": The Importance of the Body's Clock. Hannah Devlin, October 6, 2017 https://www.theguardian.com/science/2017/oct/06/western-society-is-chronically-sleep-deprived-the-importance-of-the-bodys-clock

333.   theguardian.com / Nobel Prize for Medicine Awarded for Insights into Internal Biological Clock. Nicola Davis, Ian Sample, October 2, 2017 https://www.theguardian.com/science/2017/oct/02/nobel-prize-for-medicine-awarded-for-insights-into-internal-biological-clock

334.   nejm.org / Villareal DT, et al. Weight Loss, Exercise, or Both and Physical Function in Obese Older Adults. NEJM; 2011 Mar 31; 364(13): 1218–1229 http://www.nejm.org/doi/full/10.1056/NEJMoa1008234

335.   nejm.org / Brownell KD and Koplan JP. Front-of-Package Nutrition Labeling: An Abuse of Trust by the Food Industry? NEJM; 2011 June 23; 364 (25): 2373–2375 http://www.nejm.org/doi/full/10.1056/NEJMp1101033

336.   nejm.org / Mozaffarian D, et al. Changes in Diet and Lifestyle and Long-Term Weight Gain in Women and Men; NEJM; 2011 June 23; 364 (25); 2392–2404 http://www.nejm.org/doi/full/10.1056/NEJMoa1014296

337.   nejm.org / Boggs DA, et al. General and Abdominal Obesity and Risk of Death among Black Women; NEJM; 2011 Sept 8; 365(10): 901–908 http://www.nejm.org/doi/full/10.1056/NEJMoa1104119

338.   nejm.org / Hudson KL. Genomics, Health Care, and Society; NEJM; 2011 Sept 15;365(11): 1033–1041 http://www.nejm.org/doi/full/10.1056/NEJMra1010517

339.   nejm.org / Kesselheim AS, Rajkumar R. Who Owns Federally Funded Research? The Supreme Court and the Bayh–Dole Act; NEJM; 2011 Sept 29; 365(13): 1167–1169 http://www.nejm.org/doi/full/10.1056/NEJMp1109168

340.   nejm.org / Mello MM, Messing NA. Restrictions on the Use of Prescribing Data for Drug Promotion; NEJM; 2011 Sept 29; 365(13): 12478–1254 http://www.nejm.org/doi/full/10.1056/NEJMhle1107678

341.   nejm.org / Willett WC, Ludwig DS. The 2010 Dietary Guidelines: The Best Recipe for Health? NEJM; 2011 Oct 27; 365(17): 1563–1565 http://www.nejm.org/doi/full/10.1056/NEJMp1107075

342.   nejm.org / Appel LJ, et al. Comparative Effectiveness of Weight-Loss Interventions in Clinical Practice. NEJM; 2011 Nov 24; 365(21): 1959–1968 http://www.nejm.org/doi/full/10.1056/NEJMoa1108660

343.   nejm.org / Wadden TA, et al. A Two-Year Randomized Trial of Obesity Treatment in Primary Care Practice; NEJM; 2011 Nov 24; 365(21): 1969–1979 http://www.nejm.org/doi/full/10.1056/NEJMoa1109220

344. nejm.org / Avorn J. Learning about the Safety of Drugs: A Half-Century of Evolution; NEJM; 2011 Dec 8; 365(23): 2151–2153 http://www.nejm.org/doi/full/10.1056/NEJMp1110327

345. nejm.org / Weil A. The Value of Federalism in Defining Essential Health Benefits; NEJM; 2012 Feb 23; 366(8): 679–681 http://www.nejm.org/doi/full/10.1056/NEJMp1200751

346. nejm.org / Fuchs VR. Major Trends in the U.S. Health Economy since 1950; NEJM;2012 Mar 15; 366(11) http://www.nejm.org/doi/full/10.1056/NEJMp1200478

347. nejm.org / Fineberg HV. A Successful and Sustainable Health System: How to Get There from Here; NEJM; 2012 Mar 15; 366(1): 1020–1027 http://www.nejm.org/doi/full/10.1056/NEJMsa1114777

348. nejm.org / Rejeski JW, et al; Lifestyle Change and Mobility in Obese Adults with Type 2Diabetes; NEJM; 2012 Mar 29; 366(13): 1209–1217 http://www.nejm.org/doi/full/10.1056/NEJMoa1110294

349. nejm.org / Pedersen BK. A Muscular Twist on the Fate of Fat; NEJM; 2012 Apr 19;366(16): 1544–1545 http://www.nejm.org/doi/full/10.1056/NEJMcibr1201024

350. nejm.org / Jha AK, et al. The Long-Term Effect of Premier Pay for Performance on Patient Outcomes; NEJM; 2012 Apr 26; 366(17): 1606–1615 http://www.nejm.org/doi/full/10.1056/NEJMsa1112351

351. nejm.org / Brody H. From an Ethics of Rationing to an Ethics of Waste Avoidance; NEJM; 2012 May 24; 366(21): 1949–1951 http://www.nejm.org/doi/full/10.1056/NEJMp1203365

352. nejm.org / Bloche MG. Beyond the "R Word"? Medicine's New Frugality; NEJM; May24, 2012 May 24; 366(21): 1951–1953 http://www.nejm.org/doi/full/10.1056/NEJMp1203521

353. nejm.org / Blumenthal D. Performance Improvement in Health Care: Seizing the Moment; NEJM; 2012 May 24; 366(21): 1953–1955 http://www.nejm.org/doi/full/10.1056/NEJMp1203427

354. nejm.org / Ghorob A, Bodenheimer T. Sharing the Care to Improve Access to Primary Care; NEJM; 2012 May 24; 366(21): 1955–1957 http://www.nejm.org/doi/full/10.1056/NEJMp1202775

355. nejm.org / Jones SS, et al. Unraveling the IT Productivity Paradox: Lessons for HealthCare; NEJM; 2012 Jun 14; 366(24): 2243–2245 http://www.nejm.org/doi/full/10.1056/NEJMp1204980

356. nejm.org / Laviano A, Fanelli FR. Toxicity in Chemotherapy: When Less Is More; NEJM; 2012 Jun 14; 366(24): 2319–2320 http://www.nejm.org/doi/full/10.1056/NEJMcibr1202395

357. nejm.org / Bischoff-Ferrari HA, et al. A Pooled Analysis of Vitamin D Dose Requirements for Fracture Prevention; NEJM; 2012 Jul 5; 367(1): 40–49 http://www.nejm.org/doi/full/10.1056/NEJMoa1109617

358. nejm.org / Lisa Rosenbaum L, Lamas D. Cents and Sensitivity: Teaching Physicians to Think about Costs; NEJM; 2012 Jul 12; 367(2): 99–101 http://www.nejm.org/doi/full/10.1056/NEJMp1205634

359. nejm.org / Shea SA. Obesity and Pharmacologic Control of the Body Clock; NEJM;2012 Jul 12; 367(2): 175–178 http://www.nejm.org/doi/full/10.1056/NEJMcibr1204644

360. nejm.org / Avorn J. Two Centuries of Assessing Drug Risks; NEJM; 2012 Jul 19;367(3): 193–197 http://www.nejm.org/doi/full/10.1056/NEJMp1206652

361. nejm.org / Chokshi DA, Farley TA. The Cost-Effectiveness of Environmental Approaches to Disease Prevention; NEJM; 2012 Jul 26; 367(4): 295–297 http://www.nejm.org/doi/full/10.1056/NEJMp1206268

362.   nejm.org / The ORIGIN Trial Investigators: n-3 Fatty Acids and Cardiovascular Outcomes in Patients with Dysglycemia; NEJM; 2012 Jul 26; 367(4): 309–318 http://www.nejm.org/doi/full/10.1056/NEJMoa1203859

363.   nejm.org / Barry CL, et al. Are Americans Ready to Solve the Weight of the Nation? NEJM; 2012 Aug 2; 367(5): 389–391 http://www.nejm.org/doi/full/10.1056/NEJMp1206519

364.   nejm.org / Richman BD, et al. Overbilling and Informed Financial Consent: A Contractual Solution; NEJM; 2012 Aug 2; 367(5): 396–397 http://www.nejm.org/doi/full/10.1056/NEJMp1205225

365.   nejm.org / Annas GJ. Doctors, Patients, and Lawyers: Two Centuries of Health Law; NEJM; 2012 Aug 2; 367(5): 445–450 http://www.nejm.org/doi/full/10.1056/NEJMra1108646

366.   nejm.org / Lee TH. Care Redesign: A Path Forward for Providers; NEJM; 2012 Aug 2;367(5): 466–472 http://www.nejm.org/doi/full/10.1056/NEJMhpr1204386

367.   nejm.org / Roehrig C, et al. When the Cost Curve Bent: Pre-Recession Moderation in Health Care Spending; NEJM; 2012 Aug 16; 367(7): 590–593 http://www.nejm.org/doi/full/10.1056/NEJMp1205958

368.   nejm.org. / Asch DA, Volpp KG. What Business Are We In? The Emergence of Health as the Business of Health Care; NEJM; 2012 Sept 6; 367(10): 888–889 http://www.nejm.org/doi/full/10.1056/NEJMp1206862

369.   nejm.org / Marvasti FF, Stafford RS. From Sick Care to Health Care: Reengineering Prevention into the U.S. System; NEJM; 2012 Sept 6; 367(10): 889–891 http://www.nejm.org/doi/full/10.1056/NEJMp1206230

370.   nejm.org / Barnes KA, et al. The Developing Vision of Primary Care; NEJM; 2012 Sept6; 367(10): 891–893 http://www.nejm.org/doi/full/10.1056/NEJMp1204487

371.   nejm.org / Emanuel E, et al. A Systemic Approach to Containing Health Care Spending; NEJM; 2012 Sept 6; 367(10): 949–954 http://www.nejm.org/doi/full/10.1056/NEJMsb1205901

372.   nejm.org / Antos JR, et al. Bending the Cost Curve through Market-Based Incentives; NEJM; 2012 Sept 6; 367(10): 954–958 http://www.nejm.org/doi/full/10.1056/NEJMsb1207996

373.   nejm.org / Mello MM, et al. Ethical Considerations in Studying Drug Safety: The Institute of Medicine Report; NEJM; 2012 Sept 6; 367(10): 959–964 http://www.nejm.org/doi/full/10.1056/NEJMhle1207160

374.   nejm.org / Hartzband P, Groopman J. There Is More to Life Than Death; NEJM; 2012Sept 13; 367(11): 987–989 http://www.nejm.org/doi/full/10.1056/NEJMp1207052

375.   nejm.org / Greene JA, et al. Therapeutic Evolution and the Challenge of Rational Medicine; NEJM; 2012 Sept 20; 367(12): 1077–1082 http://www.nejm.org/doi/full/10.1056/NEJMp1113570

376.   nejm.org / Outterson K. Punishing Health Care Fraud: Is the GSK Settlement Sufficient? NEJM; 2012 Sept 20; 367(12): 1082–1085 http://www.nejm.org/doi/full/10.1056/NEJMp1209249

377.   nejm.org / Kesselheim AS, et al. A Randomized Study of How Physicians Interpret Research Funding Disclosures; NEJM; 2012 Sept 20; 367(12): 1119–1127 http://www.nejm.org/doi/full/10.1056/NEJMsa1202397

378.   nejm.org / Fradkin JE, et al. What's Preventing Us from Preventing Type 2Diabetes? NEJM; 2012 Sep 27; 367(13): 1177–1179 http://www.nejm.org/doi/full/10.1056/NEJMp1208169

379.   nejm.org / Kramer DB, Kesselheim AS. User Fees and Beyond: The FDA Safety and Innovation Act of 2012; NEJM; 2012 Oct 4; 367(14): 1277–1279 http://www.nejm.org/doi/full/10.1056/NEJMp1207800

380. nejm.org / Ware JH, et al. Missing Data; NEJM; 2012 Oct 4; 367(14): 1353–1354 http://www.nejm.org/doi/full/10.1056/NEJMsm1210043

381. nejm.org / Little RJ, et al. The Prevention and Treatment of Missing Data in Clinical Trials; NEJM; 2012 Oct 4; 367(14): 1355–1360 http://www.nejm.org/doi/full/10.1056/NEJMsr1203730

382. nejm.org / Cohen DA, Babey SH. Candy at the Cash Register: A Risk Factor for Obesity and Chronic Disease; NEJM; 2012 Oct 11; 367(15): 1381–1383 http://www.nejm.org/doi/full/10.1056/NEJMp1209443

383. nejm.org / Pomeranz JL, Brownell KD. Portion Sizes and Beyond: Government's Legal Authority to Regulate Food-Industry Practices; NEJM; 2012 Oct 11; 367(15): 1383–1385 http://www.nejm.org/doi/full/10.1056/NEJMp1208167

384. nejm.org / Qi Q, et al. Sugar-Sweetened Beverages and Genetic Risk of Obesity; NEJM;2012 Oct 11; 367(15): 1387–1396 http://www.nejm.org/doi/full/10.1056/NEJMoa1203039

385. nejm.org / de Ruyter JC, et al. A Trial of Sugar-Free or Sugar-Sweetened Beverages and Body Weight in Children; NEJM; 2012 Oct 11; 367(15): 1397–1406 http://www.nejm.org/doi/full/10.1056/NEJMoa1203034

386. nejm.org / Ebbeling CB, et al. A Randomized Trial of Sugar-Sweetened Beverages and Adolescent Body Weight; NEJM; 2012 Oct 11; 367(15): 1407–1416 http://www.nejm.org/doi/full/10.1056/NEJMoa1203388

387. nejm.org / Caprio S. Calories from Soft Drinks: Do They Matter? NEJM; 2012 Oct 11;367(15): 1462–1463 http://www.nejm.org/doi/full/10.1056/NEJMe1209884

388. nejm.org / Pitts SR. Higher-Complexity ED Billing Codes: Sicker Patients, More Intensive Practice, or Improper Payments? NEJM; 2012 Dec 27; 367(26): 2465–2467 http://www.nejm.org/doi/full/10.1056/NEJMp1211315

389. nejm.org / Partridge L. Diet and Healthy Aging; NEJM; 2012 Dec 27; 367(26): 2550–551 http://www.nejm.org/doi/full/10.1056/NEJMcibr1210447

390. nejm.org / Friedmann PD. Alcohol Use in Adults; NEJM; 2013 Jan 24; 368(4): 365–373 http://www.nejm.org/doi/full/10.1056/NEJMcp1204714

391. nejm.org / van Nood E, et al. Duodenal Infusion of Donor Feces for Recurrent Clostridium Difficile; NEJM; 2013 Jan 31; 368(5): 407–415 http://www.nejm.org/doi/full/10.1056/NEJMoa1205037

392. nejm.org / Casazza K, et al. Myths, Presumptions, and Facts about Obesity; NEJM; 2013Jan 31; 368(5): 446–454 http://www.nejm.org/doi/full/10.1056/NEJMsa1208051

393. nejm.org / Ciarán PK. Fecal Microbiota Transplantation: An Old Therapy Comes of Age; NEJM; 2013 Jan 31; 368(5): 474–475 http://www.nejm.org/doi/full/10.1056/NEJMe1214816

394. nejm.org / Kotchen A, et al. Salt in Health and Disease: A Delicate Balance; NEJM; 2013 Mar 28; 368(13): 1229–1237 http://www.nejm.org/doi/full/10.1056/NEJMra1212606

395. nejm.org / Tracy SW. Something New under the Sun? The Mediterranean Diet and Cardiovascular Health.; NEJM; 2013 Apr 4; 368(14): 1274–1276 http://www.nejm.org/doi/full/10.1056/NEJMp1302616

396. nejm.org / Estruch R, et al. Primary Prevention of Cardiovascular Disease with a Mediterranean Diet; NEJM; 2013 Apr 4; 368(14): 1279–1290 http://www.nejm.org/doi/full/10.1056/NEJMoa1200303

397. nejm.org / McMichael AJ. Globalization, Climate Change, and Human Health; NEJM;2013 Apr 4; 368(14): 1335–1343 http://www.nejm.org/doi/full/10.1056/NEJMra1109341

398. nejm.org / Heyland D, et al. A Randomized Trial of Glutamine and Antioxidants in Critically Ill Patients; NEJM; 2013 Apr 18; 368(16): 1489–1497 http://www.nejm.org/doi/full/10.1056/NEJMoa1212722

399.   nejm.org / Halfon N, Conway PH. The Opportunities and Challenges of a Lifelong Health System; NEJM; 2013 Apr 25; 368(17): 1569-1571 http://www.nejm.org/doi/full/10.1056/NEJMp1215897

400.   nejm.org / Tang WHW, et al. Intestinal Microbial Metabolism of Phosphatidylcholine and Cardiovascular Risk; NEJM; 2013 Apr 25; 368(17): 1575-1584 http://www.nejm.org/doi/full/10.1056/NEJMoa1109400

401.   nejm.org / Loscalzo J. Gut Microbiota, the Genome, and Diet in Atherogenesis; NEJM;2013 Apr 25; 368(17): 1647-1649 http://www.nejm.org/doi/full/10.1056/NEJMe1302154

402.   nejm.org / Mosholder AD, et al. Cardiovascular Risks with Azithromycin and Other Antibacterial Drugs; NEJM; 2013 May 2; 368(18): 1665-1668 http://www.nejm.org/doi/full/10.1056/NEJMp1302726

403.   nejm.org / Garrett WS. Kwashiorkor and the Gut Microbiota; NEJM; 2013 May 2;368(18): 1746-1747 http://www.nejm.org/doi/full/10.1056/NEJMcibr1301297

404.   nejm.org / Bleich SN, Rutkow L. Improving Obesity Prevention at the Local Level: Emerging Opportunities; NEJM; 2013 May 9; 368(19): 1761-1763 http://www.nejm.org/doi/full/10.1056/NEJMp1301685

405.   nejm.org / Mariner WK, Annas GJ. Limiting "Sugary Drinks" to Reduce Obesity: Who Decides? NEJM; 2013 May 9; 368(19): 1763-1765 http://www.nejm.org/doi/full/10.1056/NEJMp1303706

406.   nejm.org / Fairchild AL. Half Empty or Half Full? New York's Soda Rule in Historical Perspective; NEJM; 2013 May 9; 368(19): 1765-1767 http://www.nejm.org/doi/full/10.1056/NEJMp1303698

407.   nejm.org / Frieden TR. Government's Role in Protecting Health and Safety; NEJM; 2013May 16; 368(20): 1857-1859 http://www.nejm.org/doi/full/10.1056/NEJMp1303819

408.   nejm.org / Iglehart JK. Expanding the Role of Advanced Nurse Practitioners: Risks and Rewards; NEJM; 2013 May 16; 368(20): 1935-1941 http://www.nejm.org/doi/full/10.1056/NEJMhpr1301084

409.   nejm.org / Kesselheim AS, Robe CT. Distributions of Industry Payments to Massachusetts Physicians; NEJM; 2013 May 30; 368(22): 2049-2052 http://www.nejm.org/doi/full/10.1056/NEJMp1302723

410.   nejm.org / Rosenthal MB, Mello MM. Sunlight as Disinfectant: New Rules on Disclosure of Industry Payments to Physicians; NEJM; 2013 May 30; 368(22): 2052-2054 http://www.nejm.org/doi/full/10.1056/NEJMp1305090

411.   nejm.org / Agrawal S, et al. The Sunshine Act: Effects on Physicians; NEJM; 2013 May30; 368(22): 2054-2057 http://www.nejm.org/doi/full/10.1056/NEJMp1303523

412.   nejm.org / Croskerry P. From Mindless to Mindful Practice: Cognitive Bias and Clinical Decision Making; NEJM; 2013 Jun 27; 368(26): 2445-2448 http://www.nejm.org/doi/full/10.1056/NEJMp1303712

413.   nejm.org / Smith AK, et al. Uncertainty: The Other Side of Prognosis; NEJM; 2013Jun 27; 368(26): 2448-2450 http://www.nejm.org/doi/full/10.1056/NEJMp1303295

414.   nejm.org / van der Meer JWM, Netea MG. A Salty Taste to Autoimmunity; NEJM; 2013 Jun 27; 368(26): 2520-2521 http://www.nejm.org/doi/full/10.1056/NEJMcibr1303292

415.   nejm.org / Oberlander J, Morrison M. Failure to Launch? The Independent Payment Advisory Board's Uncertain Prospects; NEJM; 2013 Jul 11; 369(2): 105-107 http://www.nejm.org/doi/full/10.1056/NEJMp1306051

416.   nejm.org / Fuchs VR. The Gross Domestic Product and Health Care Spending; NEJM; 2013 Jul 11; 369(2): 107-109 http://www.nejm.org/doi/full/10.1056/NEJMp1305298

417.   nejm.org / Neumann PJ. Communicating and Promoting Comparative-Effectiveness Research Findings; NEJM; 2013 Jul 18; 369(3): 209–211 http://www.nejm.org/doi/full/10.1056/NEJMp1300312

418.   nejm.org / Morden NE, et al. Accountable Prescribing; NEJM; 2013 Jul 25; 369(4): 299–302 http://www.nejm.org/doi/full/10.1056/NEJMp1301805

419.   nejm.org / C.W. Baugh and J.D. Schuur. Observation Care: High-Value Care or a Cost-Shifting Loophole? NEJM; 2013 Jul 25; 369(4): 302–305 http://www.nejm.org/doi/full/10.1056/NEJMp1304493

420.   nejm.org / Murray CJL, Lopez AD. Measuring the Global Burden of Disease; NEJM; 2013 Aug 1; 369(5): 448–457 http://www.nejm.org/doi/full/10.1056/NEJMra1201534

421.   nejm.org / Hochman ME, et al. Payer Agnosticism; NEJM; 2013 Aug 8; 369(6): 502–503 http://www.nejm.org/doi/full/10.1056/NEJMp1303174

422.   nejm.org / T.A. Rando and T. Finkel. Cardiac Aging and Rejuvenation: A Sense of Humors? NEJM; 2013 Aug 8; 369(6): 575–576 http://www.nejm.org/doi/full/10.1056/NEJMcibr1306063

423.   nejm.org / K. Baicker and H. Levy. Coordination versus Competition in Health Care Reform; NEJM; 2013 Aug 29; 369(9): 789–791 http://www.nejm.org/doi/full/10.1056/NEJMp1306268

424.   nejm.org / Kesselheim AS, et al. Gene Patenting: The Supreme Court Finally Speaks; NEJM; 2013 Aug 29; 369(9): 869–875 http://www.nejm.org/doi/full/10.1056/NEJMhle1308199

425.   nejm.org / Ezzati M, Riboli E. Behavioral and Dietary Risk Factors for Noncommunicable Diseases; NEJM; 2013 Sep 5; 369(10): 954–964 http://www.nejm.org/doi/full/10.1056/NEJMra1203528

426.   nejm.org / Huang J. Tracking Drugs; NEJM; 2013 Sep 19; 369(12): 1168–1169 http://www.nejm.org/doi/full/10.1056/NEJMcibr1308868

427.   nejm.org / Ross JS, Kesselheim AS. Prescription-Drug Coupons: No Such Thing as a Free Lunch; NEJM; 2013 Sep 26; 369(13): 1188–1189 http://www.nejm.org/doi/full/10.1056/NEJMp1301993

428.   nejm.org / Colbert JA, Jangi S. Training Physicians to Manage Obesity: Back to the Drawing Board; NEJM; 2013 Oct 10; 369(15): 1389–1391 http://www.nejm.org/doi/full/10.1056/NEJMp1306460

429.   nejm.org / Taqueti VR. No Easy Fixes; NEJM; 2013 Oct 10; 369(15): 1392–1393 http://www.nejm.org/doi/full/10.1056/NEJMp1303484

430.   nejm.org / Ubel PA, Aberne AP. Full Disclosure-Out-of-Pocket Costs as Side Effects; NEJM; 2013 Oct 17; 369(16): 1484–1486 http://www.nejm.org/doi/full/10.1056/NEJMp1306826

431.   nejm.org / Bettigole C. The Thousand-Dollar Pap Smear; NEJM; 2013 Oct 17; 369(16):1486–1487 http://www.nejm.org/doi/full/10.1056/NEJMp1307295

432.   nejm.org / Litvak E, Fineberg HV. Smoothing the Way to High Quality, Safety, and Economy; NEJM; 2013 Oct 24; 369(17): 1581–1583 http://www.nejm.org/doi/full/10.1056/NEJMp1307699

433.   nejm.org / Kachalia A. Improving Patient Safety through Transparency; NEJM; 2013Oct 31; 369(18): 1677–1679 http://www.nejm.org/doi/full/10.1056/NEJMp1303960

434.   nejm.org / Berenson RA, Kaye DR. Grading a Physician's Value: The Misapplication of Performance Measurement; NEJM; 2013 Nov 28; 369(22): 2079–2081 http://www.nejm.org/doi/full/10.1056/NEJMp1312287

435.   nejm.org / Gillman MW, Ludwig DS. How Early Should Obesity Prevention Start? NEJM; 2013 Dec 5; 369(23): 2173–2175 http://www.nejm.org/doi/full/10.1056/NEJMp1310577

436.   nejm.org / Archer SL. Mitochondrial Dynamics: Mitochondrial Fission and Fusion in Human Diseases; NEJM; 2013 Dec 5; 369(23): 2236–2251 http://www.nejm.org/doi/full/10.1056/NEJMra1215233

437.   nejm.org / Blumenthal D, Stremi K. Health Care Spending: A Giant Slain or Sleeping? NEJM; 2013 Dec 26; 369(26): 2551–2557 http://www.nejm.org/doi/full/10.1056/NEJMhpr1310415

438.   nejm.org / Outterson K. The Drug Quality and Security Act: Mind the Gaps; NEJM;2014 Jan 9; 370(2): 97–99 http://www.nejm.org/doi/full/10.1056/NEJMp1314691

439.   nejm.org / Baron RJ, Davis K. Accelerating the Adoption of High-Value Primary Care: A New Provider Type under Medicare? NEJM; 2014 Jan 9; 370(2): 99–101 http://www.nejm.org/doi/full/10.1056/NEJMp1314933

440.   nejm.org / Reenan R. Correcting Mutations by RNA Repair; NEJM; 2014 Jan 9; 370(2): 172–174 http://www.nejm.org/doi/full/10.1056/NEJMcibr1313514

441.   nejm.org / Lamas D. Chronic Critical Illness; NEJM; 2014 Jan 9; 370(2): 175–177 http://www.nejm.org/doi/full/10.1056/NEJMms1310675

442.   nejm.org / Dafny L. Hospital Industry Consolidation: Still More to Come? NEJM;2014 Jan 16; 370(3): 198–199 http://www.nejm.org/doi/full/10.1056/NEJMp1313948

443.   nejm.org / Tobias DK, et al. Body-Mass Index and Mortality among Adults with Incident Type 2 Diabetes; NEJM; 2014 Jan 16; 370(3): 233–244 http://www.nejm.org/doi/full/10.1056/NEJMoa1304501

444.   nejm.org / Keaney JF Jr., et al. A Pragmatic View of the New Cholesterol Treatment Guidelines; NEJM; 2014 Jan 16; 370(3): 275–278 http://www.nejm.org/doi/full/10.1056/NEJMms1314569

445.   nejm.org / Fairchild AL, et al. The Renormalization of Smoking? E-Cigarettes and the Tobacco "Endgame"; NEJM; 2014 Jan 24; 370(4): 293–295 http://www.nejm.org/doi/full/10.1056/NEJMp1313940

446.   nejm.org / Winickoff JP, et al. Tobacco 21: An Idea Whose Time Has Come; NEJM;2014 Jan 24; 370(4): 295–297 http://www.nejm.org/doi/full/10.1056/NEJMp1314626

447.   nejm.org / Cunningham SA, et al. Incidence of Childhood Obesity in the United States; NEJM; 2014 Jan 30; 370(5): 403–411 http://www.nejm.org/doi/full/10.1056/NEJMoa1309753

448.   nejm.org / Morden NE, et al. Choosing Wisely: The Politics and Economics of Labeling Low-Value Services; NEJM; 2014 Feb 13; 370(7): 589–592 http://www.nejm.org/doi/full/10.1056/NEJMp1314965

449.   nejm.org / Rosenbaum L. "Misfearing": Culture, Identity, and Our Perceptions of Health Risks; NEJM; 2014 Feb 13; 370(7): 595–597 http://www.nejm.org/doi/full/10.1056/NEJMp1314638

450.   nejm.org / Reuben DB, Tinetti ME. The Hospital-Dependent Patient; NEJM; 2014 Feb20; 370(8): 694–697 http://www.nejm.org/doi/full/10.1056/NEJMp1315568

451.   nejm.org / Darrow JJ, et al. New FDA Breakthrough-Drug Category: Implications for Patients; NEJM; 2014 Mar 27; 370(13): 1252–1258 http://www.nejm.org/doi/full/10.1056/NEJMhle1311493

452.   nejm.org / Cohen PA. Hazards of Hindsight: Monitoring the Safety of Nutritional Supplements; NEJM; 2014 Apr 3; 370(14): 1277–1280 http://www.nejm.org/doi/full/10.1056/NEJMp1315559

453.   nejm.org / Ubel PA, Jagsi R. Promoting Population Health through Financial Stewardship; NEJM; 2014 Apr 3; 370(14): 1280–1281 http://www.nejm.org/doi/full/10.1056/NEJMp1401335

454. nejm.org / Huang X, Rosenthal MB. Transforming Specialty Practice: The Patient-Centered Medical Neighborhood; NEJM; 2014 Apr 10; 370(15): 1376–1379 http://www.nejm.org/doi/full/10.1056/NEJMp1315416

455. nejm.org / Kocher R, Roberts B. The Calculus of Cures; NEJM; 2014 Apr 17; 370(16): 1473–1475 http://www.nejm.org/doi/full/10.1056/NEJMp1400868

456. nejm.org / Sarpatwari A, et al. Using a Drug-Safety Tool to Prevent Competition; NEJM;2014 Apr 17; 370(16): 1476–1478 http://www.nejm.org/doi/full/10.1056/NEJMp1400488

457. nejm.org / Brownell KD, Pomeranz JL. The Trans-Fat Ban: Food Regulation and Long-Term Health; NEJM; 2014 May 8; 370(19): 1773–1775 http://www.nejm.org/doi/full/10.1056/NEJMp1314072

458. nejm.org / Jou C. The Biology and Genetics of Obesity: A Century of Inquiries; NEJM; 2014 May 15; 370(20): 1874–1877 http://www.nejm.org/doi/full/10.1056/NEJMp1400613

459. nejm.org / Psaty BM, Breckenridge AM. Mini-Sentinel and Regulatory Science: Big Data Rendered Fit and Functional; NEJM; 2014 Jun 5; 370(23): 2165–2167 http://www.nejm.org/doi/full/10.1056/NEJMp1401664

460. nejm.org / Volkow ND, et al. Adverse Health Effects of Marijuana Use; NEJM; 2014 Jun 5; 370(23): 2219–2227 http://www.nejm.org/doi/full/10.1056/NEJMra1402309

461. nejm.org / Cathomen T, Ehl S. Translating the Genomic Revolution: Targeted Genome Editing in Primates; NEJM; 2014 Jun 12; 370(24): 2342–2345 http://www.nejm.org/doi/full/10.1056/NEJMcibr1403629

462. nejm.org / Screening an Asymptomatic Person for Genetic Risk; NEJM; 2014 Jun 19;370(25): 2442–2445 http://www.nejm.org/doi/full/10.1056/NEJMclde1311959

463. nejm.org / Anderson WH, Mackay IR. Gut Reactions: From Celiac Affection to Autoimmune Model; NEJM; 2014 Jul 3; 371(1): 6–7 http://www.nejm.org/doi/full/10.1056/NEJMp1405192

464. nejm.org / Howard DH. Drug Companies' Patient-Assistance Programs: Helping Patients or Profits? NEJM; 2014 Jul 10; 371(2): 97–99 http://www.nejm.org/doi/full/10.1056/NEJMp1401658

465. nejm.org / Chandel NS, Tuveson DA. The Promise and Perils of Antioxidants for Cancer Patients; NEJM; 2014 Jul 10; 371(2): 177–178 http://www.nejm.org/doi/full/10.1056/NEJMcibr1405701

466. nejm.org / Kessler DA. Toward More Comprehensive Food Labeling; NEJM; 2014 Jul17; 371(3): 193–195 http://www.nejm.org/doi/full/10.1056/NEJMp1402971

467. nejm.org / Sylvetsky AC, Dietz WH. Nutrient-Content Claims: Guidance or Cause for Confusion? NEJM; 2014 Jul 17; 371(3): 195–198 http://www.nejm.org/doi/full/10.1056/NEJMp1404899

468. nejm.org / Hotchkiss RS, Moldawer LL. Parallels between Cancer and Infectious Disease; NEJM; 2014 Jul 24; 371(4): 380–383 http://www.nejm.org/doi/full/10.1056/NEJMcibr1404664

469. nejm.org / Richter KP, Levy S. Big Marijuana: Lessons from Big Tobacco; NEJM;2014 Jul 31; 371(5): 399–401 http://www.nejm.org/doi/full/10.1056/NEJMp1406074

470. nejm.org / Schuster MA, P.J. Chung PJ. Time Off to Care for a Sick Child: Why Family-Leave Policies Matter; NEJM; 2014 Aug 7; 371(6): 493–495 http://www.nejm.org/doi/full/10.1056/NEJMp1404860

471. nejm.org / Laviano A. Young Blood; NEJM; 2014 Aug 7; 371(6): 573–575 http://www.nejm.org/doi/full/10.1056/NEJMcibr1407158

472. nejm.org / Shulman GI. Ectopic Fat in Insulin Resistance, Dyslipidemia, and Cardiometabolic Disease; NEJM; 2014 Sep 18; 371(12): 1131–1141 http://www.nejm.org/doi/full/10.1056/NEJMra1011035

473.   nejm.org / Behforouz HL, et al. Rethinking the Social History; NEJM; 2014 Oct 2;371(14): 1277–1279 http://www.nejm.org/doi/full/10.1056/NEJMp1404846

474.   nejm.org / Okun MS. Deep-Brain Stimulation: Entering the Era of Human Neural-Network Modulation; NEJM; 2014 Oct 9; 371(15): 1369–1373 http://www.nejm.org/doi/full/10.1056/NEJMp1408779

475.   nejm.org / Manz C, et al. Marketing to Physicians in a Digital World; NEJM; 2014 Nov13; 371(20): 1857–1859 http://www.nejm.org/doi/full/10.1056/NEJMp1408974

476.   nejm.org / Alpern JD, et al. High-Cost Generic Drugs: Implications for Patients and Policymakers; NEJM; 2014 Nov 13; 371(20): 1859–1862 http://www.nejm.org/doi/full/10.1056/NEJMp1408376

477.   nejm.org / Woo Baidal JA, Taveras EM. Protecting Progress against Childhood Obesity: The National School Lunch Program; NEJM; 2014 Nov 13; 371(20): 1862–1865 http://www.nejm.org/doi/full/10.1056/NEJMp1409353

478.   nejm.org / Simon A. Cholesterol Metabolism and Immunity; NEJM; 2014 Nov 13;371(20): 1933–1935 http://www.nejm.org/doi/full/10.1056/NEJMcibr1412016

479.   nejm.org / Pomeranz JL, Brownell KD. Can Government Regulate Portion Sizes? NEJM; 2014 Nov 20; 371(21): 1956–1958 http://www.nejm.org/doi/full/10.1056/NEJMp1410076

480.   nejm.org / Cassel CK, et al. Getting More Performance from Performance Measurement; NEJM; 2014 Dec 4; 371(23): 2145–2147 http://www.nejm.org/doi/full/10.1056/NEJMp1408345

481.   nejm.org / McGlynn EA, et al. Reimagining Quality Measurement; NEJM; 2014 Dec 4;371(23): 2150–2153 http://www.nejm.org/doi/full/10.1056/NEJMp1407883

482.   nejm.org / Harkin A. Muscling In on Depression; NEJM; 2014 Dec 11; 371(24): 2333–2334 http://www.nejm.org/doi/full/10.1056/NEJMcibr1411568

483.   nejm.org / Schwamm LH. Progesterone for Traumatic Brain Injury: Resisting the Sirens' Song; NEJM; 2014 Dec 25; 371(26): 2522–2523 http://www.nejm.org/doi/full/10.1056/NEJMe1412951

484.   nejm.org / Jess T. Microbiota, Antibiotics, and Obesity; NEJM; 2014 Dec 25; 371(26): 2526–2528 http://www.nejm.org/doi/full/10.1056/NEJMcibr1409799

485.   nejm.org / Chandra A, et al. Addressing the Challenge of Gray-Zone Medicine; NEJM;2015 Jan 15; 372(3): 203–205 http://www.nejm.org/doi/full/10.1056/NEJMp1409696

486.   nejm.org / DeCamp M, Lehmann S. Guiding Choice: Ethically Influencing Referrals in ACOs; NEJM; 2015 Jan 15; 372(3): 205–207 http://www.nejm.org/doi/full/10.1056/NEJMp1412083

487.   nejm.org / Darrow JJ, et al. Practical, Legal, and Ethical Issues in Expanded Access to Investigational Drugs; NEJM; 2015 Jan 15; 372(3): 279–286 http://www.nejm.org/doi/full/10.1056/NEJMhle1409465

488.   nejm.org / Jacobs DB, Sommers BD. Using Drugs to Discriminate: Adverse Selection in the Insurance Marketplace; NEJM; 2015 Jan 29; 372(5): 399–402 http://www.nejm.org/doi/full/10.1056/NEJMp1411376

489.   nejm.org / Roman BR. On Marginal Health Care: Probability Inflation and the Tragedy of the Commons; NEJM; 2015 Feb 5; 372(6): 572–575 http://www.nejm.org/doi/full/10.1056/NEJMms1407446

490.   nejm.org / Pizzo PA, Walker DM. Should We Practice What We Profess? Care near the End of Life; NEJM; 2015 Feb 12; 372(7): 595–598 http://www.nejm.org/doi/full/10.1056/NEJMp1413167

491.   nejm.org / Wolf SM, et al. Forty Years of Work on End-of-Life Care: From Patients' Rights to Systemic Reform; NEJM; 2015 Feb 12; 372(7): 678–682 http://www.nejm.org/doi/full/10.1056/NEJMms1410321

492.   nejm.org / Adler NE, Stead WW. Patients in Context: EHR Capture of Social and Behavioral Determinants of Health; NEJM; 2015 Feb 12; 372(7): 698–701 http://www.nejm.org/doi/full/10.1056/NEJMp1413945

493.   nejm.org / Collins FS, Varmus H. A New Initiative on Precision Medicine; NEJM; 2015Feb 26; 372(9): 793–795 http://www.nejm.org/doi/full/10.1056/NEJMp1500523

494.   nejm.org / Ozanne SE. Epigenetic Signatures of Obesity; NEJM; 2015 Mar 5; 372(10): 973–974 http://www.nejm.org/doi/full/10.1056/NEJMcibr1414707

495.   nejm.org / MacCoun RJ, Mello MM. Half-Baked: The Retail Promotion of Marijuana Edibles; NEJM; 2015 Mar 12; 372(11): 989–991 http://www.nejm.org/doi/full/10.1056/NEJMp1416014

496.   nejm.org / Ghosh TS, et al. Medical Marijuana's Public Health Lessons: Implications for Retail Marijuana in Colorado; NEJM; 2015 Mar 12; 372(11): 991–993 http://www.nejm.org/doi/full/10.1056/NEJMp1500043

497.   nejm.org / Anderson ML, et al. Compliance with Results Reporting at ClinicalTrials.gov; NEJM; 2015 Mar 12; 372(11): 1031–1039 http://www.nejm.org/doi/full/10.1056/NEJMsa1409364

498.   nejm.org / Rockey DC, et al. Fibrosis: A Common Pathway to Organ Injury and Failure; NEJM; 2015 Mar 19; 372(12): 1138–1149 http://www.nejm.org/doi/full/10.1056/NEJMra1300575

499.   nejm.org / Mouncey PR, et al. Trial of Early, Goal-Directed Resuscitation for Septic Shock; NEJM; 2015 Apr 2; 372(14): 1301–1311 http://www.nejm.org/doi/full/10.1056/NEJMoa1500896

500.   nejm.org / Frakt AB, Bagley N. Protection or Harm? Suppressing Substance-Use Data; NEJM; 2015 May 14; 372(20): 1879–1881 http://www.nejm.org/doi/full/10.1056/NEJMp1501362

501.   nejm.org / Rosenbaum L. Understanding Bias: The Case for Careful Study; NEJM; 2015 May 14; 372(20): 1959–1963 http://www.nejm.org/doi/full/10.1056/NEJMms1502497

502.   nejm.org / L. Rosenbaum. Beyond Moral Outrage: Weighing the Trade-Offs of COI (Conflicts of Interest) Regulation; NEJM; 2015 May 21; 372(21): 2064–2068 http://www.nejm.org/doi/full/10.1056/NEJMms1502498

503.   nejm.org / Dafny LS, Lee TH. The Good Merger; NEJM; 2015 May 28; 372(22): 2077–2079 http://www.nejm.org/doi/full/10.1056/NEJMp1502338

504.   nejm.org / Jameson, Longo DL. Precision Medicine: Personalized, Problematic, and Promising; NEJM; 2015 Jun 4; 372(23): 2229–2234 http://www.nejm.org/doi/full/10.1056/NEJMsb1503104

505.   nejm.org / Khullar D, et al. Behavioral Economics and Physician Compensation: Promise and Challenges; NEJM; 2015 Jun 11; 372(24): 2281–2283 http://www.nejm.org/doi/full/10.1056/NEJMp1502312

506.   nejm.org / Sarpatwari A, et al. Progress and Hurdles for Follow-on Biologics; NEJM;2015 Jun 18; 372(25): 2380–2382 http://www.nejm.org/doi/full/10.1056/NEJMp1504672

507.   nejm.org / Avorn J, Kesselheim AS. The 21st Century Cures Act: Will It Take Us Back in Time? NEJM; 2015 Jun 25; 372(26): 2473–2475 http://www.nejm.org/doi/full/10.1056/NEJMp1506964

508.   nejm.org / Ubel PA. Medical Facts versus Value Judgments: Toward Preference-Sensitive Guidelines; NEJM; 2015 Jun 25; 372(26): 2475–2477 http://www.nejm.org/doi/full/10.1056/NEJMp1504245

509.   nejm.org / Kaptchuk TJ, Miller FG. Placebo Effects in Medicine; NEJM; 2015 Jul 2;373(1): 8–9 http://www.nejm.org/doi/full/10.1056/NEJMp1504023

510.   nejm.org / Siraj ES, Williams KJ. Another Agent for Obesity: Will This Time Be Different? NEJM; 2015 Jul 2; 373(1): 82-83 http://www.nejm.org/doi/full/10.1056/NEJMe1506236

511.   nejm.org / Luzzatto L, Pandolfi PP. Causality and Chance in the Development of Cancer; NEJM; 2015 Jul 2; 373(1): 84-88 http://www.nejm.org/doi/full/10.1056/NEJMsb1502456

512.   nejm.org / Trecki J, et al. Synthetic Cannabinoid–Related Illnesses and Deaths; NEJM; 2015 Jul 9; 373(2): 103-107 http://www.nejm.org/doi/full/10.1056/NEJMp1505328

513.   nejm.org / Iglehart JK. The Expansion of Retail Clinics: Corporate Titans vs Organized Medicine; NEJM; 2015 Jul 23; 373(4): 301-303 http://www.nejm.org/doi/full/10.1056/NEJMp1506864

514.   nejm.org / Chang JE, et al. Convenient Ambulatory Care: Promise, Pitfalls, and Policy; NEJM; 2015 Jul 23; 373(4): 382-388 http://www.nejm.org/doi/full/10.1056/NEJMhpr1503336

515.   nejm.org / Chabner B, Richon V. Structural Approaches to Cancer Drug Development; NEJM; 2015 Jul 30; 373(5): 402-403 http://www.nejm.org/doi/full/10.1056/NEJMp1503567

516.   nejm.org / Rosenbaum L. The Paternalism Preference: Choosing Unshared Decision Making; NEJM; 2015 Aug 13; 373(7): 589-592 http://www.nejm.org/doi/full/10.1056/NEJMp1508418

517.   nejm.org / Asch DA, Rosin R. Innovation as Discipline, Not Fad; NEJM; 2015 Aug 13;373(7): 592-594 http://www.nejm.org/doi/full/10.1056/NEJMp1506311

518.   nejm.org / Landrigan PJ, Benbrook C. GMOs, Herbicides, and Public Health; NEJM; 2015 Aug 20; 373(8): 693-695 http://www.nejm.org/doi/full/10.1056/NEJMp1505660

519.   nejm.org / Avorn J, et al. Forbidden and Permitted Statements about Medications: Loosening the Rules; NEJM; 2015 Sep 3; 373(10): 967-973 http://www.nejm.org/doi/full/10.1056/NEJMhle1506365

520.   nejm.org / Robertson CT. New DTCA Guidance: Enough to Empower Consumers? NEJM; 2015 Sep 17; 373(12): 1085-1087 http://www.nejm.org/doi/full/10.1056/NEJMp1508548

521.   nejm.org / Greene JA, Watkins ES. The Vernacular of Risk: Rethinking Direct-to-Consumer Advertising of Pharmaceuticals; NEJM; 2015 Sep 17; 373(12): 1087-1089 http://www.nejm.org/doi/full/10.1056/NEJMp1507924

522.   nejm.org / Resnik DB, McCann DJ. Deception by Research Participants; NEJM; 2015 Sep 24; 373(13): 1192-1193 http://www.nejm.org/doi/full/10.1056/NEJMp1506985

523.   nejm.org / Skinner AC, et al. Cardiometabolic Risks and Severity of Obesity in Children and Young Adults; NEJM; 2015 Oct 1; 373(14): 1307-1317 http://www.nejm.org/doi/full/10.1056/NEJMoa1502821

524.   nejm.org / Rosenbaum L. Scoring No Goal: Further Adventures in Transparency; NEJM; 2015 Oct 8; 373(15): 1385-1388 http://www.nejm.org/doi/full/10.1056/NEJMp1510094

525.   nejm.org / Helleday T. Poisoning Cancer Cells with Oxidized Nucleosides; NEJM; 2015Oct 15; 373(16): 1570-1571 http://www.nejm.org/doi/full/10.1056/NEJMcibr1510335

526.   nejm.org / Rosenbaum L. Transitional Chaos or Enduring Harm? The EHR and the Disruption of Medicine; NEJM; 2015 Oct 22; 373(17): 1585-1588 http://www.nejm.org/doi/full/10.1056/NEJMp1509961

527.   nejm.org / Nikpay SS, Ayanian JZ. Hospital Charity Care: Effects of New Community-Benefit Requirements; NEJM; 2015 Oct 29; 373(18): 1687-1690 http://www.nejm.org/doi/full/10.1056/NEJMp1508605

528.   nejm.org / Frieden TR. The Future of Public Health; NEJM; 2015 Oct 29; 373(18): 1748–1754 http://www.nejm.org/doi/full/10.1056/NEJMsa1511248

529.   nejm.org / Drazen JM. Fifteen Years; NEJM; 2015 Oct 29; 373(18): 1774–1775 http://www.nejm.org/doi/full/10.1056/NEJMe1512739

530.   nejm.org / Bach PB. New Math on Drug Cost-Effectiveness; NEJM; 2015 Nov 5; 373(19): 1797–1799 http://www.nejm.org/doi/full/10.1056/NEJMp1512750

531.   nejm.org / Chin WW. A Delicate Balance: Pharmaceutical Innovation and Access; NEJM; 2015 Nov 5; 373(19): 1799–1801 http://www.nejm.org/doi/full/10.1056/NEJMp1513227

532.   nejm.org / Lauer MS, Nakamura R. Reviewing Peer Review at the NIH; NEJM; 2015 Nov 12; 373(20): 1893–1895 http://www.nejm.org/doi/full/10.1056/NEJMp1507427

533.   nejm.org / Halpern SD. Toward Evidence-Based End-of-Life Care; NEJM; 2015 Nov 19; 373(21): 2001–2003 http://www.nejm.org/doi/full/10.1056/NEJMp1509664

534.   nejm.org / Rosenbaum JT. The Immune Response: Learning to Leave Well Enough Alone; NEJM; 2015 Dec 10; 373(24): 2378–2379 http://www.nejm.org/doi/full/10.1056/NEJMcibr1511284

535.   nejm.org / Haug CJ. Peer-Review Fraud: Hacking the Scientific Publication Process; NEJM; 2015 Dec 17; 373(25): 2393–2395 http://www.nejm.org/doi/full/10.1056/NEJMp1512330

536.   nejm.org / Sommers BD. Health Care Reform's Unfinished Work: Remaining Barriers to Coverage and Access; NEJM; 2015 Dec 17; 373(25): 2395–2397 http://www.nejm.org/doi/full/10.1056/NEJMp1509462

537.   nejm.org / Lee TH, et al. Leading the Transformation of Health Care Delivery: The Launch of NEJM Catalyst; NEJM; 2015 Dec 17; 373(25): 2468–2469 http://www.nejm.org/doi/full/10.1056/NEJMe1515517

538.   nejm.org / Khullar D, et al. Reducing Diagnostic Errors: Why Now? NEJM; 2015 Dec 24; 373(26): 2491–2493 http://www.nejm.org/doi/full/10.1056/NEJMp1508044

539.   nejm.org / Singh H, Graber ML. Improving Diagnosis in Health Care: The Next Imperative for Patient Safety; NEJM; 2015 Dec 24; 373(26): 2493–2495 http://www.nejm.org/doi/full/10.1056/NEJMp1512241

540.   nejm.org / Holt PG, Sly PD. Environmental Microbial Exposure and Protection against Asthma; NEJM; 2015 Dec 24; 373(26): 2576–2578 http://www.nejm.org/doi/full/10.1056/NEJMcibr1511291

541.   nejm.org / Young RC. Value-Based Cancer Care; NEJM; 2015 Dec 31; 373(27): 2593–2595 http://www.nejm.org/doi/full/10.1056/NEJMp1508387

542.   nejm.org / Neumann PJ, Cohen JT. Measuring the Value of Prescription Drugs; NEJM; 2015 Dec 31; 373(27): 2595–2597 http://www.nejm.org/doi/full/10.1056/NEJMp1512009

543.   nejm.org / Ward JW, Mermin JH. Simple, Effective, but Out of Reach? Public Health Implications of HCV Drugs; NEJM; 2015 Dec 31; 373(27): 2678–2680 http://www.nejm.org/doi/full/10.1056/NEJMe1513245

544.   nejm.org / Alley DE, et al. Accountable Health Communities: Addressing Social Needs through Medicare and Medicaid; NEJM; 2016 Jan 7; 374(1): 8–11 http://www.nejm.org/doi/full/10.1056/NEJMp1512532

545.   nejm.org / Fried TR. Shared Decision Making: Finding the Sweet Spot; NEJM; 2016 Jan 14; 374(2): 104–106 http://www.nejm.org/doi/full/10.1056/NEJMp1510020

546.   nejm.org / Hartzband P, Groopman J. Medical Taylorism; NEJM; 2016 Jan 14; 374(2): 106–108 http://www.nejm.org/doi/full/10.1056/NEJMp1512402

547.   nejm.org / Gainty C. Mr. Gilbreth's Motion Pictures: The Evolution of Medical Efficiency; NEJM; 2016 Jan 14; 374(2): 109–111 http://www.nejm.org/doi/full/10.1056/NEJMp1514048

548.   nejm.org / Inge TH, et al. Weight Loss and Health Status 3 Years after Bariatric Surgery in Adolescents; NEJM; 2016 Jan 14; 374(2): 113–123 http://www.nejm.org/doi/full/10.1056/NEJMoa1506699

549.   nejm.org / Compton WM, et al. Relationship between Nonmedical Prescription-Opioid Use and Heroin Use; NEJM; 2016 Jan 14; 374(2): 154–163 http://www.nejm.org/doi/full/10.1056/NEJMra1508490

550.   nejm.org / Apovian CM. The Obesity Epidemic: Understanding the Disease and the Treatment; NEJM; 2016 Jan 14; 374(2): 177–179 http://www.nejm.org/doi/full/10.1056/NEJMe1514957

551.   nejm.org / Podolsky SH, Kesselheim AS. Regulating Homeopathic Products: A Century of Dilute Interest; NEJM; 2016 Jan 21; 374(3): 201–203 http://www.nejm.org/doi/full/10.1056/NEJMp1513393

552.   nejm.org / Powers BW, Chaguturu SK. ACOs and High-Cost Patients; NEJM; 2016 Jan21; 374(3): 203–205 http://www.nejm.org/doi/full/10.1056/NEJMp1511131

553.   nejm.org / Mandl KD, Kohane IS. Time for a Patient-Driven Health Information Economy? NEJM; 2016 Jan 21; 374(3): 205–208 http://www.nejm.org/doi/full/10.1056/NEJMp1512142

554.   nejm.org / Volkow ND, et al. Neurobiologic Advances from the Brain Disease Model of Addiction; NEJM; 2016 Jan 28; 374(4): 363–371 http://www.nejm.org/doi/full/10.1056/NEJMra1511480

555.   nejm.org / Porter ME, et al. Standardizing Patient Outcomes Measurement; NEJM; 2016 Feb 11; 374(6): 504–506 http://www.nejm.org/doi/full/10.1056/NEJMp1511701

556.   nejm.org / Asch DA, et al. Asymmetric Thinking about Return on Investment; NEJM; 2016 Feb 18; 374(7): 606–608 http://www.nejm.org/doi/full/10.1056/NEJMp1512297

557.   nejm.org / Conti RM, Rosenthal MB. Pharmaceutical Policy Reform: Balancing Affordability with Incentives for Innovation; NEJM; 2016 Feb 25; 374(8): 703–706 http://www.nejm.org/doi/full/10.1056/NEJMp1515068

558.   nejm.org / Rosen ED. Burning Fat by Bugging the System; NEJM; 2016 Mar 3; 374(9): 885–887 http://www.nejm.org/doi/full/10.1056/NEJMcibr1515457

559.   nejm.org / Charo RA. On the Road (to a Cure?): Stem-Cell Tourism and Lessons for Gene Editing; NEJM; 2016 Mar 10; 374(10): 901–903 http://www.nejm.org/doi/full/10.1056/NEJMp1600891

560.   nejm.org / Fisher ES, Lee PV. Toward Lower Costs and Better Care: Averting a Collision between Consumer- and Provider-Focused Reforms; NEJM; 2016 Mar 10; 374(10): 903–906 http://www.nejm.org/doi/full/10.1056/NEJMp1514921

561.   nejm.org / Agrawal S, Brown D. The Physician Payments Sunshine Act: Two Years of the Open Payments Program; NEJM; 2016 Mar 10; 374(10): 906–909 http://www.nejm.org/doi/full/10.1056/NEJMp1509103

562.   nejm.org / Dreischulte T, et al. Safer Prescribing: A Trial of Education, Informatics, and Financial Incentives; NEJM; 2016 Mar 17; 374(11): 1053–1064 http://www.nejm.org/doi/full/10.1056/NEJMsa1508955

563.   nejm.org / Fivez T, et al. Early versus Late Parenteral Nutrition in Critically Ill Children; NEJM; 2016 Mar 24; 374(12): 1111–1122 http://www.nejm.org/doi/full/10.1056/NEJMoa1514762

564.   nejm.org / Mehta NM. Parenteral Nutrition in Critically Ill Children; NEJM; 2016 Mar 24; 374(12): 190–1192 http://www.nejm.org/doi/full/10.1056/NEJMe1601140

565.   nejm.org / Casarett D. The Science of Choosing Wisely: Overcoming the Therapeutic Illusion; NEJM; 2016 Mar 31; 374(13): 1203–1205 http://www.nejm.org/doi/full/10.1056/NEJMp1516803

566.   nejm.org / Lo B, Barnes M. Federal Research Regulations for the 21st Century; NEJM; 2016 Mar 31; 374(13): 1205–1207 http://www.nejm.org/doi/full/10.1056/NEJMp1600511

567.   nejm.org / Farley TA. When Is It Ethical to Withhold Prevention? NEJM; 2016 Apr 7; 374(14): 1303–1306 http://www.nejm.org/doi/full/10.1056/NEJMp1516534

568.   nejm.org / Berenson RA, Goodson JD. Finding Value in Unexpected Places: Fixing the Medicare Physician Fee Schedule; NEJM; 2016 Apr 7; 374(14): 1306–1309 http://www.nejm.org/doi/full/10.1056/NEJMp1600999

569.   nejm.org / Kernan WN, et al. Pioglitazone after Ischemic Stroke or Transient Ischemic Attack; NEJM; 2016 Apr 7; 374(14): 1321–1331 http://www.nejm.org/doi/full/10.1056/NEJMoa1506930

570.   nejm.org / Du H, et al. Fresh Fruit Consumption and Major Cardiovascular Disease in China; NEJM; 2016 Apr 7; 374(14): 1332–1343 http://www.nejm.org/doi/full/10.1056/NEJMoa1501451

571.   nejm.org / Blendon RJ, et al. The Public and the Gene-Editing Revolution; NEJM; 2016 Apr 14; 374(15): 1406–1411 http://www.nejm.org/doi/full/10.1056/NEJMp1602010

572.   nejm.org / Karpe F, Lindgren CM. Obesity: On or Off? NEJM; 2016 Apr 14; 374(15): 1486–1488 http://www.nejm.org/doi/full/10.1056/NEJMcibr1601693

573.   nejm.org / Mechanic RE. When New Medicare Payment Systems Collide; NEJM; 2016 May 5; 374(18): 1706–1709 http://www.nejm.org/doi/full/10.1056/NEJMp1601464

574.   nejm.org / Alpern JD, et al. Essential Medicines in the United States: Why Access Is Diminishing; NEJM; 2016 May 19; 374(20): 1904–1907 http://www.nejm.org/doi/full/10.1056/NEJMp1601559

575.   nejm.org / Bonham VL, et al. Will Precision Medicine Move Us beyond Race? NEJM; 2016 May 26; 374(21): 2003–2005 http://www.nejm.org/doi/full/10.1056/NEJMp1511294

576.   nejm.org / Sarpatwari A, et al. State Initiatives to Control Medication Costs: Can Transparency Legislation Help? NEJM; 2016 Jun 16; 374(24): 2301–2304 http://www.nejm.org/doi/full/10.1056/NEJMp1605100

577.   nejm.org / Dale SB, et al. Two-Year Costs and Quality in the Comprehensive Primary Care Initiative; NEJM; 2016 Jun 16; 374(24): 2345–2356 http://www.nejm.org/doi/full/10.1056/NEJMsa1414953

578.   nejm.org / Ayanian JZ, Hamel MB. Transforming Primary Care: We Get What We Pay For; NEJM; 2016 Jun 16; 374(24): 2390–2392 http://www.nejm.org/doi/full/10.1056/NEJMe1603778

579.   nejm.org / Jones DS, et al. "Ethics and Clinical Research": The 50th Anniversary of Beecher's Bombshell; NEJM; 2016 Jun 16; 374(24): 2393–2398 http://www.nejm.org/doi/full/10.1056/NEJMms1603756

580.   nejm.org / Twig G, et al. Body-Mass Index in 2.3 Million Adolescents and Cardiovascular Death in Adulthood; NEJM; 2016 Jun 23; 374(25): 2430–2440 http://www.nejm.org/doi/full/10.1056/NEJMoa1503840

581.   nejm.org / Tilg H. A Gut Feeling about Thrombosis; NEJM; 2016 Jun 23; 374(25): 2494–2496 http://www.nejm.org/doi/full/10.1056/NEJMcibr1604458

582.   nejm.org / Dorsey ER, Topol EJ. State of Telehealth; NEJM; 2016 Jul 14; 375(2): 154–161 http://www.nejm.org/doi/full/10.1056/NEJMra1601705

583.   nejm.org / Hunter DJ. Uncertainty in the Era of Precision Medicine; NEJM; 2016 Aug 25; 375(8): 711–713 http://www.nejm.org/doi/full/10.1056/NEJMp1608282

584.   nejm.org / Lauby-Secretan B, et al. Body Fatness and Cancer: Viewpoint of the IARC Working Group; NEJM; 2016 Aug 25; 375(8): 794–798 http://www.nejm.org/doi/full/10.1056/NEJMsr1606602

585. nejm.org / Lucia A, Ramírez M. Muscling in on Cancer; NEJM; 2016 Sep 1; 375(9): 892–894 http://www.nejm.org/doi/full/10.1056/NEJMcibr1606456

586. nejm.org / Blumenthal D, et al. Caring for High-Need, High-Cost Patients: An Urgent Priority; NEJM; 2016 Sep 8; 375(10): 909–911 http://www.nejm.org/doi/full/10.1056/NEJMp1608511

587. nejm.org / Kocher KE, Ayanian JZ. Flipping the Script: A Patient-Centered Approach to Fixing Acute Care; NEJM; 2016 Sep 8; 375(10): 915–917 http://www.nejm.org/doi/full/10.1056/NEJMp1601899

588. nejm.org / Pocock SJ, Stone GW. The Primary Outcome Is Positive: Is That Good Enough? NEJM; 2016 Sep 8; 375(10): 971–979 http://www.nejm.org/doi/full/10.1056/NEJMra1601511

589. nature.com / Enck P, et al. The Placebo Response in Medicine: Minimize, Maximize or Personalize? Nature Reviews Drug Discovery; 2013; 12: 191–204 https://www.nature.com/articles/nrd3923

590. nejm.org / Gunderman R. Hospitalists and the Decline of Comprehensive Care; NEJM; 2016 Sep 15; 375(11): 1011–1013 http://www.nejm.org/doi/full/10.1056/NEJMp1608289

591. nejm.org / Bodenheimer T, Bauer L. Rethinking the Primary Care Workforce: An Expanded Role for Nurses; NEJM; 2016 Sep 15; 375(11): 1015–1017 http://www.nejm.org/doi/full/10.1056/NEJMp1606869

592. nejm.org / Yeh JS, et al. Obesity and Management of Weight Loss; NEJM; 2016 Sep 22; 375(12): 1187–1189 http://www.nejm.org/doi/full/10.1056/NEJMclde1515935

593. nejm.org / Obermeyer Z, Emanuel EJ. Predicting the Future: Big Data, Machine Learning, and Clinical Medicine; NEJM; 2016 Sep 29; 375(13): 1216–1219 http://www.nejm.org/doi/full/10.1056/NEJMp1606181

594. nejm.org / Tannock IF, Hickman JA. Limits to Personalized Cancer Medicine; NEJM; 2016 Sep 29; 375(13): 1289–1294 http://www.nejm.org/doi/full/10.1056/NEJMsb1607705

595. nejm.org / Manson JE, et al. Vitamin D Deficiency: Is There Really a Pandemic? NEJM; 2016 Nov 10; 375(19): 1817–1820 http://www.nejm.org/doi/full/10.1056/NEJMp1608005

596. nejm.org / Kaplan RS, et al. Adding Value by Talking More; NEJM; 2016 Nov 17; 375(20): 1918–1920 http://www.nejm.org/doi/full/10.1056/NEJMp1607079

597. nejm.org / Zarin DA, et al. Trial Reporting in ClinicalTrials.gov: The Final Rule; NEJM; 2016 Nov 17; 375(20): 1998–2004 http://www.nejm.org/doi/full/10.1056/NEJMsr1611785

598. nejm.org / Dafny LS, et al. Undermining Value-Based Purchasing: Lessons from the Pharmaceutical Industry; NEJM; 2016 Nov 24; 375(21): 2013–2015 http://www.nejm.org/doi/full/10.1056/NEJMp1607378

599. nejm.org / Schwartz JL. Fifty Years of Expert Advice: Pharmaceutical Regulation and the Legacy of the Drug Efficacy Study; NEJM; 2016 Nov 24; 375(21): 2015–2017 http://www.nejm.org/doi/full/10.1056/NEJMp1609763

600. nejm.org / Robertson C, Kesselheim AS. Regulating Off-Label Promotion: A Critical Test; NEJM; 2016 Dec 15; 375(24): 2313–2315 http://www.nejm.org/doi/full/10.1056/NEJMp1611755

601. nejm.org / Khera AV, et al. Genetic Risk, Adherence to a Healthy Lifestyle, and Coronary Disease; NEJM; 2016 Dec 15; 375(24): 2349–2358 http://www.nejm.org/doi/full/10.1056/NEJMoa1605086

602. nejm.org / Lynch SV, Pedersen O. The Human Intestinal Microbiome in Health and Disease; NEJM; 2016 Dec 15; 375(24): 2369–2379 http://www.nejm.org/doi/full/10.1056/NEJMra1600266

603.   nejm.org / Califf RM, et al. Transforming Evidence Generation to Support Health and Health Care Decisions; NEJM; 2016 Dec 15; 375(24): 2395–2400 http://www.nejm.org/doi/full/10.1056/NEJMsb1610128

604.   nejm.org / Asch DA, Rosin R. Engineering Social Incentives for Health; NEJM; 2016 Dec 29; 375(26): 2511–2513 http://www.nejm.org/doi/full/10.1056/NEJMp1603978

605.   nejm.org / Wolff JL, et al. Supporting Family Caregivers of Older Americans; NEJM; 2016 Dec 29; 375(26): 2513–2515 http://www.nejm.org/doi/full/10.1056/NEJMp1612351

606.   nejm.org / Khvorova A. Oligonucleotide Therapeutics: A New Class of Cholesterol-Lowering Drugs; NEJM; 2017 Jan 5; 376(1): 4–7 http://www.nejm.org/doi/full/10.1056/NEJMp1614154

607.   nejm.org / Rosenblatt M. The Large Pharmaceutical Company Perspective; NEJM; 2017 Jan 5; 376(1): 52–60 http://www.nejm.org/doi/full/10.1056/NEJMra1510069

608.   nejm.org / Levin AA. Targeting Therapeutic Oligonucleotides; NEJM; 2017 Jan 5; 376(1): 86–88 http://www.nejm.org/doi/full/10.1056/NEJMcibr1613559

609.   nejm.org / Heymsfield SB, Wadden TA. Mechanisms, Pathophysiology, and Management of Obesity; NEJM; 2017 Jan 19; 376(3): 254–266 http://www.nejm.org/doi/full/10.1056/NEJMra1514009

610.   nejm.org / Moon S. Powerful Ideas for Global Access to Medicines; NEJM; 2017 Feb 9; 376(6): 505–507 http://www.nejm.org/doi/full/10.1056/NEJMp1613861

611.   nejm.org / Buntin MB, Ayanian JZ. Social Risk Factors and Equity in Medicare Payment; NEJM; 2017 Feb 9; 376(6): 507–510 http://www.nejm.org/doi/full/10.1056/NEJMp1700081

612.   nejm.org / Joynt KE, et al. Others. Should Medicare Value-Based Purchasing Take Social Risk into Account? NEJM; 2017 Feb 9; 376(6): 510–513 http://www.nejm.org/doi/full/10.1056/NEJMp1616278

613.   nejm.org / Finkelstein A, et al. Adjusting Risk Adjustment: Accounting for Variation in Diagnostic Intensity; NEJM; 2017 Feb 16; 376(7): 608–610 http://www.nejm.org/doi/full/10.1056/NEJMp1613238

614.   nejm.org / Gassman AL, et al. FDA Regulation of Prescription Drugs; NEJM; 2017 Feb 16; 376(7): 674–682 http://www.nejm.org/doi/full/10.1056/NEJMra1602972

615.   nejm.org / Kilmer B. Recreational Cannabis: Minimizing the Health Risks from Legalization; NEJM; 2017 Feb 23; 376(8): 705–707 http://www.nejm.org/doi/full/10.1056/NEJMp1614783

616.   nejm.org / Schneider EC, Hall JC. Improve Quality, Control Spending, Maintain Access: Can the Merit-Based Incentive Payment System Deliver? NEJM; 2017 Feb 23; 376(8): 708–710 http://www.nejm.org/doi/full/10.1056/NEJMp1613876

617.   nejm.org / Lieu TA, Platt R. Applied Research and Development in Health Care: Time for a Frameshift; NEJM; 2017 Feb 23; 376(8): 710–713 http://www.nejm.org/doi/full/10.1056/NEJMp1611611

618.   nejm.org / McWilliams JM, Schwartz AL. Focusing on High-Cost Patients: The Key to Addressing High Costs? NEJM; 2017 Mar 2; 376(9): 807–809 http://www.nejm.org/doi/full/10.1056/NEJMp1612779

619.   nejm.org / Landon BE. Tipping the Scale: The Norms Hypothesis and Primary Care Physician Behavior; NEJM; 2017 Mar 2; 376(9): 810–811 http://www.nejm.org/doi/full/10.1056/NEJMp1510923

620.   nejm.org / McCoy MS, et al. Conflicts of Interest for Patient-Advocacy Organizations; NEJM; 2017 Mar 2; 376(9): 880–885 http://www.nejm.org/doi/full/10.1056/NEJMsr1610625

621.   nejm.org / Goodman-Bacon AJ, Nikpay SS. Per Capita Caps in Medicaid: Lessons from the Past; NEJM; 2017 Mar 16; 376(11): 1005–1007 http://www.nejm.org/doi/full/10.1056/NEJMp1615696

622.   nejm.org / Ederhof M, Ginsburg PB. Improving Hospital Incentives with Better Cost Data; NEJM; 2017 Mar 16; 376(11): 1010–1011 http://www.nejm.org/doi/full/10.1056/NEJMp1613181

623.   nejm.org / Serrano M. Understanding Aging; NEJM; 2017 Mar 16; 376(11): 1083–1085 http://www.nejm.org/doi/full/10.1056/NEJMcibr1615878

624.   nejm.org / Chaiyachati KH, et al. Patient Inducements: High Graft or High Value? NEJM; 2017 Mar 23; 376(12): 1107–1109 http://www.nejm.org/doi/full/10.1056/NEJMp1613274

625.   nejm.org / Najafzadeh M, Schneeweiss S. From Trial to Target Populations: Calibrating Real-World Data; NEJM; 2017 Mar 30; 376(13): 1203–1205 http://www.nejm.org/doi/full/10.1056/NEJMp1614720

626.   nejm.org / Bleich SN, et al. U.S. Nutrition Assistance, 2018: Modifying SNAP to Promote Population Health; NEJM; 2017 Mar 30; 376(13): 1205–1207 http://www.nejm.org/doi/full/10.1056/NEJMp1613222

627.   nejm.org / Feldman R, Wang C. A Citizen's Pathway Gone Astray: Delaying Competition from Generic Drugs; NEJM; 2017 Apr 20; 376(16): 1499–1501 http://www.nejm.org/doi/full/10.1056/NEJMp1700202

628.   nejm.org / Parikh RB, et al. Beyond Genes and Molecules: A Precision Delivery Initiative for Precision Medicine; NEJM; 2017 Apr 27; 376(17): 1609–1612 http://www.nejm.org/doi/full/10.1056/NEJMp1613224

629.   nejm.org / Dafny LS. Good Riddance to Big Insurance Mergers; NEJM; 2017 May 11; 376(19): 1804–1806 http://www.nejm.org/doi/full/10.1056/NEJMp1616553

630.   nejm.org / Connolly C, Lee TH. The Committed Perspective: Policy Principles for Regional Health Plans; NEJM; 2017 May 18; 376(20): 1903–1905 http://www.nejm.org/doi/full/10.1056/NEJMp1700461

631.   nejm.org / Gellad WF, Kesselheim AS. Accelerated Approval and Expensive Drugs: A Challenging Combination; NEJM; 2017 May 25; 376(21): 2001–2004 http://www.nejm.org/doi/full/10.1056/NEJMp1700446

632.   nejm.org / Goroll AH. Emerging from EHR Purgatory: Moving from Process to Outcomes; NEJM; 2017 May 25; 376(21): 2004–2006 http://www.nejm.org/doi/full/10.1056/NEJMp1700601

633.   nejm.org / Newhouse JP, Normand S.-LT. Health Policy Trials; NEJM; 2017 Jun 1; 376(22): 2160–2167 http://www.nejm.org/doi/full/10.1056/NEJMra1602774

634.   nejm.org / Rosenbaum L. Bridging the Data-Sharing Divide: Seeing the Devil in the Details, Not the Other Camp; NEJM; 2017 Jun 8; 376(23): 2201–2203 http://www.nejm.org/doi/full/10.1056/NEJMp1704482

635.   nejm.org / Haug CJ. Whose Data Are They Anyway? Can a Patient Perspective Advance the Data-Sharing Debate? NEJM; 2017 Jun 8; 376(23): 2203–2205 http://www.nejm.org/doi/full/10.1056/NEJMp1704485

636.   nejm.org / Burns NS, Miller PW. Learning What We Didn't Know: The SPRINT Data Analysis Challenge; NEJM; 2017 Jun 8; 376(23): 2205–2207 http://www.nejm.org/doi/full/10.1056/NEJMp1705323

637.   nejm.org / Welch HG, Fisher ES. Income and Cancer Overdiagnosis: When Too Much Care Is Harmful; NEJM; 2017 Jun 8; 376(23): 2208–2209 http://www.nejm.org/doi/full/10.1056/NEJMp1615069

638.   nejm.org / Taichman DB, et al. Data Sharing Statements for Clinical Trials: A Requirement of the International Committee of Medical Journal Editors; NEJM; 2017 Jun 8; 376(23): 2277–2279 http://www.nejm.org/doi/full/10.1056/NEJMe1705439

639.   nejm.org / Ryu J, Lee TH. The Waiting Game: Why Providers May Fail to Reduce Wait Times; NEJM; 2017 Jun 15; 376(24): 2309–2311 http://www.nejm.org/doi/full/10.1056/NEJMp1704478

640.   nejm.org / Ryan AM, et al. Changes in Hospital Quality Associated with Hospital Value-Based Purchasing; NEJM; 2017 Jun 15; 376(24): 2358–2366 http://www.nejm.org/doi/full/10.1056/NEJMsa1613412

641.   nejm.org / Aronson L. A Tale of Two Doctors: Structural Inequalities and the Culture of Medicine; NEJM; 2017 Jun 15; 376(24): 2390–2393 http://www.nejm.org/doi/full/10.1056/NEJMms1702140

642.   nejm.org / Griffiths EP. Effective Legislative Advocacy: Lessons from Successful Medical Trainee Campaigns; NEJM; 2017 Jun 22; 376(25): 2409–2411 http://www.nejm.org/doi/full/10.1056/NEJMp1704120

643.   nejm.org / Chen JH, Asch SM. Machine Learning and Prediction in Medicine: Beyond the Peak of Inflated Expectations; NEJM; 2017 Jun 29; 376(26): 2507–2509 http://www.nejm.org/doi/full/10.1056/NEJMp1702071

644.   nejm.org / Brunoni AR, et al. Trial of Electrical Direct-Current Therapy versus Escitalopram for Depression; NEJM; 2017 Jun 29; 376(26): 2523–2533 http://www.nejm.org/doi/full/10.1056/NEJMoa1612999

645.   nejm.org / Ford AC, et al. Irritable Bowel Syndrome; NEJM; 2017 Jun 29; 376(26): 2566–2578 http://www.nejm.org/doi/full/10.1056/NEJMra1607547

646.   nejm.org / Lisanby SH. Noninvasive Brain Stimulation for Depression: The Devil Is in the Dosing; NEJM; 2017 Jun 29; 376(26): 2593–2594 http://www.nejm.org/doi/full/10.1056/NEJMe1702492

647.   nejm.org / Barnett ML, et al. Home-to-Home Time: Measuring What Matters to Patients and Payers; NEJM; 2017 Jul 6; 377(1): 4–6 http://www.nejm.org/doi/full/10.1056/NEJMp1703423

648.   nejm.org / Baumhauer JF. Patient-Reported Outcomes: Are They Living Up to Their Potential? NEJM; 2017 Jul 6; 377(1): 6–9 http://www.nejm.org/doi/full/10.1056/NEJMp1702978

649.   nejm.org / The GBD 2015 Obesity Collaborators. Health Effects of Overweight and Obesity in 195 Countries over 25 Years; NEJM; 2017 Jul 6; 377(1): 13–27 http://www.nejm.org/doi/full/10.1056/NEJMoa1614362

650.   nejm.org / Gregg EW, Shaw JE. Global Health Effects of Overweight and Obesity; NEJM; 2017 Jul 6; 377(1): 80–81 http://www.nejm.org/doi/full/10.1056/NEJMe1706095

651.   nejm.org / Greene JA, Padula WV. Targeting Unconscionable Prescription-Drug Prices: Maryland's Anti-Price-Gouging Law; NEJM; 2017 Jul 13; 377(2): 101–103 http://www.nejm.org/doi/full/10.1056/NEJMp1704907

652.   nejm.org / Chandra A, Garthwaite C. The Economics of Indication-Based Drug Pricing; NEJM; 2017 Jul 13; 377(2): 103–106 http://www.nejm.org/doi/full/10.1056/NEJMp1705035

653.   nejm.org / Sotos-Prieto M, et al. Association of Changes in Diet Quality with Total and Cause-Specific Mortality; NEJM; 2017 Jul 13; 377(2): 143–153 http://www.nejm.org/doi/full/10.1056/NEJMoa1613502

654.   nejm.org / Rosenbaum L. The March of Science: The True Story; NEJM; 2017 Jul 13; 377(2): 188–191 http://www.nejm.org/doi/full/10.1056/NEJMms1706087

655.   nejm.org / Schwarze ML, Taylor LJ. Managing Uncertainty: Harnessing the Power of Scenario Planning; NEJM; 2017 Jul 20; 377(3): 206–208 http://www.nejm.org/doi/full/10.1056/NEJMp1704149

656.   nejm.org / Ginsburg PB, Patel KK. Physician Payment Reform: Progress to Date; NEJM; 2017 Jul 20; 377(3): 285–292 http://www.nejm.org/doi/full/10.1056/NEJMhpr1606353

657.   nejm.org / Fralick M, et al. The Price of Crossing the Border for Medications; NEJM; 2017 Jul 27; 377(4): 311–313 http://www.nejm.org/doi/full/10.1056/NEJMp1704489

658.   nejm.org / Sommers BD, et al. Health Insurance Coverage and Health: What the Recent Evidence Tells Us; NEJM; 2017 Aug 10; 377(6): 586–593 http://www.nejm.org/doi/full/10.1056/NEJMsb1706645

659.   nejm.org / Schwartzstein RM, Roberts DH. Saying Goodbye to Lectures in Medical School: Paradigm Shift or Passing Fad? NEJM; 2017 Aug 17; 377(7): 605–607 http://www.nejm.org/doi/full/10.1056/NEJMp1706474

660.   nejm.org / Wenzel RP. Medical Education in the Era of Alternative Facts; NEJM; 2017 Aug 17; 377(7): 607–609 http://www.nejm.org/doi/full/10.1056/NEJMp1706528

661.   nejm.org / Robinson JC, et al. Association of Reference Pricing with Drug Selection and Spending; NEJM; 2017 Aug 17; 377(7): 658–665 http://www.nejm.org/doi/full/10.1056/NEJMsa1700087

662.   nejm.org / Gordon WJ, et al. Threats to Information Security: Public Health Implications; NEJM; 2017 Aug 24; 377(8): 707–709 http://www.nejm.org/doi/full/10.1056/NEJMp1707212

663.   nejm.org / Dow A, Thibault G. Interprofessional Education: A Foundation for a New Approach to Health Care; NEJM; 2017 Aug 31; 377(9): 803–805 http://www.nejm.org/doi/full/10.1056/NEJMp1705665

664.   nejm.org / Schneider EC, Squires D. From Last to First: Could the U.S. Health Care System Become the Best in the World? NEJM; 2017 Sep 7; 377(10): 901–904 http://www.nejm.org/doi/full/10.1056/NEJMp1708704

665.   nejm.org / Choudhry NK. Randomized, Controlled Trials in Health Insurance Systems; NEJM; 2017 Sep 7; 377(10): 957–964 http://www.nejm.org/doi/full/10.1056/NEJMra1510058

666.   nejm.org / Lozano AM. Waving Hello to Noninvasive Deep-Brain Stimulation; NEJM; 2017 Sep 14; 377(11): 1096–1098 http://www.nejm.org/doi/full/10.1056/NEJMcibr1707165

667.   nejm.org / Woloshin S, et al. The Fate of FDA Post Approval Studies; NEJM; 2017 Sep 21; 377(12): 1114–1117 http://www.nejm.org/doi/full/10.1056/NEJMp1705800

668.   nejm.org / Jones SM, Burks AW. Food Allergy; NEJM; 2017 Sep 21; 377(12): 1168–1176 http://www.nejm.org/doi/full/10.1056/NEJMcp1611971

669.   nejm.org / Obermeyer Z, Lee TH. Lost in Thought: The Limits of the Human Mind and the Future of Medicine; NEJM; 2017 Sep 28; 377(13): 1209–1211 http://www.nejm.org/doi/full/10.1056/NEJMp1705348

670.   nejm.org / Landon BE, Mechanic RE. The Paradox of Coding: Policy Concerns Raised by Risk-Based Provider Contracts; NEJM; 2017 Sep 28; 377(13): 1211–1213 http://www.nejm.org/doi/full/10.1056/NEJMp1708084

671.   nejm.org / Richardson HS, et al. When Ancillary Care Clashes with Study Aims; NEJM; 2017 Sep 28; 377(13): 1213–1215 http://www.nejm.org/doi/full/10.1056/NEJMp1702651

672.   nejm.org / Dzau V, et al. Investing in Global Health for Our Future; NEJM; 2017 Sep 28; 377(13): 1292–1296 http://www.nejm.org/doi/full/10.1056/NEJMsr1707974

673.   nejm.org / Rotenstein LS, et al. Making Patients and Doctors Happier: The Potential of Patient-Reported Outcomes; NEJM; 2017 Oct 5; 377(14): 1309–1312 http://www.nejm.org/doi/full/10.1056/NEJMp1707537

674.   nejm.org / Mauri L, D'Agostino, Sr. RB. Challenges in the Design and Interpretation of Noninferiority Trials; NEJM; 2017 Oct 5; 377(14): 1357–1367 http://www.nejm.org/doi/full/10.1056/NEJMra1510063

675.   nejm.org / Hernán MA, Robins JM. Per-Protocol Analyses of Pragmatic Trials; NEJM; 2017 Oct 5; 377(14): 1391–1398 http://www.nejm.org/doi/full/10.1056/NEJMsm1605385

676.   nejm.org / Asch DA, et al. Misdirections in Informed Consent: Impediments to Health Care Innovation; NEJM; 2017 Oct 12; 377(15): 1412–1414 http://www.nejm.org/doi/full/10.1056/NEJMp1707991

677.   nejm.org / Tuckson RV, et al. Telehealth; NEJM; 2017 Oct 19; 377(16): 1585–1592 http://www.nejm.org/doi/full/10.1056/NEJMsr1503323

678.   ncbi.nlm.nih.gov / Hallman CA, et al. More Than 75 Percent Decline over 27 Years in Total Flying Insect Biomass in Protected Areas; PLOS One; 2017 Oct 18; 12(10): e0185809. DOI: 10.1371/journal.pone.0185809 https://www.ncbi.nlm.nih.gov/pmc/articles/PMC5646769/

679.   ncbi.nlm.nih.gov / Fairbrother A, et al. Risks of Neonicotinoid Insecticides to Honeybees; Environmental Toxicology and Chemistry; 2014 Apr; 33(4): 719–731 DOI: 10.1002/etc.2527 https://www.ncbi.nlm.nih.gov/pmc/articles/PMC4312970/

680.   nature.com / Peeters K, et al. Fructose-1,6-Biphosphate Couples Glycolytic Flux to Activation of Ras; Nature Communications; 2017 Oct 13; 8: 922 DOI: 10.1038/s41467-017-01019-z https://www.ncbi.nlm.nih.gov/pmc/articles/PMC5640605/

681.   businessinsider.com / Google Built a New Trojan Horse to Get inside Every Aspect of Your Life. Steve Kovach, October 21, 2017 http://www.businessinsider.com/google-hardware-plan-trojan-horse-2017-10

682.   niddk.nih.gov / Health Information / Health Statistics / Overweight & Obesity Statistics https://www.niddk.nih.gov/health-information/health-statistics/overweight-obesity

683.   cdc.gov / Chronic Disease Prevention and Health Promotion https://www.cdc.gov/chronicdisease/index.htm

684.   niddk.nih.gov / Strategic Plans Reports / Burden of Digestive Diseases in the United States Report https://www.niddk.nih.gov/about-niddk/strategic-plans-reports/burden-of-digestive-diseases-in-united-states/burden-of-digestive-diseases-in-the-united-states-report

685.   academic.oup.com / Johnson RJ, et al. Potential Role of Sugar (Fructose) in the Epidemic of Hypertension, Obesity and the Metabolic Syndrome, Diabetes, Kidney Disease, and Cardiovascular Disease; The American Journal of Clinical Nutrition; 2007 October 1; 86(4): 899–906 https://doi.org/10.1093/ajcn/86.4.899; https://academic.oup.com/ajcn/article/86/4/899/4649308

686.   washingtonpost.com / Wonkblog / How the American Diet Has Failed. Roberto A. Ferdman, June 18, 2014 https://www.washingtonpost.com/news/wonk/wp/2014/06/18/the-rise-of-processed-and-fast-foods-and-the-ever-expanding-american-waistline/?noredirect=on&utm_term=.d9e6503d3c76

687.   usgovernmentspending.com / Government Debt Chart https://www.usgovernmentspending.com/federal_debt_chart.html

688.   kff.org / KFF Henry J Kaiser Family Foundation / 10 Essential Facts about Medicare and Prescription Drug Spending. November 10, 2017 https://www.kff.org/infographic/10-essential-facts-about-medicare-and-prescription-drug-spending/

689.   healthcare.mckinsey.com / McKinsey Center for U.S. Health System Reform / Accounting for the Cost of U.S. Health Care / Pre-reform Trends and the Impact of the Recession. Jesse W. Bradford, et al. December 2011 https://healthcare.mckinsey.com/sites/default/files/793268__Accounting_for_the_Cost_of_US_Health_Care__Prereform_Trends_and_the_Impact_of_the_Recession.pdf

690.   huffingtonpost.com / Business / Why U.S. Health Care Is Obscenely Expensive, in 12 Charts. Katy Hall and Jan Diehm, October 3, 2013, Updated December 6, 2017 https://www.huffingtonpost.com/2013/10/03/health-care-costs-_n_3998425.html

691.   blogs.reuters.com / Macroscope / The U.S. Productivity Farce. Pedro da Costa, May 4, 2012 http://blogs.reuters.com/macroscope/2012/05/04/the-u-s-productivity-farce/

692.   epi.org / Wage Stagnation in Nine Charts. Lawrence Mishel, Elise Gould, and Josh Bivens, January 6, 2015 https://www.epi.org/publication/charting-wage-stagnation/

693.   stateofworkingamerica.org / Economic Policy Institute / The State of Working America / Charts & Tables / Trends http://stateofworkingamerica.org/subjects/overview/

694.   stateofworkingamerica.org / Economic Policy Institute / The State of Working America / Charts & Tables / Trends / Productivity and Real Median Family Income Growth, 1948–2013 http://www.stateofworkingamerica.org/charts/productivity-an d-real-median-family-income-growth-1947-2009/

695.   theatlantic.com / Corporate Profits Are Eating the Economy. Derek Thompson, March 4, 2013 https://www.theatlantic.com/business/archive/2013/03/ corporate-profits-are-eating-the-economy/273687/

696.   motherjones.com / Overworked America: 12 Charts That Will Make Your Blood Boil / Why "Efficiency" and "Productivity" Really Mean More Profits for Corporations and Less Sanity for You. Dave Gilson, July/August 2011 https://www.motherjones.com/ politics/2011/05/speedup-americans-working-harder-charts/

697.   motherjones.com / It's the Inequality, Stupid / Eleven Charts That Explain What's Wrong with America. Dave Gilson and Carolyn Perot, March/April 2011 https://www. motherjones.com/politics/2011/02/income-inequality-in-america-chart-graph/

698.   forbes.com / Pharma & Healthcare / 2012—The Year in Healthcare Charts. Dan Munro, December 30, 2012 https://www.forbes.com/sites/danmunro/2012/12/30/2 012-the-year-in-healthcare-charts/#679d7d9f6c8c

699.   slideshare.net / USA Inc. / A Basic Summary of America's Financial Statements. Mary Meeker, February 2011 https://www.slideshare.net/kleinerperkins/usa-in c-a-basic-summary-of-americas-financial-statements http://www.kpcb.com/ blog/2011-usa-inc-full-report

700.   brookings.edu / Upfront / The Hutchins Center Explains: Prescription Drug Spending. Peter Olson and Louise Sheiner, April 26, 2017 https://www.brookings.edu/blog/ up-front/2017/04/26/the-hutchins-center-explains-prescription-drug-spending/

701.   iqvia.com / Medicines Use and Spending in the U.S.: A Review of 2016 and Outlook to 2021. Institute Report, May 4, 2017 https://www.iqvia.com/institute/reports/ medicines-use-and-spending-in-the-us-a-review-of-2016

702.   acrabstracts.org / Tatangelo M, et al. Temporal Trends in Drug Prescription, Utilization and Costs among Rheumatoid Arthritis (RA) Patients Show Wide Regional Variation Despite Universal Drug Coverage; Meeting: 2015 ACR/ARHP Annual Meeting [abstract]. Arthritis Rheumatol. 2015; 67 (suppl 10) https://acrabstracts.org/abstract/ temporal-trends-in-drug-prescription-utilization-and-costs-among-rheumatoid-arth ritis-ra-patients-show-wide-regional-variation-despite-universal-drug-coverage/

703.   ers.usda.gov / US Department of Agriculture Economic Research Service Food Choices & Health / Food Consumption & Demand / Food Away from Home https:// www.ers.usda.gov/topics/food-choices-health/food-consumption-demand/ food-away-from-home.aspx

704.   ers.usda.gov / US Department of Agriculture Economic Research Service Data Products / Ag and Food Statistics: Charting the Essentials / Food Prices and Spending https://www.ers.usda.gov/data-products/ag-and-food-statistics-charting-the-essen tials/food-prices-and-spending/

705.   annals.org / Grande D. Editorial: Prescriber Profiling; Time to Call It Quits; Annals of Internal Medicine; 2007 May 15; 146(10): 751–752 http://annals.org/aim/ article-abstract/734744

706.   nationalgeographic.com / Zimmer C. Secrets of the Brain: National Geographic; 2014 Feb; 225(2): 28–57 https://www.nationalgeographic.com/magazine/2014/02/ brain/

707.   nationalgeographic.com / Finkel M. Star Eater; National Geographic; 2014 Mar; 225(3): 88–103 https://www.nationalgeographic.com/magazine/2014/03/black-holes-einstein-star-eaters/

708.   nationalgeographic.com / Foley J. Feeding Nine Billion: A Five-Step Plan to Feed the World; National Geographic; 2014 May; 225(5): 26–59 https://www.nationalgeographic.com/foodfeatures/feeding-9-billion/

709.   gutmicrobes.org / Conferences 2015, 2016, 2017. Huntington Beach, CA

710.   thelancet.com / Ajiboye AB, et al. Restoration of Reaching and Grasping Movements through Brain-Controlled Muscle Stimulation in a Person with Tetraplegia: A Proof-of-Concept Demonstration; The Lancet; 2017 May 6; 389(10081): 1821–1830 https://dx.doi.org/10.1016/S0140-6736(17)30601-3

711.   Sun AJ, Eisenberg ML. Association between Marijuana Use and Sexual Frequency in the United States: A Population-Based Study; The Journal of Sexual Medicine; 2017 Nov; 14(11): 1342–1347 https://dx.doi.org/10.1016/j.jsxm.2017.09.005

712.   sciencedaily.com / Novel Diet Therapy Helps Children with Crohn's Disease and Ulcerative Colitis Reach Remission. Seattle Children's Hospital, December 28, 2016 https://www.sciencedaily.com/releases/2016/12/161228171130.htm

713.   ncbi.nlm.nih.gov / Suskind DL, et al. Clinical and Fecal Microbial Changes with Diet Therapy in Active Inflammatory Bowel Disease. Journal of Clinical Gastroenterology; 2018 Feb; 52(2): 155–163 (Published online 2016 Dec 27) DOI: 10.1097/MCG.0000000000000772 https://www.ncbi.nlm.nih.gov/pubmed/28030510 https://www.ncbi.nlm.nih.gov/pmc/articles/PMC5484760/

714.   ncbi.nlm.nih.gov / Govender M, et al. A Review of the Advancements in Probiotic Delivery: Conventional vs. Non-conventional Formulations for Intestinal Flora Supplementation; AAPS PharmSciTech; 2014 Feb; 15(1): 29–43 DOI: 10.1208/s12249-013-0027-1 https://www.ncbi.nlm.nih.gov/pmc/articles/PMC3909163/

715.   axios.com / Sean Parker Unloads on Facebook "Exploiting" Human Psychology. Mike Allen, November 9, 2017 https://www.axios.com/sean-parker-unloads-on-facebook-god-only-knows-what-its-doing-to-our-childrens-brains-1513306792-f855e7b4-4e99-4d60-8d51-2775559c2671.html

716.   businessinsider.com / Billionaire Ex-Facebook President Sean Parker Unloads on Mark Zuckerberg and Admits He Helped Build a Monster. Rob Price, November 9, 2017 https://www.businessinsider.com/ex-facebook-president-sean-parker-social-network-human-vulnerability-2017-11

717.   independent.co.uk / Facebook's First President Sean Parker Says App Has Secretly Snared Billions of People into Using It; The app Has Been Purposefully Getting People Hooked and Potentially Destroying Society as It Does So. Andrew Griffin, November 9, 2017 http://www.independent.co.uk/life-style/gadgets-and-tech/news/facebook-sean-parker-mark-zuckerberg-instagram-secrets-why-keep-using-it-app-website-a8045816.html

718.   salon.com / Facebook's Co-Founder Blasts Social Media: "It Literally Changes Your Relationship with Society." Matthew Rozsa, November 9, 2017 https://www.salon.com/2017/11/09/facebooks-co-founder-blasts-social-media-it-literally-changes-your-relationship-with-society/

719.   npr.org / What the Industry Knew about Sugar's Health Effects but Didn't Tell Us. Allison Aubrey, November 21, 2017, All Things Considered; https://www.npr.org/sections/thesalt/2017/11/21/565766988/what-the-industry-knew-about-sugars-health-effects-but-didnt-tell-us

720.   journals.plos.org / Kearns CE, et al. Sugar Industry Sponsorship of Germ-Free Rodent Studies Linking Sucrose to Hyperlipidemia and Cancer: An Historical Anal-

ysis of Internal Documents; PLOS Biology; 15(11); 2017 Nov 21: Online Nov 17, 2017 e2003460 https://doi.org/10.1371/journal.pbio.2003460

721. medicalnewstoday.com / Cancer: 42 Percent of Cases Down to Risk Factors You Can Change. Ana Sandoiu, November 21, 2017 https://www.medicalnewstoday.com/articles/320121.php

722. onlinelibrary.wiley.com / Islami F, et al. Proportion and Number of Cancer Cases and Deaths Attributable to Potentially Modifiable Risk Factors in the United States; CA: A Cancer Journal for Clinicians; 2017 Nov 21; DOI: https://doi.org/10.3322/caac.21440; https://onlinelibrary.wiley.com/doi/full/10.3322/caac.21440

723. ns.umich.edu / Cinnamon Turns Up the Heat on Fat Cells. Emily Kagey, November 21, 2017 https://ns.umich.edu/new/releases/25273-cinnamon-turns-up-the-heat-on-fat-cells

724. Metabolismjournal.com / Jiang J, et al. Cinnamaldehyde Induces Fat Cell-Autonomous thermogenesis and Metabolic Reprogramming; Metabolism Clinical and Experimental; 2017 Dec; 77: 58–64 DOI: http://dx.doi.org/10.1016/j.metabol.2017.08.006

725. livescience.com / How Much Water Do You Really Need to Drink? Brandon Specktor, January 7, 2018 https://www.livescience.com/61353-how-much-water-you-really-need-drink.html

726. ncbi.nlm.nih.gov / Palma L, et al. Dietary Water Affects Human Skin Hydration and Biomechanics; Clinical, Cosmetic and Investigational Dermatology; 2015 Aug; 8: 413–421 DOI: 10.2147/CCID.S86822 https://www.ncbi.nlm.nih.gov/pmc/articles/PMC4529263/

727. humanetech.com / problem / Our Society Is Being Hijacked by Technology. What Began as a Race to Monetize Our Attention Is Now Eroding the Pillars of Our Society: Mental Health, Democracy, Social Relationships, and Our Children. Center for Humane Technology. February 5, 2018 https://humanetech.com/problem/

728. nytimes.com / Early Facebook and Google Employees Form Coalition to Fight What They Built. Nellie Bowles, February 4, 2018 https://www.nytimes.com/2018/02/04/technology/early-facebook-google-employees-fight-tech.html

729. businessinsider.com / A Group of Former Facebook and Apple Employees Are Teaming Up to Warn Kids about Tech Addiction. Chris Weller, February 5, 2018 http://www.businessinsider.com/ex-facebook-and-google-employees-launch-anti-tech-addiction-campaign-2018-2

730. chicagobusiness.com / Largest Hospitals in Chicago Area Brought in Nearly $17 billion in Patient Revenue in 2016. November 10, 2017 http://www.chicagobusiness.com/article/20171110/ISSUE01/171109882/largest-hospitals-in-chicago-area-brought-in-nearly-17-billion-in-patient-revenue-in-2016; http://www.chicagobusiness.com/article/99999999/DATA/50001633

731. thehealthcareblog.com / The Fairy Tale of a Non-Profit Hospital. Niran al-Agba, MD, April 25, 2017 http://thehealthcareblog.com/blog/2017/04/25/the-fairy-tale-of-a-non-profit-hospital/

732. revcycleintelligence.com / 2017 Hospital Merger Activity Likely to Beat 102 Deals in 2016. The Industry Has Seen 87 Health System and Hospital Merger Deals So Far in 2017 and That Number Is Likely to Exceed the 102 Deals Announced in 2016, an Analysis Uncovered. Jacqueline LaPointe, October 18, 2017 https://revcycleintelligence.com/news/2017-hospital-merger-activity-likely-to-beat-102-deals-in-2016

733. healthcarefinancenews.com / Healthcare Mergers, Acquisitions and Joint Ventures in 2017: Running List. Healthcare Finance Staff https://www.healthcarefinancenews.com/slideshow/healthcare-mergers-and-acquisitions-2017-running-list?p=9

734. mlive.com / Michigan Medicine Program Criticized for Allowing Patients to "Jump the Line." Martin Slagter, March 9, 2018 https://www.mlive.com/news/ann-arbor/index.ssf/2018/03/michigan_medicine_concierge_ca.html

735. wsj.com / CVS to Buy Aetna for $69 Billion, Combining Major Health-Care Players. Deal Is Latest and Most Dramatic Sign of How the Lines between Traditional Segments in Health Care Are Blurring. Sharon Terlep, Anna Wilde Mathews and Dana Cimilluca, December 3, 2017 https://www.wsj.com/articles/cvs-to-buy-aetna-for-69-billion-1512325099

736. washingtonpost.com / Doctor Bought Jet and Maserati from Proceeds of Unnecessary Chemotherapy, Authorities Say. Alex Horton, May 17, 2018 https://www.washingtonpost.com/news/to-your-health/wp/2018/05/17/doctor-bought-jet-and-maserati-from-proceeds-of-unnecessary-chemotherapy-authorities-say/?noredirect=on&utm_term=.cb7e43541704

737. washingtonpost.com / NIH Halts $100 Million Study of Moderate Drinking That Is Funded by Alcohol Industry. Joel Achenbach, May 18, 2018 https://www.washingtonpost.com/news/to-your-health/wp/2018/05/17/nih-halts-controversial-study-of-moderate-drinking/?utm_term=.bc7c2022cb6d

738. washingtonpost.com / NIH Will Examine Ethics of Its Study on the Health Effects of a Daily Glass of Wine. Amy Goldstein, March 20, 2018 https://www.washingtonpost.com/national/health-science/nih-will-examine-ethics-of-its-study-on-the-health-effects-of-a-daily-glass-of-wine/2018/03/20/db8f2806-2c78-11e8-b0b0-f706877db618_story.html?utm_term=.5009e55b1c51

739. statnews.com / NIH Abruptly Changes Course on Industry Opioids Partnership after Ethics Flags Raised. Lev Facher, April 19, 2018 https://www.statnews.com/2018/04/19/nih-industry-partnership-ethics-opioids/

740. statnews.com / NIH Says Dozens of Drug Makers Interested in Partnering to Develop Drugs to Address Opioid Epidemic. Lev Facher, March 20, 2018 https://www.statnews.com/2018/03/20/nih-drug-makers-opioid-partnership/

741. cgfa.ilga.gov / An Evaluation of Illinois' Certificate of Need Program: Prepared for: State of Illinois Commission on Government Forecasting and Accountability. The Lewin Group, February 15, 2007 http://cgfa.ilga.gov/Upload/LewinGroupEvalCertOfNeed.pdf

742. usatoday.com / Wealth of Millionaires Surges 10.6% to Top $70 Trillion for the First Time. David Carrig, June 19, 2018 https://www.usatoday.com/story/money/nation-now/2018/06/19/wealthy-millionaires-global-stocks/711875002/

743. capgemini.com / World Wealth Report 2018 https://www.capgemini.com/us-en/service/world-wealth-report-2018/

744. usatoday.com / Vast Majority of New Wealth Last Year Went to Top 1%. Kim Hjelmgaard, January 21, 2018 https://www.usatoday.com/story/money/2018/01/22/vast-majority-new-wealth-last-year-went-top-1/1051947001/

745. usatoday.com / One-Third of Adults in U.S. Taking Drugs That May Cause Depression, Study Finds. Brett Molina, June 13, 2018 https://www.usatoday.com/story/news/nation-now/2018/06/13/prescription-drugs-may-cause-depression/697354002/

746. today.uic.edu / One-Third of US Adults May Unknowingly Use Medications That Can Cause Depression. June 12, 2018 https://today.uic.edu/one-third-of-us-adults-may-unknowingly-use-medications-that-can-cause-depression

747. jamanetwork.com / Qato DM, et al. Prevalence of Prescription Medications with Depression as a Potential Adverse Effect among Adults in the United States; JAMA; 2018 Jun 12; 319(22): 2289–2298 DOI:10.1001/jama.2018.6741 https://jamanetwork.com/journals/jama/article-abstract/2684607

748.   theguardian.com / Revealed: 50 Million Facebook Profiles Harvested for Cambridge Analytica in Major Data Breach. Carole Cadwalladr and Emma Graham-Harrison, March 17, 2018 https://www.theguardian.com/news/2018/mar/17/cambridge-analytica-facebook-influence-us-election

749.   scientificamerican.com / Does TV Rot Your Brain? Scientists Have Linked TV Viewing to Antisocial Behavior, Lowered Verbal IQ and Altered Brain Structure—but a New Study Raises Questions. R. Douglas Fields, January 1, 2016 https://www.scientificamerican.com/article/does-tv-rot-your-brain/

750.   ncbi.nlm.nih.gov / Tucker LA, Bagwell M. Television Viewing and Obesity in Adult Females. American Journal of Public Health; 1991 Jul; 81(7): 908–911 https://www.ncbi.nlm.nih.gov/pmc/articles/PMC1405200/

751.   hsph.harvard.edu / Television Watching and "Sit Time" https://www.hsph.harvard.edu/obesity-prevention-source/obesity-causes/television-and-sedentary-behavior-and-obesity/

752.   academic.oup.com / Cleland VJ, et al. Television Viewing and Abdominal Obesity in Young Adults: Is the Association Mediated by Food and Beverage Consumption during Viewing Time or Reduced Leisure-Time Physical Activity? The American Journal of Clinical Nutrition; 2008 May 1; 87(5): 1148–1155 https://doi.org/10.1093/ajcn/87.5.1148

753.   jamanetwork.com / Hoang TD, et al. Effect of Early Adult Patterns of Physical Activity and Television Viewing on Midlife Cognitive Function; JAMA Psychiatry; 2016 Jan; 73(1): 73–79 DOI:10.1001/jamapsychiatry.2015.2468 https://jamanetwork.com/journals/jamapsychiatry/fullarticle/2471270

754.   independent.co.uk / Watching Lots of TV "Makes You Stupid," Say Researchers at Universities of California and San Francisco. Emma Henderson, December 3, 2015 https://www.independent.co.uk/news/science/watching-lots-of-tv-makes-you-stupid-says-american-universities-a6759026.html

755.   engadget.com / Study Finds over 3,300 Android Apps Improperly Tracking Kids: They May Be Violating a US Law Protecting Kids' Privacy. Jon Fingas, April 15, 2018 https://www.engadget.com/2018/04/15/study-finds-over-3300-android-apps-improperly-tracking-kids/

756.   petsymposium.org / Reyes I, et al. "Won't Somebody Think of the Children?": Examining COPPA Compliance at Scale; Proceedings on Privacy Enhancing Technologies; 2018; (3): 63–83 DOI 10.1515/popets-2018–0021 https://petsymposium.org/2018/files/papers/issue3/popets-2018-0021.pdf; https://www.degruyter.com/dg/viewarticle/j$002fpopets.2018.2018.issue-3$002fpopets-2018–0021$002fpopets-2018-0021.xml

757.   engadget.com / Websites Settle with New York over Online Child Tracking; They'll Have to Rethink Their Sites after Illegally Scooping Up Personal Data. Jon Fingas, September 13, 2016 https://www.engadget.com/2016/09/13/new-york-settlement-over-online-child-tracking/

758.   engadget.com / Lawsuit claims Disney Illegally Collected Data in Kids Apps: The Suit Names 42 Apps That Allegedly Tracked and Sold Personal Information. Mallory Locklear, August 9, 2017 https://www.engadget.com/2017/08/09/disney-illegally-collected-data-kids-apps/

759.   ftc.gov / Children's Online Privacy Protection Rule ("COPPA"). 16 CFR Part 312 Children's Online Privacy Protection Act of 1998, 15 U.S.C. 6501–6505 Children's Privacy https://www.ftc.gov/enforcement/rules/rulemaking-regulatory-reform-proceedings/childrens-online-privacy-protection-rule

760.   tomsguide.com / Google Responds to Troubling Report of Apps Tracking Kids. Henry T. Casey, April 17, 2018 https://www.tomsguide.com/us/android-apps-tracking-kids-google-play,news-26983.html

761. thesun.co.uk / Search Alert: Google Collects Enough Data on You to Fill an 8ft Stack of Paper Every Two Weeks . . . Then It Flogs the Info to the Highest Bidder: Over 12 Months the Company Reportedly Stores Enough Browsing Data to Fill 569,555 Pages of A4 Paper. Charlie Parker, April 22, 2018 https://www.thesun.co.uk/news/6114042/google-collects-enough-data-on-you-to-fill-an-8ft-stack-of-paper-every-two-weeks-then-it-flogs-the-info-to-the-highest-bidder/

762. wsj.com / Who Has More of Your Personal Data Than Facebook? Try Google. Christopher Mims, April 22, 2018 https://www.wsj.com/articles/who-has-more-of-your-personal-data-than-facebook-try-google-1524398401

763. theverge.com / Google Maps Is Getting Augmented Reality Directions and Recommendation Features. Chaim Gartenberg, May 8, 2018 https://www.theverge.com/2018/5/8/17332480/google-maps-augmented-reality-directions-walking-ar-street-view-personalized-recommendations-voting

764. wraltechwire.com / "Gaming Disorder": WHO Declares Compulsive Playing a Mental Health Problem (+ video). Staff, wire reports, June 18, 2018 https://www.wraltechwire.com/2018/06/18/gaming-disorder-who-declares-compulsive-playing-a-mental-health-problem-video/

765. techcrunch.com / "Gaming Disorder" Is Officially Recognized by the World Health Organization. Brian Heater, June 18, 2018 https://techcrunch.com/2018/06/18/gaming-disorder-is-officially-recognized-by-the-world-health-organization/

766. bmj.com / Fiolet T, et al. Consumption of Ultra-Processed Foods and Cancer Risk: Results from NutriNet-Santé Prospective Cohort; BMJ; 2018 Feb 14; 360: k322 DOI: https://doi.org/10.1136/bmj.k322 https://www.bmj.com/content/360/bmj.k322

767. jaha.ahajournals.org / Saint-Maurice PF, et al. Moderate-to-Vigorous Physical Activity and All-Cause Mortality: Do Bouts Matter? Journal of the American Heart Association. 2018; 7: e007678 Originally published March 22, 2018 https://doi.org/10.1161/JAHA.117.007678; http://jaha.ahajournals.org/content/7/6/e007678

768. forbes.com / Short Bursts of Exercise May Be as Beneficial as Regular Workouts in Extending Life. Bruce Y. Lee, March 25, 2018 https://www.forbes.com/sites/brucelee/2018/03/25/short-bursts-may-prevent-death-too-this-changes-how-you-view-exercise/#446159fc5a39

769. livescience.com / 1 in 12 Deaths Worldwide Could Be Prevented with Regular Physical Activity. Rachael Rettner, September 21, 2017 https://www.livescience.com/60490-physical-activity-prevent-deaths.html

770. thelancet.com / Lear SA, et al. The Effect of Physical Activity on Mortality and Cardiovascular Disease in 130 000 People from 17 High-Income, Middle-Income, and Low-Income Countries: The PURE Study; The Lancet; 2017 Dec 16; 390(10113):2643–2654 DOI: https://doi.org/10.1016/S0140-6736(17)31634-3; https://www.thelancet.com/journals/lancet/article/PIIS0140-6736(17)31634-3/fulltext?elsca1=tlpr

771. physoc.onlinelibrary.wiley.com / Shibata S, et al. The Effect of Lifelong Exercise Frequency on Arterial Stiffness; The Journal of Physiology; 2018 May 20: https://doi.org/10.1113/JP275301; https://physoc.onlinelibrary.wiley.com/doi/full/10.1113/JP275301

772. qz.com / Scientists Have Figured Out Exactly How Much You Need to Exercise to Slow Your Heart's Aging Process. Chase Purdy, May 21, 2018 https://qz.com/1284072/the-right-exercise-to-slow-down-heart-disease-according-to-a-new-study/

773. ncbi.nlm.nih.gov / Kennedy PJ, et al. Irritable Bowel Syndrome: A Microbiome-Gut-Brain Axis Disorder? World Journal of Gastroenterology; 2014 Oct

21; 20(39): 14105–14125 DOI: 10.3748/wjg.v20.i39.14105 https://www.ncbi.nlm.nih.gov/pmc/articles/PMC4202342/

774.   thoracic.org / Svanes O, et al. Cleaning at Home and at Work in Relation to Lung Function Decline and Airway Obstruction; http://www.thoracic.org/about/news-room/press-releases/resources/women-cleaners-lung-function.pdf

775.   eurekalert.org / Women Who Clean at Home or Work Face Increased Lung Function Decline. American Thoracic Society. Feb 16, 2018 https://eurekalert.org/pub_releases/2018-02/ats-wwc021318.php

776.   livescience.com / No, Drinking Alcohol Won't Make You Live Past 90. Brandon Specktor, February 21, 2018 https://www.livescience.com/61824-drinking-alcohol-longer-life-explainer.html

777.   pediatrics.aappublications.org / Cockrell Skinner A, et al. Prevalence of Obesity and Severe Obesity in US Children, 1999–2016; Pediatrics; 2018 Mar; 141(3) http://pediatrics.aappublications.org/content/early/2018/02/22/peds.2017-3459; http://pediatrics.aappublications.org/content/pediatrics/early/2018/02/22/peds.2017-3459.full.pdf

778.   cdc.gov / National Health and Nutrition Examination Survey https://www.cdc.gov/nchs/nhanes/index.htm

779.   cdc.gov / Multistate Outbreak of Salmonella Infections Linked to Kratom (Final Update). May 24, 2018 https://www.cdc.gov/salmonella/kratom-02-18/index.html

780.   ucsf.edu / E-Cigarette Use Exposes Teens to Toxic Chemicals: Toxic Byproducts Are Found Even in Adolescents Who Use E-cigarettes without Nicotine. Elizabeth Fernandez, March 5, 2018 https://www.ucsf.edu/news/2018/03/409946/e-cigarette-use-exposes-teens-toxic-chemicals

781.   pediatrics.aappublications.org / Rubinstein ML, et al. Adolescent Exposure to Toxic Volatile Organic Chemicals from E-Cigarettes; Pediatrics; 2018 April; 141(4) http://pediatrics.aappublications.org/content/early/2018/03/01/peds.2017-3557; http://pediatrics.aappublications.org/content/pediatrics/early/2018/03/01/peds.2017-3557.full.pdf

782.   wsj.com / Something's Brewing: Coca-Cola Plans Its First Alcoholic Drink: Coke to Experiment with Its First Alcoholic Product: In Japan. Suryatapa Bhattacharya and Cara Lombardo, March 7, 2018 https://www.wsj.com/articles/somethings-brewing-coca-cola-plans-its-first-alcoholic-drink-1520423751

783.   foxnews.com / Human Tooth Found in Bag of Planters Cashews, Woman Says. Nicole Darrah, March 7, 2018 http://www.foxnews.com/us/2018/03/07/human-tooth-found-in-bag-planters-cashews-woman-says.html

784.   federalregister.gov / Tobacco Product Standard for Nicotine Level of Combusted Cigarettes: A Proposed Rule by the Food and Drug Administration on 3/16/2018; Administration Federal Register; 2018 Mar 16; 83(52) https://www.federalregister.gov/documents/2018/03/16/2018-05345/tobacco-product-standard-for-nicotine-level-of-combusted-cigarettes

785.   healio.com / Kanny D, et al. CDC: Adult Binge Drinkers Collectively Consume 17.5 Billion Drinks a Year. American Journal of Preventive Medicine; 2018; DOI: 10.1016/j.amepre.2017.12.021, March 16, 2018 https://www.healio.com/family-medicine/addiction/news/online/%7Bf392e9fa-1413-41e0-87da-b21b79b5d748%7D/cdc-adult-binge-drinkers-collectively-consume-175-billion-drinks-a-year

786.   ajpmonline.org / Hingson RW, et al. Drinking Beyond the Binge Threshold: Predictors, Consequences, and Changes in the U.S.; American Journal of Preventive Medicine; 2017 Jun; 52(6): 717–727 DOI: https://doi.org/10.1016/j.amepre.2017.02.014 https://www.ajpmonline.org/article/S0749-3797(17)30161-7/fulltext

787. cdc.gov / CDC Newsroom: During Binges, U.S. Adults Have 17 Billion Drinks a Year: More Than Half of Those Drinks Are by Adults Ages 35 Years and Older. March 16, 2018 https://www.cdc.gov/media/releases/2018/p0316-binge-drinking.html

788. ajpmonline.org / Kanny D, et al. Annual Total Binge Drinks Consumed by U.S. Adults, 2015; American Journal of Preventive Medicine; 2018 April; 54(4): 486–496 DOI: https://doi.org/10.1016/j.amepre.2017.12.021 https://www.ajpmonline.org/article/S0749–3797(17)30753–5/fulltext

789. today.com / Grilling Meat May Raise Risk of High Blood Pressure, Study Finds. A. Pawlowski and Lauren Dunn, March 21, 2018 https://www.today.com/health/grilling-meat-may-raise-risk-high-blood-pressure-study-t125532

790. today.com / 7 Things You Need to Know When You Barbecue. Natalie Azar, June 6, 2017 https://www.today.com/health/grilled-meats-7-things-you-need-know-when-you-barbecue-t112371

791. nbcnews.com / Ham, Sausages Cause Cancer; Red Meat Probably Does, Too, WHO Group Says. Maggie Fox, October 26, 2015 https://www.nbcnews.com/health/cancer/processed-meat-causes-cancer-red-meat-probably-does-group-says-n451396

792. thelancet.com / Bouvard V, et al. Carcinogenicity of Consumption of Red and Processed Meat; The Lancet Oncology; 2015 December 2015; 16(16): 1599–1600 DOI: https://doi.org/10.1016/S1470–2045(15)00444-1; https://www.thelancet.com/journals/lanonc/article/PIIS1470-2045(15)00444-1/fulltext

793. accuweather.com / You're Likely Gulping a Mouthful of Microplastics If You Drink Bottled Water, New Study Reveals. Ashley Williams, March 27, 2018 https://www.accuweather.com/en/weather-news/youre-likely-gulping-a-mouthful-of-microplastics-if-you-drink-bottled-water-new-study-reveals/70004515

794. orbmedia.org / Plus Plastic: Microplastics Found in Global Bottled Water. Christopher Tyree and Dan Morrison. https://orbmedia.org/stories/plus-plastic/text

795. publichealth.gwu.edu / Fast Food May Expose Consumers to Harmful Chemicals Called Phthalates https://publichealth.gwu.edu/content/fast-food-may-expose-consumers-harmful-chemicals-called-phthalates

796. ncbi.nlm.nih.gov / Zota AR, et al. Recent Fast Food Consumption and Bisphenol A and Phthalates Exposures among the U.S. Population in NHANES, 2003–2010; Environmental Health Perspectives; 2016 Oct; 124(10): 1521–1528 DOI: 10.1289/ehp.1510803 https://www.ncbi.nlm.nih.gov/pmc/articles/PMC5047792/

797. sciencedirect.com / Varshavsky JR, et al. Dietary Sources of Cumulative Phthalates Exposure among the U.S. General Population in NHANES 2005–2014; 2018 June; 115: 417–429 https://doi.org/10.1016/j.envint.2018.02.029; https://www.sciencedirect.com/science/article/pii/S0160412017314666?via%3Dihub

798. dph.illinois.gov / Synthetic Cannabinoids http://dph.illinois.gov/topics-services/prevention-wellness/medical-cannabis/synthetic-cannabinoids

799. cnn.com / A Kroger Supplier Recalls Ground Beef Because It Might Be Contaminated with Bits of Plastic. Doug Criss, May 3, 2018 https://www.cnn.com/2018/05/03/health/ground-beef-recall-trnd/index.html

800. who.int / WHO Plan to Eliminate Industrially-Produced Trans-Fatty Acids from Global Food Supply. May 14, 2018 http://www.who.int/news-room/detail/14-05-2018-who-plan-to-eliminate-industrially-produced-trans-fatty-acids-from-global-food-supply

801. usnews.com / As ADHD Diagnoses Increased, So Did Calls to Poison Control. Gaby Galvin, May 21, 2018 https://www.usnews.com/news/healthiest-communities/articles/2018-05-21/study-shows-surge-in-calls-to-poison-control-for-adhd-meds

802.   pediatrics.aappublications.org / King SA, et al. Pediatric ADHD Medication Exposures Reported to US Poison Control Centers; Pediatrics; 2018 June; 141(6) http://pediatrics.aappublications.org/content/141/6/e20173872

803.   wnep.com / FDA Warns Teething Medicines Unsafe, Wants Them Off Shelves. CNN wire, May 23, 2018 https://wnep.com/2018/05/23/fda-warns-teething-medicines-unsafe-wants-them-off-shelves/

804.   washingtonpost.com / Five Dead, Nearly 200 Sick in E. coli Outbreak from Lettuce. And Investigators Are Stumped. Kristine Phillips, June 2, 2018 https://www.washingtonpost.com/news/to-your-health/wp/2018/06/02/five-dead-nearly-200-sick-in-e-coli-outbreak-from-lettuce-and-investigators-are-stumped/?noredirect=on&utm_term=.12ee9434b6b9

805.   foxnews.com / Salmonella Found in Pre-cut Melon Sickens 60 People, CDC Says. Katherine Lam, June 10, 2018 http://www.foxnews.com/health/2018/06/10/salmonella-found-in-pre-cut-melon-sickens-60-people-cdc-says.html

806.   jsonline.com / Cyclospora Illness Outbreak Tied to Kwik Trip Vegetable Trays Grows in Wisconsin and Minnesota. Rick Barrett, June 15, 2018 https://www.jsonline.com/story/money/2018/06/15/cyclospora-illness-outbreak-kwik-trip-vegetable-trays-worsens/704446002/

807.   npr.org / Kellogg's Honey Smacks Recalled Amid Salmonella Outbreak Investigation. Cameron Jenkins, June 15, 2018 https://www.npr.org/2018/06/15/620382377/kelloggs-honey-smacks-recalled-amid-salmonella-outbreak-investigation

808.   bbc.com / BBC News: Health: Cannabis: What Are the Risks of Recreational Use? June 19, 2018 https://www.bbc.com/news/health-44532417

809.   jamanetwork.com / Gardner CD, et al. Effect of Low-Fat vs Low-Carbohydrate Diet on 12-Month Weight Loss in Overweight Adults and the Association with Genotype Pattern or Insulin Secretion: The DIETFITS Randomized Clinical Trial; JAMA; 2018 Feb 20; 319(7): 667–679 DOI: 10.1001/jama.2018.0245 https://jamanetwork.com/journals/jama/article-abstract/2673150?redirect=true

810.   straitstimes.com / Taking a Closer Look at Dietary Fads and What They Actually Accomplish. Chris Chan, March 13, 2018 https://www.straitstimes.com/lifestyle/food/taking-a-closer-look-at-dietary-fads-and-what-they-actually-accomplish

811.   mailman.columbia.edu / Food Policy and Obesity: What Is the Best Way to Measure Obesity? The Humble and Much-Maligned Body Mass Index Takes the Cake. December 27, 2012 https://www.mailman.columbia.edu/public-health-now/news/what-best-way-measure-obesity

812.   sciencedirect.com / Mooney SJ, et al. Comparison of Anthropometric and Body Composition Measures as Predictors of Components of the Metabolic Syndrome in a Clinical Setting; Obesity Research & Clinical Practice; 2013 January–February; 7(1): e55-e66 https://www.sciencedirect.com/science/article/pii/S1871403X12002657

813.   nature.com / O'Keefe SJD, et al. Fat, Fibre and Cancer Risk in African Americans and Rural Africans; Nature Communications; 2015 Apr 28; 6: 6342 https://www.nature.com/articles/ncomms7342#affil-auth

814.   sciencealert.com / Here's What Happens When Rural Africans Eat an American Diet for 2 Weeks. Fiona Macdonald, March 28, 2018 https://www.sciencealert.com/what-happens-when-rural-africans-eat-an-american-diet-for-2-weeks

815.   news-medical.net / Single High-Fat Meal Can Set the Stage for Cardiovascular Disease. March 29, 2018 https://www.news-medical.net/news/20180329/Single-high-fat-meal-can-set-the-stage-for-cardiovascular-disease.aspx

816.   jagwire.augusta.edu / Just One High-Fat Meal Sets the Perfect Stage for Heart Disease. Toni Baker, March 29, 2018 http://jagwire.augusta.edu/archives/52420

817.   nature.com / Benson TW, et al. A Single High-Fat Meal Provokes Pathological Erythrocyte Remodeling and Increases Myeloperoxidase Levels: Implications for Acute Coronary Syndrome. Laboratory Investigation; 2018 Mar 23 DOI: https://doi.org/10.1038/s41374-018-0038-3 https://www.nature.com/articles/s41374-018-0038-3

818.   business-standard.com / Is Your Belly Putting Your Heart at Risk? April 21, 2018 https://www.business-standard.com/article/news-ani/is-your-belly-putting-your-heart-at-risk-118042100087_1.html

819.   medicalxpress.com / A fat Belly Is Bad for Your Heart. European Society of Cardiology, April 20, 2018 https://medicalxpress.com/news/2018-04-fat-belly-bad-heart.html

820.   scienceblog.com / Why Zero-Calorie Sweeteners Can Still Lead to Diabetes, Obesity. April 22, 2018 https://scienceblog.com/500456/why-zero-calorie-sweeteners-can-still-lead-to-diabetes-obesity/

821.   plan.core-apps.com / Hoffman B, et al. The Influence of Sugar and Artificial Sweeteners on Vascular Health during the Onset and Progression of Diabetes; EB Experimental Biology 2018; Board # / Pub #: A322 603.20 https://plan.core-apps.com/eb2018/abstract/382e0c7eb95d6e76976fbc663612d58a

822.   thedenverchannel.com / Research: Curbing Salt Intake Could Add Years to Your Life. CNN, April 26, 2018 https://www.thedenverchannel.com/news/health/research-curbing-salt-intake-could-add-years-to-your-life

823.   journals.plos.org / Pearson-Stuttard J, et al. Estimating the Health and Economic Effects of the Proposed US Food and Drug Administration Voluntary Sodium Reformulation: Microsimulation Cost-Effectiveness Analysis; PLOS Medicine; 2019 Apr 10; http://journals.plos.org/plosmedicine/article?id=10.1371/journal.pmed.1002551 https://doi.org/10.1371/journal.pmed.1002551

824.   circ.ahajournals.org / Cook NR, et al. Lower Levels of Sodium Intake and Reduced Cardiovascular Risk; Circulation; 2014 Mar 3; 129(9): 981–989 https://circ.ahajournals.org/content/129/9/981; https://doi.org/10.1161/circulationaha.113.006032

825.   health.gov / Dietary Guidelines 2015–2020: Executive Summary https://health.gov/dietaryguidelines/2015/guidelines/executive-summary/#footnote-4

826.   news.llu.edu / New studies Show Dark Chocolate Consumption Reduces Stress and Inflammation, While Improving Memory, Immunity and Mood: Data Represent First Human Trials Examining the Impact of Dark Chocolate Consumption on Cognition and Other Brain Functions. Loma Linda, CA, April 24, 2018 https://news.llu.edu/for-journalists/press-releases/new-studies-show-dark-chocolate-consumption-reduces-stress-and-inflammation-while-improving-memory-immunity-and-mood

827.   fda.gov / US Food & Drug Administration: Food Additives & Ingredients: Final Determination Regarding Partially Hydrogenated Oils (Removing Trans Fat) https://www.fda.gov/Food/IngredientsPackagingLabeling/FoodAdditivesIngredients/ucm449162.htm

828.   reuters.com / Egg a Day Tied to Lower Risk of Heart Disease. Lisa Rapaport, May 21, 2018 https://www.reuters.com/article/us-health-heart-eggs/egg-a-day-tied-to-lower-risk-of-heart-disease-idUSKCN1IM2G9

829.   heart.bmj.com / Qin C, et al. Associations of Egg Consumption with Cardiovascular Disease in a Cohort Study of 0.5 Million Chinese Adults; BMJ Heart: 2018 May 21; 0: 1–8 DOI: 10.1136/heartjnl-2017–312651 https://heart.bmj.com/content/heartjnl/early/2018/04/17/heartjnl-2017-312651.full.pdf

830.   journals.lww.com / Suskind DL, et al. Nutritional Therapy in Pediatric Crohn Disease: The Specific Carbohydrate Diet; JPGN; 2014 Jan; 58(1): 87–91 DOI: 10.1097/

MPG.0000000000000103 https://journals.lww.com/jpgn/Fulltext/2014/01000/Nutritional_Therapy_in_Pediatric_Crohn_Disease__.22.aspx

831.   journals.lww.com / Cohen, SA, et al. Clinical and Mucosal Improvement with Specific Carbohydrate Diet in Pediatric Crohn Disease; 2014 October; 59(4): 516–521 DOI: 10.1097/MPG.0000000000000449 https://journals.lww.com/jpgn/Fulltext/2014/10000/Clinical_and_Mucosal_ImprovementWith_Specific.20.aspx

832.   techtimes.com / Toddlers Consume More "Added Sugar" Than the Recommended Amount for Adults. Sami Ghanmi, June 11, 2018 https://www.techtimes.com/articles/229867/20180611/toddlers-consume-more-added-sugar-than-the-recommended-amount-for-adults.htm

833.   abcnews.go.com / Toddlers Consuming Too Much Added Sugar, Study Finds. Karine Tawagi, June 10, 2018 https://abcnews.go.com/Health/toddlers-consuming-added-sugar-study-finds/story?id=55719076

834.   qz.com / American Toddlers Are Eating More Sugar Than the Maximum Amount Recommended for Adults. Annabelle Timsit, June 11, 2018 https://qz.com/1302201/american-toddlers-are-eating-more-sugar-than-the-amount-recommended-for-adults/

835.   eventscribe.com / Herrick K. Consumption of Added Sugars among U.S. Infants Aged 6–23 Months, 2011–2014; Nutrition 2018; June 10, 2018 https://www.eventscribe.com/2018/Nutrition2018/fsPopup.asp?Mode=presInfo&PresentationID=405508

836.   sciencemag.org / Following Charges of Flawed Statistics, Major Medical Journal Sets the Record Straight. Jennifer Couzin-Frankel, June 13, 2018 http://www.sciencemag.org/news/2018/06/following-charges-flawed-statistics-major-medical-journal-sets-record-straight

837.   newscientist.com / Your Brain Absolutely Cannot Resist Doughnuts: Here's Why. Alison George, June 14, 2018 https://www.newscientist.com/article/2171695-your-brain-absolutely-cannot-resist-doughnuts-heres-why/

838.   cell.com / DiFeliceantonio AG, et al. Supra-Additive Effects of Combining Fat and Carbohydrate on Food Reward; Cell Metabolism; 2018 Jul 3; 28: 1–12 DOI: https://doi.org/10.1016/j.cmet.2018.05.018; https://www.cell.com/cell-metabolism/fulltext/S1550-4131(18)30325-5

839.   medicalxpress.com / Exercise Can Slow the Aging Process: A Professor Explains How. Janet M. Lord, March 9, 2018 https://medicalxpress.com/news/2018-03-aging-professor.html

840.   onlinelibrary.wiley.com / Duggal NA, et al. Major Features of Immunesenescence, Including Reduced Thymic Output, Are Ameliorated by High Levels of Physical Activity in Adulthood; Aging Cell; 2018 Mar 8; https://doi.org/10.1111/acel.12750; https://onlinelibrary.wiley.com/doi/full/10.1111/acel.12750; https://onlinelibrary.wiley.com/doi/epdf/10.1111/acel.12750

841.   sciencedirect.com / Martin A, et al. Does Active Commuting Improve Psychological Wellbeing? Longitudinal Evidence from Eighteen Waves of the British Household Panel Survey; Preventive Medicine; 2014 December 2014, 69: 296–303 https://doi.org/10.1016/j.ypmed.2014.08.023; https://www.sciencedirect.com/science/article/pii/S0091743514003144

842.   americanscientist.org / How Animals Communicate via Pheromones. Tristram Wyatt https://www.americanscientist.org/article/how-animals-communicate-via-pheromones

843.   livescience.com / Freezing This Nerve Could Trick Your Body into Losing Weight. Tereza Pultarova, March 22, 2018 https://www.livescience.com/62095-hunger-nerve-freezing-weight-loss.html

844.   latimes.com / Surprise! Scientists Find Signs of New Brain Cells in Adults as Old as 79. Deborah Netburn, April 5, 2018 http://www.latimes.com/science/sciencenow/la-sci-sn-new-brain-cells-20180405-story.html

845.   cell.com / Boldrini M, et al. Human Hippocampal Neurogenesis Persists throughout Aging; Cell Stem Cell; 2018 Apr 5; 22(4): 589–599.e5 DOI: https://doi.org/10.1016/j.stem.2018.03.015 https://www.cell.com/cell-stem-cell/fulltext/S1934-5909(18)30121-8

846.   sfgate.com / SF Scientists Erase Alzheimer-Causing Gene in Human Brain. Michelle Robertson, April 12, 2018 https://www.sfgate.com/science/article/alzheimer-cure-human-sf-gladstone-brain-gene-12822737.php

847.   thelancet.com / Wood AM, et al. Risk Thresholds for Alcohol Consumption: Combined Analysis of Individual-Participant Data for 599 912 Current Drinkers in 83 Prospective Studies; The Lancet; 2018 Apr 14; 391(10129): 1513–1523 DOI: https://doi.org/10.1016/S0140-6736(18)30134-X; https://www.thelancet.com/journals/lancet/article/PIIS0140-6736(18)30134-X/fulltext

848.   livescience.com / Too Much Sitting May Shrink the Part of Your Brain Tied to Memory. Samantha Mathewson, April 13, 2018 https://www.livescience.com/62299-sitting-sedentary-shrinks-brain-memory.html

849.   journals.plos.org / Siddarth P, et al. Sedentary Behavior Associated with Reduced Medial Temporal Lobe Thickness in Middle-Aged and Older Adults; PLOS; 2018 Apr 12; https://doi.org/10.1371/journal.pone.0195549; http://journals.plos.org/plosone/article?id=10.1371/journal.pone.0195549

850.   ksat.com / Baboons Used Barrel to Escape Enclosure at Texas Biomedical Research Institute. Julie Moreno, April 16, 2018 https://www.ksat.com/news/baboons-used-a-barrel-to-escape-their-enclosure-at-the-texas-biomedical-research-institute

851.   ncbi.nlm.nih.gov / Derikx JP, et al. Non-invasive Markers of Gut Wall Integrity in Health and Disease; World Journal of Gastroenterology; 2010 Nov 14; 16(42): 5272–5279 DOI: 10.3748/wjg.v16.i42.5272 https://www.ncbi.nlm.nih.gov/pmc/articles/PMC2980675/

852.   en.wikipedia.org / Intestinal Permeability. https://en.wikipedia.org/wiki/Intestinal_permeability

853.   microbiomejournal.biomedcentral.com / Fan X, et al. Drinking Alcohol Is Associated with Variation in the Human Oral Microbiome in a Large Study of American Adults; Microbiome; 2018 Apr 24; 6(59); https://doi.org/10.1186/s40168-018-0448-x; https://microbiomejournal.biomedcentral.com/articles/10.1186/s40168-018-0448-x

854.   bmj.com / Richardson K, et al. Anticholinergic Drugs and Risk of Dementia: Case-Control Study; British Medical Journal; 2018 Apr 25; 360: k1315 DOI: https://doi.org/10.1136/bmj.k1315; https://www.bmj.com/content/361/bmj.k1315 https://www.bmj.com/content/bmj/361/bmj.k1315.full.pdf

855.   ncbi.nlm.nih.gov / Socci V, et al. Enhancing Human Cognition with Cocoa Flavonoids; Frontiers in Nutrition; online 2017 May 6; 4(19) DOI: 10.3389/fnut.2017.00019 https://www.ncbi.nlm.nih.gov/pmc/articles/PMC5432604/

856.   studyfinds.org / Study: Multivitamins, Other Common Supplements Have No Health Benefits. May 29, 2018 https://www.studyfinds.org/multivitamins-common-supplements-no-health-benefits/

857.   eurekalert.org / Most Popular Vitamin and Mineral Supplements Provide No Health Benefit, Study Finds. May 28, 2018 https://www.eurekalert.org/pub_releases/2018-05/smh-mpv052518.php

858.   onlinejacc.org / Jenkins DJ, et al. Supplemental Vitamins and Minerals for CVD Prevention and Treatment; Journal of the American College of Cardiology;

2018 Jun; 71(22) DOI: 10.1016/j.jacc.2018.04.020 http://www.onlinejacc.org/content/71/22/2570 file:///C:/Users/George/Downloads/2570.full.pdf

859.   ketv.com / Cockroach Milk Anyone? It May Be the Next Big Superfood. Chelsea Robinson, May 29, 2018 http://www.ketv.com/article/cockroach-milk-anyone-it-may-be-the-next-big-superfood/20950351

860.   washingtonpost.com / New Report Finds No Evidence That Having Sex with Robots Is Healthy. Ben Guarino, June 4, 2018 https://www.washingtonpost.com/news/speaking-of-science/wp/2018/06/04/theres-no-evidence-that-having-sex-with-robots-is-healthy-new-report-finds/?noredirect=on&utm_term=.85521823a30b

861.   bmj.com / Facchin F, et al. Sex Robots: The Irreplaceable Value of Humanity; BMJ; 2017 Aug 15; 358: j3790 DOI: https://doi.org/10.1136/bmj.j3790; https://www.bmj.com/content/358/bmj.j3790.long

862.   medicaldaily.com / Loneliness Is an Invisible Epidemic Affecting Physical and Mental Health. Sadhana Bharanidharan, April 27, 2018 https://www.medicaldaily.com/loneliness-invisible-epidemic-affecting-physical-and-mental-health-423814

863.   news.sfsu.edu / Digital Addiction Increases Loneliness, Anxiety and Depression. Lisa Owens Viani, April 10, 2018 https://news.sfsu.edu/news-story/digital-addiction-increases-loneliness-anxiety-and-depression

864.   cell.com / Cacioppo JT, Hawkley LC. Review: Perceived Social Isolation and Cognition; Trends in Cognitive Sciences; 2009 Oct; 13(10): 447–454 DOI: https://doi.org/10.1016/j.tics.2009.06.005 https://www.cell.com/trends/cognitive-sciences/fulltext/S1364-6613(09)00147–8

865.   ncbi.nlm.nih.gov / Mushtag R, et al. Relationship between Loneliness, Psychiatric Disorders and Physical Health? A Review on the Psychological Aspects of Loneliness; Journal of Clinical & Diagnostic Research; 2014 Sep; 8(9): WE01–WE04 DOI: 10.7860/JCDR/2014/10077.4828 https://www.ncbi.nlm.nih.gov/pmc/articles/PMC4225959/#!po=39.2857

866.   medicaldaily.com / 5 Health Benefits of Being Silent for Your Mind and Body. Lizette Borreli, September 2, 2016 https://www.medicaldaily.com/5-health-benefits-being-silent-your-mind-and-body-396934

867.   srh.bmj.com / Cox-George C, Bewley S. Editorial: I, Sex Robot: The Health Implications of the Sex Robot Industry; BMJ Sexual & Reproductive Health; Online 2018 Jun 4; DOI: 10.1136/bmjsrh-2017–200012 http://srh.bmj.com/content/early/2018/04/24/bmjsrh-2017-200012

868.   prnewswire.com / New Cigna Study Reveals Loneliness at Epidemic Levels in America. May 1, 2018 https://www.prnewswire.com/news-releases/new-cigna-study-reveals-loneliness-at-epidemic-levels-in-america-300639747.html; https://www.multivu.com/players/English/8294451-cigna-us-loneliness-survey/; https://www.multivu.com/players/English/8294451-cigna-us-loneliness-survey/docs/IndexReport_1524069371598-173525450.pdf

869.   latimes.com / These Five Healthy Habits Could Extend Your Life by a dozen Years or More, Study Says. Karen Kaplan, April 30, 2018 http://www.latimes.com/science/sciencenow/la-sci-sn-five-health-habits-20180430-story.html

870.   circ.ahajournals.org / Li Y, et al. Impact of Healthy Lifestyle Factors on Life Expectancies in the US Population; Circulation; 2018 Jun 19; 137(25) https://doi.org/10.1161/CIRCULATIONAHA.117.032047; http://circ.ahajournals.org/content/early/2018/04/25/CIRCULATIONAHA.117.032047

871.   onlinelibrary.wiley.com / Akerstedt T, et al. Sleep Duration and Mortality: Does Weekend Sleep Matter? Journal of Sleep Research; 2018; e12712. https://doi.org/10.1111/jsr.12712; https://onlinelibrary.wiley.com/doi/epdf/10.1111/jsr.12712

872.   nytimes.com / How Nighttime Tablet and Phone Use Disturbs Sleep. Nicholas Baka-
        lar, May 23, 2018 https://www.nytimes.com/2018/05/23/well/mind/how-nighttim
        e-tablet-and-phone-use-disturbs-sleep.html

873.   arstechnica.com / How You End Up Sleep-Deprived Matters. John Timmer, May
        23, 2018 https://arstechnica.com/science/2018/05/sleep-deprivation-is-probabl
        y-more-complicated-than-it-feels/

874.   physoc.onlinelibrary.wiley.com / Chinoy ED, et al. Unrestricted Evening Use of
        Light-Emitting Tablet Computers Delays Self-Selected Bedtime and Disrupts Circa-
        dian Timing and Alertness; Physiological Reports; 2018 May 22; 6(10); e13692 https://
        doi.org/10.14814/phy2.13692; https://physoc.onlinelibrary.wiley.com/doi/10.14814/
        phy2.13692; https://physoc.onlinelibrary.wiley.com/doi/epdf/10.14814/phy2.13692

875.   pnas.org / McHill AW, et al. Chronic Sleep Curtailment, Even without Extended
        (>16-h) Wakefulness, Degrades Human Vigilance Performance; PNAS May 21, 2018.
        201706694; published ahead of print https://doi.org/10.1073/pnas.1706694115

876.   health.usnews.com / A Lonely Heart Poses a Big Health Risk. Mary Elizabeth Dallas,
        May 23, 2018 https://health.usnews.com/health-care/articles/2018-05-23/a-lonely-
        heart-poses-a-big-health-risk

877.   jaha.ahajournals.org / Manemann SM, et al. Perceived Social Isolation and
        Outcomes in Patients with Heart Failure; Journal of the American Heart Association;
        2018 Jun 5; 7(11): e008069 DOI: https://doi.org/10.1161/JAHA.117.008069 http://
        jaha.ahajournals.org/content/7/11/e008069

878.   arstechnica.com / "I Don't F—Ing Care": In Wooing $67M from Big Alcohol, NIH
        Nixed Critical Study; The NIH Is Already Investigating the Matter as More Unseemly
        Details Emerge. Beth Mole, April 3, 2018 https://arstechnica.com/science/2018/0
        4/i-dont-f-ing-care-in-wooing-67m-from-big-alcohol-nih-nixed-critical-study/

879.   arstechnica.com / NIH Shuts Down Controversial $100M Drinking Study Backed by
        Big Alcohol; Study Leaders Wooed Industry and Biased Scientific Framing to Favor
        Daily Drinking. Beth Mole, June 15, 2018 https://arstechnica.com/science/2018/06/
        nih-shuts-down-controversial-100m-drinking-study-backed-by-big-alcohol/

880.   nih.gov / News Releases; NIH to End Funding for Moderate Alcohol and Cardiovas-
        cular Health Trial. June 15, 2018 https://www.nih.gov/news-events/news-releases/
        nih-end-funding-moderate-alcohol-cardiovascular-health-trial

881.   academic.oup.com / Johnson RJ, et al. Potential Role of Sugar (Fructose) in the
        Epidemic of Hypertension, Obesity and the Metabolic Syndrome, Diabetes, Kidney
        Disease, and Cardiovascular Disease; The American Journal of Clinical Nutrition;
        2007 Oct 1; 86(4): 899–906 https://doi.org/10.1093/ajcn.86.4.899; https://academic.
        oup.com/ajcn/article/86/4/899/4649308

882.   wasingtonpost.com / Wonkblog; How the American Diet Has Failed. Roberto
        A. Ferdman, June 18, 2014 https://www.washingtonpost.com/news/wonk/
        wp/2014/06/18/the-rise-of-processed-and-fast-foods-and-the-ever-expandin
        g-american-waistline/?noredirect=on&utm_term=.cab535aa38b0

883.   aswathdamodaran.blogspot.com / Musings on Markets: My Not-So-Profound
        Thoughts about Valuation, Corporate Finance and the News of the Day! Aswath
        Damodaran, November 10, 2015 http://aswathdamodaran.blogspot.com/2015/11/
        divergence-in-drug-businesses.html

884.   marketsize.net / Editorial Code and Data, Inc. An Editorial Subcontractor for Proj-
        ects Large and Small. Pharmacy & Drug Stores. April 4, 2012 http://marketsize.net/
        category/drugs/

885.   healthline.com / 11 Graphs That Show Everything That Is Wrong with the Modern
        Diet. https://www.healthline.com/nutrition/11-graphs-that-show-what-is-
        wrong-with-modern-diet

886. gizmodo.com / Controversial Study Suggests There's No Limit to Human Aging. George Dvorsky, June 28, 2018 https://gizmodo.com/controversial-stud y-suggests-there-s-no-limit-to-human-1827207011

887. science.sciencemag.org / Barbi E, et al. The Plateau of Human Mortality: Demography of Longevity Pioneers; Science; 2018 Jun 29; 360(6396): 1459–1461 DOI: 10.1126/ science.aat3119 http://science.sciencemag.org/content/360/6396/1459

888. bbc.com / Seeing the Same Doctor over Time "Lowers Death Rates." June 29, 2018 https://www.bbc.com/news/health-44643607

889. bmjJopen.bmj.com / Pereira Gray DJ, et al. Continuity of Care with Doctors: A Matter of Life and Death? A Systematic Review of Continuity of Care and Mortality; BMJ Open 2018; 8: e021161. DOI: 10.1136/bmjopen-2017-021161 https://bmjopen.bmj. com/content/8/6/e021161

890. genome.gov / National Human Genome Research Institute / Knockout Mice https:// www.genome.gov/12514551/knockout-mice-fact-sheet/

891. geeksta.net / Daily Calorie Intake in the US from 1970–2010 https://geeksta.net/visu-alizations/calories-us/

892. pewresearch.org / What's on Your Table? How America's Diet Has Changed over the Decades. Drew Desilver, December 13, 2016 http://www.pewresearch.org/ fact-tank/2016/12/13/whats-on-your-table-how-americas-diet-has-changed -over-the-decades/

893. morningconsult.com / IMS Institute for Healthcare Informatics / April 2016: Medi-cines Use and Spending in the U.S.: A Review of 2015 and Outlook to 2020 https:// morningconsult.com/wp-content/uploads/2016/04/IMS-Institute-US-Drug-Spend-ing-2015.pdf

894. cms.gov / History of Health Spending in the United States, 1960–2013. Aaron C. Catlin and Cathy A. Cowan, November 19, 2015 https://www.cms.gov/ Research-Statistics-Data-and-Systems/Statistics-Trends-and-Reports/NationalHeal-thExpendData/Downloads/HistoricalNHEPaper.pdf

895. en.wikipedia.org / S&P 500 Index https://en.wikipedia.org/wiki/S%26P_500_Index

896. consumeraffairs.com / Most Consumers Wash Hands Incorrectly, USDA Study Finds: Researchers Found That Study Participants Failed to Wash Their Hands Correctly 97 Percent of the Time. Sarah D. Young, June 29, 2018 https://www. consumeraffairs.com/news/most-consumers-wash-hands-incorrectly-usda-study -finds-062918.html

897. usda.gov / Study Shows Most People Are Spreading Dangerous Bacteria around the Kitchen and Don't Even Realize It. June 28, 2018 https://www.usda.gov/media/ press-releases/2018/06/28/study-shows-most-people-are-spreading-danger-ous-bacteria-around

898. fsis.usda.gov / Food Safety Consumer Research Project: Meal Preparation Exper-iment Related to Thermometer Use. Executive Summary May 2018 https://www. fsis.usda.gov/wps/wcm/connect/1fe5960e-c1d5–4bea-bccc-20b07fbfde50/ Observational-Study-Addendum.pdf?MOD=AJPERES

899. cdc.gov / Handwashing: Clean Hands Save Lives / When & How to Wash Your Hands https://www.cdc.gov/handwashing/when-how-handwashing.html

900. theguardian.com / Electrical Brain Stimulation May Help Reduce Violent Crime in Future: Study. Ian Sample, July 2, 2018 https://www.theguardian.com/science/2018/ jul/02/electrical-brain-stimulation-may-help-reduce-violent-in-future-study

901. jneurosci.org / Choy O, et al. Stimulation of the Prefrontal Cortex Reduces Intentions to Commit Aggression: A Randomized, Double-Blind, Placebo-Controlled, Stratified, Parallel-Group Trial; The Journal of Neuroscience; 2018 Jul 18; 38(29): 6505–6512

DOI: https://doi.org/10.1523/JNEUROSCI.3317-17.2018 http://www.jneurosci.org/content/38/29/6505

902. irishexaminer.com / These Five Healthy Habits for Mothers Can 'Substantially' Cut Risk of Child Obesity. Irish Examiner, July 5, 2018 https://www.irishexaminer.com/breakingnews/world/these-five-healthy-habits-for-mothers-can-substantially-cut-risk-of-child-obesity-853176.html

903. bmj.com / Dhana K, et al. Association between Maternal Adherence to Healthy Lifestyle Practices and Risk of Obesity in Offspring: Results from Two Prospective Cohort Studies of Mother-Child Pairs in the United States; The British Medical Journal; 2018 July 4; 362: k2486 DOI: https://doi.org/10.1136/bmj.k2486 https://www.bmj.com/content/362/bmj.k2486

904. dailymail.co.uk / Common High Blood Pressure and Heart Drugs Are Recalled amid Fears They Could Cause Cancer. Stephen Matthews, July 5, 2018 http://www.dailymail.co.uk/health/article-5922015/Common-heart-drug-recalled-amid-fears-cause-CANCER.html

905. nypost.com / OxyContin Maker Placed Profits Over People. Lawsuit Reveals. Associated Press, July 6, 2018 https://nypost.com/2018/07/06/oxycontin-maker-placed-profits-over-people-lawsuit-reveals/

906. wsj.com / California Shields Big Soda from Local Taxes. Alejandro Lazo, June 29, 2018 https://www.wsj.com/articles/california-shields-big-soda-from-local-taxes-1530273603

907. foxnews.com / California governor signs soda tax ban into law. Kimberly Leonard, June 29, 2018 http://www.foxnews.com/politics/2018/06/29/california-governor-signs-soda-tax-ban-into-law.html

908. politico.com / Sources: EPA Blocks Warnings on Cancer-Causing Chemical: Burying the Formaldehyde Study Is Part of an Effort by Pruitt and Aides to Undermine EPA's Research Program, Current and Former Officials Tell POLITICO. Annie Snider, July 6, 2018 https://www.politico.com/story/2018/07/06/epa-formaldehyde-warnings-blocked-696628

909. ktla.com / Over 200 People Sick from Parasite in Del Monte Vegetable Tray Recall Impacting Midwest States. CNN wire, July 6, 2018 https://ktla.com/2018/07/06/more-than-200-people-sick-from-parasite-in-del-monte-vegetable-tray-recall/

910. cdc.gov / Multistate Outbreak of Cyclosporiasis Linked to Del Monte Fresh Produce Vegetable Trays: United States, July 5, 2018 https://www.cdc.gov/parasites/cyclosporiasis/outbreaks/2018/a-062018/index.html

911. newsroom.ucla.edu / Spacing Out after Staying Up Late? Here's Why. Elaine Schmidt, November 6, 2017 http://newsroom.ucla.edu/releases/spacing-out-after-staying-up-late

912. ncbi.nlm.nih.gov / Nir Y, et al. Selective Neuronal Lapses Precede Human Cognitive Lapses Following Sleep Deprivation; Nature Medicine; 2017 Nov 6; 23(12): 1474–1480; DOI: 10.1038/nm.4433 https://www.ncbi.nlm.nih.gov/pmc/articles/PMC5720899/

913. coloradoan.com / Colorado: No Edible Pot Shaped as People, Animals or Fruit. Kathleen Foody, October 1, 2017 https://www.coloradoan.com/story/news/local/colorado/2017/10/01/colorado-no-edible-pot-shaped-people-animals-fruit/721964001/

914. ascopubs.org / LoConte NK, et al. Alcohol and Cancer: A Statement of the American Society of Clinical Oncology; Journal of Clinical Oncology; 2018 Jan 1; 36(1): 83–93 DOI: 10.1200/JCO.2017.76.1155 http://ascopubs.org/doi/full/10.1200/JCO.2017.76.1155

915. gizmodo.com / America's Obesity Problem Is Getting Even Worse. Ed Cara, September 14, 2018 https://gizmodo.com/americas-obesity-problem-is-getting-even-worse-1829068201

916. tfah.org / 2018 The State of Obesity: Better Policies for a Healthier America. Trust for America's Health, Robert Wood Johnson Foundation https://www.tfah.org/wp-content/uploads/2018/09/TFAH-2018-ObesityReport-FINAL.pdf

917. jamanetwork.com / Dieleman JL, et al. US Spending on Personal Health Care and Public Health, 1996–2013; Journal of the American Medical Association; 2016 Dec 27; 316(24): 2627–2646 DOI: 10.1001/jama.2016.16885 https://jamanetwork.com/journals/jama/fullarticle/2594716

918. bloomberg.com / Coca-Cola Is Eyeing the Cannabis Market. Jen Skerritt and Craig Giammona, September 17, 2018 https://www.bloomberg.com/news/articles/2018-09-17/coca-cola-eyes-cannabis-market-in-push-beyond-sluggish-sodas

919. ers.usda.gov / USDA: United States Department of Agriculture Economic Research Service / Chart Gallery https://www.ers.usda.gov/data-products/chart-gallery/gallery/?page=95&topicId=0

920. chicagotribune.com / Rat poison likely to blame for deadly side effects of synthetic pot in Illinois. Elvia Malagon, April 6, 2018 http://www.chicagotribune.com/news/ct-met-synthetic-marijuana-problems-history-20180406-story.html

921. hawaiinewsnow.com / Lawmakers OK ban on sale of sunscreens linked to coral damage. Mahealani Richardson, May 1, 2018 http://www.hawaiinewsnow.com/story/38085118/lawmakers-ok-ban-on-sale-of-sunscreens-linked-to-coral-damage/

922. fsis.usda.gov / USDA: United States Department of Agriculture Food Safety and Inspection Service / JBS USA, Inc. Recalls Ground Beef Products Due to Possible Foreign Matter Contamination. News Release, May 2, 2018 www.fsis.usda.gov/wps/portal/fsis/topics/recalls-and-public-health-alerts/recall-case-archive/archive/2018/recall-035-2018-release

923. abc13.com / HEALTH & FITNESS: Student warns about 'Juuling' trend in eye-opening video. May 03, 2018 https://abc13.com/health/student-warns-about-juuling-trend-in-eye-opening-video/3426544/

924. who.int / World Health Organization / News / WHO plan to eliminate industrially-produced trans-fatty acids from global food supply. News Release, May 14, 2018 http://www.who.int/news-room/detail/14-05-2018-who-plan-to-eliminate-industrially-produced-trans-fatty-acids-from-global-food-supply

925. ewg.org / The Trouble With Ingredients in Sunscreens. www.ewg.org/sunscreen/report/the-trouble-with-sunscreen-chemicals/#.WwTsFO4vyJA

926. thehill.com / Don't fall for the false claims — US sunscreens sufficiently protect your skin. Janet Hill Prystowsky, June 2, 2018 https://thehill.com/opinion/healthcare/390251-dont-fall-for-the-false-claims-us-sunscreens-sufficiently-protect-your

927. wsj.com / Frequent Technology Use Linked to ADHD Symptoms in Teens, Study Finds. Daniela Hernandez and Betsy Morris, July 17, 2018 https://www.wsj.com/articles/frequent-technology-use-linked-to-adhd-symptoms-in-teens-study-1531839628

928. jamanetwork.com / Editorial / Digital Media and Symptoms of Attention-Deficit/Hyperactivity Disorder in Adolescents. Jenny Radesky, July 17, 2018 https://jamanetwork.com/journals/jama/article-abstract/2687840

929. jamanetwork.com / Ra CK, et al. Association of Digital Media Use With Subsequent Symptoms of Attention-Deficit/Hyperactivity Disorder Among Adolescents; Journal of the American Medical Association; 2018 Jul 17; 320(3): 255–263. DOI: 10.1001/jama.2018.8931 https://jamanetwork.com/journals/jama/article-abstract/2687861

930. theguardian.com / Why we must legalise cannabis now for the sake of public health. Jeff Smith, June 2, 2018 https://www.theguardian.com/society/2018/jun/02/why-we-must-legalise-cannabis-public-health

931. thisisinsider.com /America has been hit by a 'crazy' amount of food-poisoning outbreaks in 2018. Here's one expert's theory why. Kate Taylor, July 27, 2018 https://www.thisisinsider.com/food-poisoning-news-on-the-rise-why-2018-7

932. komonews.com / Unregulated food additives could harm children, UW study says. Karina Mazhukhina, July 29th 2018 https://komonews.com/news/local/100 0-food-additives-dont-require-approval-from-the-fda-uw-study-says

933. pediatrics.aappublications.org / Trasande L, et al. Food Additives and Child Health; Pediatrics; 2018 Aug; 142(2) DOI: 10.1542/peds.2018-1408 http://pediatrics.aappublications.org/content/142/2/e20181408

934. qz.com / Humans have depleted the Earth's natural resources with five months still to go in 2018. Michael J. Coren, August 1, 2018 https://qz.com/1345205/humans-have-depleted-the-earths-natural-resources-with-five-months-still-to-go-in-2018/ https://data.footprintnetwork.org/#/

935. npr.org / Some Bacteria Are Becoming 'More Tolerant' Of Hand Sanitizers, Study Finds. Melody Schreiber, August 2, 2018 https://www.npr.org/sections/goatsand-soda/2018/08/02/635017716/some-bacteria-are-becoming-more-tolerant-of-hand-sanitizers-study-finds

936. arstechnica.com / Hospital superbugs are evolving to survive hand sanitizers. Beth Mole, August 5, 2018 https://arstechnica.com/science/2018/08/hospital-superbugs-are-evolving-to-survive-hand-sanitizers/

937. stm.sciencemag.org / Pidot SJ, et al. Increasing tolerance of hospital Enterococcus faecium to handwash alcohols; Science Translational Medicine; 2018 Aug 01; 10(452): eaar6115 DOI: 10.1126/scitranslmed.aar6115 http://stm.sciencemag.org/content/10/452/eaar6115

938. medicalnewstoday.com / Even low air pollution may cause you serious heart problems. Ana Sandoiu, August 5, 2018 https://www.medicalnewstoday.com/articles/322680.php

939. ahajournals.org / Aung N, et al. Association Between Ambient Air Pollution and Cardiac Morpho-Functional Phenotypes; Circulation; 2018 Aug 3; 138. https://www.ahajournals.org/doi/pdf/10.1161/CIRCULATIONAHA.118.034856

940. fox2now.com / No amount of alcohol is good for your overall health, global study says. CNN Wires, August 23, 2018 https://fox2now.com/2018/08/23/no-amount-of-alcohol-is-good-for-your-overall-health-global-study-says/

941. thelancet.com / GBD 2016 Alcohol Collaborators. Alcohol use and burden for 195 countries and territories, 1990–2016: a systematic analysis for the Global Burden of Disease Study 2016; The Lancet; 2018 Sep 22; 392(10152): 1015–1035 DOI: https://doi.org/10.1016/S0140-6736(18)31310-2 https://www.thelancet.com/journals/lancet/article/PIIS0140-6736(18)31310-2/fulltext#%20

942. theguardian.com / Alcohol causes one in 20 deaths worldwide, says WHO. Nicola Davis, September 21, 2018 https://www.theguardian.com/society/2018/sep/21/5-of-all-deaths-due-to-alcohol-who-says

943. who.int / WHO: Management of substance abuse; Global status report on alcohol and health 2018 http://www.who.int/substance_abuse/publications/global_alcohol_report/en/ http://www.who.int/substance_abuse/publications/global_alcohol_report/gsr_2018/en/

944. pediatrics.aappublications.org / Ryan SA, et al. Marijuana Use During Pregnancy and Breastfeeding: Implications for Neonatal and Childhood Outcomes; Pediatrics; 2018 Sept; 142(3): e20181889 http://pediatrics.aappublications.org/content/pediatrics/early/2018/08/23/peds.2018-1889.full.pdf

945. newsweek.com / Household cleaning products might be making your children fat. Kahmira Gander, September 17, 2018 https://www.newsweek.com/household-cleaning-products-linked-children-being-overweight-1121651

946.   cnn.com / Household disinfectants could be making kids overweight, study says. Susan Scutti, September 17, 2018 https://www.cnn.com/2018/09/17/health/disinfectants-baby-gut-microbiota-bmi-study/index.html

947.   cmaj.ca / Tun MH, et al. Postnatal exposure to household disinfectants, infant gut microbiota and subsequent risk of overweight in children; Canadian Medical Association Journal; 2018 Sept 17; 190(37): E1097-E1107 DOI: https://doi.org/10.1503/cmaj.170809 http://www.cmaj.ca/content/190/37/E1097

948.   nature.com / Turnbaugh, PJ, et al. A core gut microbiome in obese and lean twins; Nature; 2009 Jan; 457: 480–485 DOI: 10.1038/nature07540 https://www.nature.com/articles/nature07540.epdf https://www.nature.com/articles/nature07540.epdf

949.   forbes.com / How Sleep Deprivation Messes With Your Memory: Study. Alice G. Walton, October 2, 2018 https://www.forbes.com/sites/alicegwalton/2018/10/02/sleep-deprivation-makes-it-harder-to-deal-with-distractions/#371a3ad5788d

950.   psycnet.apa.org / Fenn ME, et al. Effects of sleep deprivation on procedural errors; Journal of Experimental Psychology: General; 2018 Sept 27 http://psycnet.apa.org/doiLanding?doi=10.1037%2Fxge0000495

951.   woodtv.com / Bye bye bugs? Scientists fear non-pest insects are declining. Seth Borenstein, September 20, 2018 https://www.woodtv.com/news/national/bye-bye-bugs-scientists-fear-non-pest-insects-are-declining/1461552524

952.   youtube.com / Are flying insects dying off? Scientists fear so. www.youtube.com/watch?v=A4do3i0qr_8

953.   npr.org / Study: Roundup Weed Killer Could Be Linked To Widespread Bee Deaths. Vanessa Romo, September 25, 2018 https://www.npr.org/2018/09/25/651618685/study-roundup-weed-killer-could-be-linked-to-widespread-bee-deaths

954.   pnas.org / Motta EVS, et al. Glyphosate perturbs the gut microbiota of honey bees; PNAS; 2018 Sep 24 https://doi.org/10.1073/pnas.1803880115 http://www.pnas.org/content/early/2018/09/18/1803880115.full

955.   futurism.com / Scientists wiped out a mosquito population by hacking their DNA with CRISPR. Kristin Houser, September 25, 2018 https://futurism.com/the-byte/gene-drive-mosquitos-crispr

956.   newsweek.com / Malaria and CRISPR: gene editing causes complete collapse of mosquito population in 'major breakthrough' for disease eradication. Hannah Osborne, September 24, 2018 https://www.newsweek.com/malaria-gene-editing-crispr-mosquitoes-1135871

957.   nature.com / Kyrou K, et al. A CRISPR–Cas9 gene drive targeting doublesex causes complete population suppression in caged Anopheles gambiae mosquitoes; Nature Biotechnology; 2018 Sept 24 https://www.nature.com/articles/nbt.4245 https://www.nature.com/articles/nbt.4245.epdf

958.   phys.org / PCB pollution threatens to wipe out killer whales. Aarhus University, September 27, 2018 https://phys.org/news/2018-09-pcb-pollution-threatens-killer-whales.html

959.   science.sciencemag.org / Desforges JP, et al. Predicting global killer whale population collapse from PCB pollution; Science; 2018 Sep 28; 361(6409): 1373–1376 DOI:10.1126/science.aat1953 http://science.sciencemag.org/content/361/6409/1373

960.   cspinet.org / FDA Removes 7 Carcinogenic Flavorings from Approved Food Additives List: Statement of CSPI Policy Director Laura MacCleery. October 5, 2018 https://cspinet.org/news/fda-removes-7-carcinogenic-flavorings-approved-food-additives-list-20181005

961.   fda.gov / FDA: U.S. Food & Drug Administration / FDA Removes 7 Synthetic Flavoring Substances from Food Additives List. October 5, 2018 https://www.fda.gov/Food/NewsEvents/ConstituentUpdates/ucm622475.htm

962.   femaflavor.org / FEMA Addresses FDA Decision on NGO Petition on 7 Synthetic Substances. October 5, 2018 https://www.femaflavor.org/fda-announces-decision-ngo-petition-7-synthetic-substances

963.   newsweek.com / Full-fat milk could cut risk of stroke, heart attack, study says. Kashmira Gander, July 16, 2018 https://www.newsweek.com/full-fat-milk-could-cut-risk-stroke-heart-attack-study-says-1025069

964.   academic.oup.com / Otto MC, et al. Serial measures of circulating biomarkers of dairy fat and total and cause-specific mortality in older adults: the Cardiovascular Health Study; The American Journal of Clinical Nutrition; 2018 Sep; 108(3): 476–484 https://doi.org/10.1093/ajcn/nqy117 https://academic.oup.com/ajcn/article/108/3/476/5052139?guestAccessKey=c18b1acf-2778-42b9-8d72-878c0e-86cdbf#118685082

965.   wsoctv.com / Study says eating fat is the only cause of weight gain. Najja Parker, July 17,2018 https://www.wsoctv.com/news/trending-now/eating-fat-is-the-only-cause-of-weight-gain-study-finds/792147273

966.   sciencedirect.com / Hu S, et al. Dietary Fat, but Not Protein or Carbohydrate, Regulates Energy Intake and Causes Adiposity in Mice; Cell Metabolism; 2018 Sep; 28(3): 415–431.e4 https://doi.org/10.1016/j.cmet.2018.06.010 https://www.sciencedirect.com/science/article/pii/S1550413118303929?via%3Dihub

967.   thisisinsider.com / These are the real 'superfoods' you should be eating more of, according to science. Erin Brodwin, August 4, 2018 https://www.thisisinsider.com/healthy-food-list-2018-8

968.   deccanchronicle.com / Adding crickets to your diet can be good for your gut: Study. August 5, 2018 https://www.deccanchronicle.com/lifestyle/health-and-wellbeing/050818/adding-crickets-to-your-diet-can-be-good-for-your-gut-study.html

969.   nature.com / Stull VJ, et al. Impact of Edible Cricket Consumption on Gut Microbiota in Healthy Adults, a Double-blind, Randomized Crossover Trial; Scientific Reports; 2018 Jul 17; 8(10762) https://www.nature.com/articles/s41598-018-29032-2

970.   cjhp.org / Kruger J, et al. The Drunchies Hangover: Heavy Episodic Drinking and Dietary Choices while Drinking and on the Following Day; Journal of Health Promotion; 2018; 16(1): 79–90 http://www.cjhp.org/volume16Issue1_2018/documents/79-90_CJHP2018Issue1_Kruger.pdf

971.   theguardian.com / Not just a fad: the surprising, gut-wrenching truth about gluten. Joanna Blythman, August 7, 2018 https://www.theguardian.com/lifeandstyle/2018/aug/07/not-just-a-fad-the-surprising-gut-wrenching-truth-about-gluten

972.   inc.com / McDonald's Is Giving Away a 'Gold Card' That Gives You Free McDonald's for Life. Here's the Catch. Bill Murphy Jr., August 10, 2018 https://www.inc.com/bill-murphy-jr/mcdonalds-is-giving-away-a-gold-card-that-gives-you-free-mcdonalds-for-life-heres-how-to-enter-without-buying-anything.html

973.   usatoday.com / Low-carb diet linked to early death, medical study suggests. Ashley May, August 20, 2018 https://www.usatoday.com/story/news/nation-now/2018/08/20/low-carb-diet-linked-early-death-study/1017131002/

974.   thelancet.com / Seidelmann SB, et al. Dietary carbohydrate intake and mortality: a prospective cohort study and meta-analysis; The Lancet; 2018 Sep 1; 3(9): PE419-E428 DOI: https://doi.org/10.1016/S2468-2667(18)30135-X https://www.thelancet.com/journals/lanpub/article/PIIS2468-2667(18)30135-X/fulltext

975.   wsj.com / Beyond Soda: How and Why Your Beverage Options Are Exploding; Drink makers create new products, like alcoholic kombucha, seeking sales growth but causing confusion among consumers and grocers. Jennifer Maloney and Julie Jargon, August 26, 2018 https://www.wsj.com/articles/beyond-soda-how-and-why-your-beverage-options-are-exploding-1535284800

976. thelancet.com / Mente A, Yusuf S. Evolving evidence about diet and health; The Lancet; 2018 Sep 1; 3(9): PE408-E409 DOI: https://doi.org/10.1016/S2468-2667(18)30160-9 https://www.thelancet.com/journals/lanpub/article/PIIS2468-2667(18)30160-9/fulltext

977. arstechnica.com / Big nutrition research scandal sees 6 more retractions, purging popular diet tips. Beth Mole, September 20, 2018 https://arstechnica.com/science/2018/09/six-new-retractions-for-now-disgraced-researcher-purges-common-diet-tips/

978. jamanetwork.com / Editorial: Notice of Retraction: Wansink B, Cheney MM. Super Bowls: Serving Bowl Size and Food Consumption; JAMA; 2005; 293(14): 1727–1728. Howard Bauchner, September 19, 2018 https://jamanetwork.com/journals/jama/fullarticle/2703449

979. ers.usda.gov / USDA: United States Department of Agriculture: Economic Research Service / Wheat's Role in the U.S. Diet https://www.ers.usda.gov/topics/crops/wheat/wheats-role-in-the-us-diet.aspx

980. ers.usda.gov / USDA: United States Department of Agriculture: Economic Research Service / ERS Charts of Note https://www.ers.usda.gov/data-products/charts-of-note/charts-of-note/?topicId=14882

981. ers.usda.gov / USDA: United States Department of Agriculture: Economic Research Service / Economic Information Bulletin No. (EIB-166) 38 pp / U.S. Trends in Food Availability and a Dietary Assessment of Loss-Adjusted Food Availability, 1970–2014. Jeanine Bentley, January 2017 https://www.ers.usda.gov/publications/pub-details/?pubid=82219

982. ers.usda.gov / USDA: United States Department of Agriculture: Economic Research Service / Food Availability (Per Capita) Data System https://www.ers.usda.gov/data-products/food-availability-per-capita-data-system/food-availability-per-capita-data-system/#Loss-Adjusted%20Food%20Availability

983. foodsystemprimer.org / Johns Hopkins Center for a Livable Future / Food System Primer / Diet and Health / Food & Nutrition http://www.foodsystemprimer.org/food-and-nutrition/diet-and-health/index.html

984. foxnews.com / More than 1 in 3 American adults eat fast food on a given day, CDC survey finds. Alexandra Deabler, October 3, 2018 https://www.foxnews.com/food-drink/more-than-1-in-3-american-adults-eat-fast-food-on-a-given-day-cdc-survey-finds

985. cdc.gov / CDC: Centers for Disease control and Prevention / National Center for Health Statistics / Fryar, CD, et al. Fast Food Consumption Among Adults in the United States, 2013–2016; NCHS Data Brief No. 322, October 2018 https://www.cdc.gov/nchs/products/databriefs/db322.htm

986. livescience.com / How Bad Is Bacon for You, Really? Leslie Nemo, October 7, 2018 https://www.livescience.com/63769-bacon-cancer-health.html

987. onlinelibrary.wiley.com / Farvid MS, et al. Consumption of red and processed meat and breast cancer incidence: A systematic review and meta-analysis of prospective studies; International Journal of Cancer; 2018 Sep 5; 0(0) https://doi.org/10.1002/ijc.31848 https://onlinelibrary.wiley.com/doi/abs/10.1002/ijc.31848

988. theguardian.com / Electrical brain stimulation may help reduce violent crime in future – study. Ian Sample, July 2, 2018 https://www.theguardian.com/science/2018/jul/02/electrical-brain-stimulation-may-help-reduce-violent-in-future-study

989. washingtonpost.com / Zapping the brain appears to decrease aggressive intentions, new study says. Amy Ellis Nutt, July 2 , 2018 https://www.washingtonpost.com/news/to-your-health/wp/2018/07/02/zapping-the-brain-appear

s-to-decrease-aggressive-intentions-new-study-says/?noredirect=on&utm_term=.7da6b1185962

990. jneurosci.org / Choy O, et al. Stimulation of the Prefrontal Cortex Reduces Intentions to Commit Aggression: A Randomized, Double-Blind, Placebo-Controlled, Stratified, Parallel-Group Trial; Journal of Neuroscience; 2018 Jul 18; 38(29): 6505–6512 DOI: https://doi.org/10.1523/JNEUROSCI.3317-17.2018 http://www.jneurosci.org/content/38/29/6505

991. scientificamerican.com / CRISPR Makes Cancer Cells Turncoats That Attack Their Tumor. Sharon Begley, July 12, 2018 https://www.scientificamerican.com/article/crispr-makes-cancer-cells-turncoats-that-attack-their-tumor/

992. nature.com / Roth TL, et al. Reprogramming human T cell function and specificity with non-viral genome targeting; Nature; 2018 Jul 19; 559: 405–409 https://www.nature.com/articles/s41586-018-0326-5

993. sciencenews.org / Cancer cells engineered with CRISPR slay their own kin. Laurel Hamers, July 11, 2018 https://www.sciencenews.org/article/cancer-cells-engineered-crispr-slay-their-own-kin

994. stm.sciencemag.org / Reinshagen C, et al. CRISPR-enhanced engineering of therapy-sensitive cancer cells for self-targeting of primary metastatic tumors; Science Translational Medicine; 2018 Jul 11; 10(449): eaao3240 DOI: 10.1126/scitranslmed.aao3240 http://stm.sciencemag.org/content/10/449/eaao3240

995. gizmodo.com / UK Ethics Council Says It's 'Morally Permissible' to Create Genetically Modified Babies. George Dvorsky, July 17, 2018 https://gizmodo.com/uk-ethics-council-says-it-s-morally-permissible-to-cr-1827655873

996. livescience.com / Gut Bacteria Enzyme Can Transform a Blood Cell's Type. Stephanie Pappas, August 21, 2018 https://www.livescience.com/63394-gut-bacteria-enzyme-change-blood-type.html

997. eurekalert.org / Gut bacteria provide key to making universal blood (video). American Chemical Society, Public Release: August 21, 2018 https://www.eurekalert.org/pub_releases/2018-08/acs-gbp071218.php

998. nature.com / Wang L, et al. The coding of valence and identity in the mammalian taste system; Nature; 2018 May 30; 558: 127–131 https://www.nature.com/articles/s41586-018-0165-4

999. medicalnewstoday.com / Research reveals four distinct personality clusters. Maria Cohut, September 18, 2018 https://www.medicalnewstoday.com/articles/323092.php

1000. nature.com / Gerlach M, et al. A robust data-driven approach identifies four personality types across four large data sets; Nature human Behaviour; 2018 Sep 17; 2: 735–742 https://www.nature.com/articles/s41562-018-0419-z

1001. phys.org / Microplastics may enter foodchain through mosquitoes. September 19, 2018 https://phys.org/news/2018-09-microplastics-foodchain-mosquitoes.html

1002. newscientist.com / Mosquitoes are eating plastic and spreading it to new food chains. Yvaine Ye, September 19, 2018 https://www.newscientist.com/article/2180055-mosquitoes-are-eating-plastic-and-spreading-it-to-new-food-chains/

1003. rsbl.royalsocietypublishing.org / Al-Jaibachi R, et al. Up and away: ontogenic transference as a pathway for aerial dispersal of microplastics; Biology Letters; 2018 Sep; 14(9) DOI: 10.1098/rsbl.2018.0479 http://rsbl.royalsocietypublishing.org/content/14/9/20180479

1004. theverge.com / Two people with paralysis walk again using an implanted device. Rachel Becker, September 24, 2018 https://www.theverge.com/2018/9/24/17896720/paralysis-spinal-cord-implant-walking-epidural-stimulation-device

1005.   nejm.org / Angeli CA, et al. Recovery of Over-Ground Walking after Chronic Motor Complete Spinal Cord Injury; NEJM; 2018 Sep 27; 379 DOI: 10.1056/NEJMoa1803588 https://www.nejm.org/doi/full/10.1056/NEJMoa1803588

1006.   nature.com / Gill ML, et al. Neuromodulation of lumbosacral spinal networks enables independent stepping after complete paraplegia; Nature Medicine; 2018 Sep 24 https://www.nature.com/articles/s41591-018-0175-7

1007.   urbanmoonshine.com / Bitter taste receptors: new insight and applications. Guido Masé, October 13, 2017 https://www.urbanmoonshine.com/blogs/blog/bitter-taste-receptors-new-insight-and-applications

1008.   ncbi.nlm.nih.gov / Lu P, et al. Extraoral bitter taste receptors in health and disease; The Journal of General Physiology; 2017 Feb; 149(2): 181–197 DOI: 10.1085/jgp.201611637. Epub 2017 Jan 4. https://www.ncbi.nlm.nih.gov/pubmed/28053191 https://www.ncbi.nlm.nih.gov/pmc/articles/PMC5299619/

1009.   nature.com / Roper SD, Chaudhari N. Taste buds: cells, signals and synapses; Nature Reviews Neuroscience; 2017 Jun 29;18: 485–497 https://www.nature.com/articles/nrn.2017.68

1010.   techtimes.com / Study Finds That People Are Not Properly Washing Their Hands 97 Percent Of The Time. Elyse Johnson, June 29, 2018 https://www.techtimes.com/articles/231476/20180629/study-finds-that-people-are-not-properly-washing-their-hands-97-percent-of-the-time.htm

1011.   consumeraffairs.com / Researchers found that study participants failed to wash their hands correctly 97 percent of the time. Sarah D. Young, June 29, 2018 https://www.consumeraffairs.com/news/most-consumers-wash-hands-incorrectly-usda-study-finds-062918.html

1012.   forbes.com / Study Shows How Bad People Are At Washing Their Hands. Bruce Y. Lee, June 30, 2018 https://www.forbes.com/sites/brucelee/2018/06/30/study-shows-how-bad-people-are-at-washing-their-hands/#783887d92481

1013.   fsis.usda.gov / Food Safety Consumer Research Project: Meal Preparation Experiment Related to Thermometer Use. Executive Summary, May 2018 https://www.fsis.usda.gov/wps/wcm/connect/1fe5960e-c1d5-4bea-bccc-20b07fbfde50/Observational-Study-Addendum.pdf?MOD=AJPERES

1014.   msutoday.msu.edu / Borchgrevink CP, et al. Hand Washing Practices in a College Town Environment; Journal of Environmental Health; 2013 Apr; 75(8): 18–24 https://msutoday.msu.edu/_/pdf/assets/2013/hand-washing-study.pdf

1015.   cdc.gov / CDC: Centers for Disease Control and Prevention / CDC Features / Wash your Hands https://www.cdc.gov/features/handwashing/index.html

1016.   cdc.gov / CDC: Centers for Disease Control and Prevention / Handwashing: Clean Hands Save Lives / Show Me the Science-How to Wash Your Hands https://www.cdc.gov/handwashing/show-me-the-science-handwashing.html

1017.   npr.org / Medical Errors Are No. 3 Cause Of U.S Deaths, Researchers Say. Marshall Allen and Olga Pierce, May 3, 2016 https://www.npr.org/sections/health-shots/2016/05/03/476636183/death-certificates-undercount-toll-of-medical-errors

1018.   bmj.com / Makary, MA, Daniel, M. Medical error—the third leading cause of death in the US; BMJ; 2016 May 3; 353: i2139 DOI: https://doi.org/10.1136/bmj.i2139 https://www.bmj.com/content/353/bmj.i2139

1019.   consumer.healthday.com / Doctor Burnout Widespread, Helps Drive Many Medical Errors. Alan Mozes, July 9, 2018 https://consumer.healthday.com/general-health-information-16/doctor-news-206/doctor-burnout-widespread-helps-drive-many-medical-errors-735560.html

1020.   mayoclinicproceedings.org / Tawfik, DS, et al. Physician Burnout, Well-being, and Work Unit Safety Grades in Relationship to Reported Medical Errors; Mayo Clinic

Proceedings; 2018 July 9 online DOI: https://doi.org/10.1016/j.mayocp.2018.05.014 https://www.mayoclinicproceedings.org/article/S0025-6196(18)30372-0/fulltext

1021.   bloomberg.com / Altria Thinks Low-Nicotine Cigarettes Could Lead to About a Million Lost Jobs. Uliana Pavlova, July 17, 2018 https://www.bloomberg.com/news/articles/2018-07-17/altria-sees-low-nicotine-smokes-eating-about-a-million-u-s-jobs

1022.   bmj.com / Tapper EB, Parikh ND. Mortality due to cirrhosis and liver cancer in the United States, 1999–2016: observational study; BMJ; 2018 July 18; 362: k2817 DOI: https://doi.org/10.1136/bmj.k2817 https://www.bmj.com/content/362/bmj.k2817

1023.   businesstimes.com.sg / "Too little too late": bankruptcy booms among older Americans. NY Times, August 6, 2018 https://www.businesstimes.com.sg/banking-finance/%E2%80%98too-little-too-late%E2%80%99-bankruptcy-booms-among-older-americans

1024.   cnn.com / Instagram worst social media app for young people's mental health. Kara Fox, May 19, 2017 https://www.cnn.com/2017/05/19/health/instagram-worst-social-network-app-young-people-mental-health/index.html

1025.   rsph.org.uk / #StatusofMind https://www.rsph.org.uk/our-work/campaigns/status-of-mind.html

1026.   edition.cnn.com / Teens: This is how social media affects your brain. Susie East, August 1, 2016 https://edition.cnn.com/2016/07/12/health/social-media-brain/

1027.   cnn.com / Social media filters mess with our perceptions so much, there's now a name for it. AJ Willingham, August 10, 2018 https://www.cnn.com/2018/08/10/health/snapchat-dysmorphia-cosmetic-surgery-social-media-trend-trnd/index.html

1028.   thehill.com / Plastic surgeons say more patients coming in with 'Snapchat dysmorphia'. Avery Anapol, August 6, 2018 https://thehill.com/policy/technology/400510-plastic-surgeons-say-more-patients-coming-in-with-snapchat-dysmorphia

1029.   jamanetwork.com / Rajanala S, et al. Selfies—Living in the Era of Filtered Photographs; JAMA Facial Plastic Surgery; 2018 August 2 online DOI: 10.1001/jamafacial.2018.0486 https://jamanetwork.com/journals/jamafacialplasticsurgery/article-abstract/2688763

1030.   drinkaware.co.uk / What is an alcohol unit? https://www.drinkaware.co.uk/alcohol-facts/alcoholic-drinks-units/what-is-an-alcohol-unit/

1031.   ahajournals.org / Barnett TA, et al. Sedentary Behaviors in Today's Youth: Approaches to the Prevention and Management of Childhood Obesity: A Scientific Statement From the American Heart Association; Circulation; 2018 Aug 6; 138: e142–e159 https://www.ahajournals.org/doi/10.1161/CIR.0000000000000591

1032.   bustle.com / 19 Signs Your Work Environment Is Toxic & Affecting You Negatively. Raven Ishak, July 8 2016 https://www.bustle.com/articles/170826-19-signs-your-work-environment-is-toxic-affecting-you-negatively

1033.   apa.org / American Psychological Association / 2015 Stress in America / Stress Snapshot https://www.apa.org/news/press/releases/stress/2015/snapshot.aspx

1034.   time.com / Preventable Heart Problems Killed 415,000 People in 2016. Here's How to Keep Your Heart Healthy. Jamie Ducharme, September 6, 2018 http://time.com/5388659/how-to-keep-your-heart-healthy/

1035.   mindbodygreen.com / This Is How Many Hours Of Lost Sleep It Takes To Negatively Affect Blood Sugar, According To Science. Lindsay Kellner, September 6, 2018 https://www.mindbodygreen.com/articles/losing-sleep-can-predispose-you-to-pre-diabetes-new-research-suggests

1036.   eurekalert.org / Losing just six hours of sleep could increase diabetes risk, study finds: Sleep deprivation alters liver metabolism and fat content. American Physiological Society, Public Release: September 5, 2018 https://www.eurekalert.org/pub_releases/2018-09/aps-ljs090418.php

1037. physiology.org / Shigiyama F, et al. Mechanisms of sleep deprivation-induced hepatic steatosis and insulin resistance in mice; American Journal of Physiology Endocrinology and Metabolism; 2018 Jul 10 online https://doi.org/10.1152/ajpendo.00072.2018 https://www.physiology.org/doi/abs/10.1152/ajpendo.00072.2018

1038. bls.gov / USDA Bureau of Labor Statistics / Labor Force Statistics from the Current Population Survey / Earnings https://www.bls.gov/cps/earnings.htm

1039. theguardian.com / Revealed: 50 million Facebook profiles harvested for Cambridge Analytica in major data breach. Carole Cadwalladr and Emma Graham-Harrison, March 17, 2018 https://www.theguardian.com/news/2018/mar/17/cambridge-analytica-facebook-influence-us-election

1040. chicagotribune.com / Commentary: I'm in an abusive relationship with Facebook, and it's becoming too much. Joseph Holt, March 21, 2018 http://www.chicagotribune.com/news/opinion/commentary/ct-perspec-facebook-cambridge-analytica-personal-data-0322-20180321-story.html

1041. independent.co.uk / Email security is unsafe and cannot be easily fixed, researchers say: Even old messages could be exposed by the bug, say experts. Andrew Griffin, May 14, 2018 https://www.independent.co.uk/life-style/gadgets-and-tech/news/email-security-s-mime-pgp-encryption-latest-broken-not-working-fix-how-to-a8351116.html

1042. wraltechwire.com / 'Gaming Disorder:' WHO declares compulsive playing a mental health problem (+ video). WRAL Tech Wire Staff, June 18, 2018 https://www.wraltechwire.com/2018/06/18/gaming-disorder-who-declares-compulsive-playing-a-mental-health-problem-video/

1043. techcrunch.com / 'Gaming disorder' is officially recognized by the World Health Organization. Brian Heater, October 2018 https://techcrunch.com/2018/06/18/gaming-disorder-is-officially-recognized-by-the-world-health-organization/

1044. bbc.com / News / Technology / Facebook and Google use 'dark patterns' around privacy settings, report says. June 28, 2018 https://www.bbc.com/news/technology-44642569

1045. tomshardware.com / Google, Facebook Accused of Using UI 'Dark Patterns' to Get Users' Data. Lucian Armasu, June 28, 2018 https://www.tomshardware.com/news/google-facebook-dark-patterns-report,37380.html

1046. tomsguide.com / These Android Apps Could Secretly Be Recording Your Screen. Monica Chin, July 5, 2018 https://www.tomsguide.com/us/android-apps-secretly-recording-you,news-27557.html

1047. foxnews.com / Is your Android phone watching you? Study of more than 17,000 popular apps reveals 'disturbing practice'. Jennifer Earl, July 5, 2018 https://www.foxnews.com/tech/is-your-android-phone-watching-you-study-of-more-than-17000-popular-apps-reveals-disturbing-practice

1048. recon.meddle.mobi / Pan E, et al. Panoptispy: Characterizing Audio and Video Exfiltration from Android Applications; Proceedings on Privacy Enhancing Technologies 2018; 18 (4): 1–18 https://recon.meddle.mobi/papers/panoptispy18pets.pdf

1049. en.wikipedia.org / Connectivity (media) https://en.wikipedia.org/wiki/Connectivity_(media)

1050. slate.com / Repeat After Me: Facebook Is an Ad Business. April Glaser, July 19, 2018 https://slate.com/technology/2018/07/zuckerberg-called-trump-to-congratulate-him-after-winning-the-election-because-facebook-is-an-ad-u.html

1051. thevisualcommunicationguy.com / Personal/Emotional Appeal (advertising). Curtis Newbold, September 28, 2017 http://thevisualcommunicationguy.com/2017/09/28/personalemotional-appeal-advertising/

1052. smallbusiness.chron.com / How Is Emotional Appeal Used to Persuade? George Boykin, June 30, 2018 https://smallbusiness.chron.com/emotional-appeal-used-persuade-56346.html

1053. koeppeldirect.com / Using emotional appeal in marketing. Peter Koeppel, November 10, 2016 https://www.koeppeldirect.com/business/using-emotional-appeal-marketing/

1054. slideshare.net / Emotional Appeal In Advertising. Pandya Riva, April 3, 2017 https://www.slideshare.net/rivapandya/emotional-appeal-in-advertising

1055. nationalgeographic.com / Fast food logos unconsciously trigger fast behaviour. Ed Young, March 22, 2010 https://www.nationalgeographic.com/science/phenomena/2010/03/22/fast-food-logos-unconsciously-trigger-fast-behaviour/

1056. journals.sagepub.com / Zhong CB, DeVoe SE. You Are How You Eat Fast Food and Impatience; Psychological Science; 2010 Mar 19 https://doi.org/10.1177/0956797610366090 http://journals.sagepub.com/doi/abs/10.1177/0956797610366090?journalCode=pssa

1057. qz.com / The strange, Freudian design of McDonald's golden arches. Olivia Goldhill, July 30, 2016 https://qz.com/745681/the-strange-freudian-design-of-mcdonalds-golden-arches/

1058. hbr.org / An Emotional Connection Matters More than Customer Satisfaction. Alan Zorfas and Daniel Leemon, August 29, 2016 https://hbr.org/2016/08/an-emotional-connection-matters-more-than-customer-satisfaction

1059. hbr.org / The New Science of Customer Emotions. Scott Magids, Alan Zorfas, and Daniel Leemon, November 2015 https://hbr.org/2015/11/the-new-science-of-customer-emotions

1060. engadget.com / Google Maps' location sharing now includes your battery life: Your mom won't panic if you don't pick up if she knows you're out of battery. Mariella Moon, August 3, 2018 https://www.engadget.com/2018/08/03/google-map-location-sharing-battery-life/

1061. thenextweb.com / Facebook recently started asking banks for your financial data. Rachel Kaser, August 6, 2018 https://thenextweb.com/facebook/2018/08/07/facebook-recently-started-asking-banks-for-your-financial-data/

1062. wsj.com / Facebook to Banks: Give Us Your Data, We'll Give You Our Users. Emily Glazer, Deepa Seetharaman and AnnaMaria Andriotis, August 6, 2018 https://www.wsj.com/articles/facebook-to-banks-give-us-your-data-well-give-you-our-users-1533564049

1063. wsj.com / Google Says It Continues to Allow Apps to Scan Data From Gmail Accounts. John D. McKinnon and Douglas MacMillan, September 20, 2018 https://www.wsj.com/articles/google-says-it-continues-to-allow-apps-to-scan-data-from-gmail-accounts-1537459989

1064. fortune.com / Google Admits That It Lets Outside Services Share Your Gmail Data. David Meyer, September 21, 2018 http://fortune.com/2018/09/21/google-gmail-privacy-data-third-parties/

1065. npr.org / Teens Sleeping Too Much, Or Not Enough? Parents Can Help. April Fulton, September 23, 2018 https://www.npr.org/sections/health-shots/2018/09/23/650452971/teens-sleeping-too-much-or-not-enough-parents-can-help

1066. nypost.com / OxyContin maker placed profits over people, lawsuit reveals. Associated press, July 6, 2018 https://nypost.com/2018/07/06/oxycontin-maker-placed-profits-over-people-lawsuit-reveals/

1067. forbes.com / An Aspirin A Day? Not So Fast. Steven Salzberg, Jul 16, 2018 https://www.forbes.com/sites/stevensalzberg/2018/07/16/an-aspirin-a-day-not-so-fast/#-1c0a7af47e17

1068. thelancet.com / Rothwell PM, et al. Effects of aspirin on risks of vascular events and cancer according to bodyweight and dose: analysis of individual patient data from randomised trials; The Lancet; 2018 Aug 4; 392(10145): 387–399 DOI: https://doi.org/10.1016/S0140-6736(18)31133-4 https://www.thelancet.com/journals/lancet/article/PIIS0140-6736(18)31133-4/fulltext

1069. npr.org / Study: A Daily Baby Aspirin Has No Benefit For Healthy Older People. Rob Stein, September 16, 2018 https://www.npr.org/sections/health-shots/2018/09/16/647415462/study-a-daily-baby-aspirin-has-no-benefit-for-healthy-older-people

1070. nejm.org / McNeil JJ, et al. Effect of Aspirin on Disability-free Survival in the Healthy Elderly; NEJM; 2018 Oct 18; 379(16): 1499–1508 DOI: 10.1056/NEJMoa1800722 https://www.nejm.org/doi/full/10.1056/NEJMoa1800722

1071. nejm.org / McNeil JJ, et al. Effect of Aspirin on Cardiovascular Events and Bleeding in the Healthy Elderly; NEJM; 2018 Oct 18; 379(16): 1509–1518 DOI: 10.1056/NEJMoa1805819 https://www.nejm.org/doi/full/10.1056/NEJMoa1805819

1072. nejm.org / McNeil JJ, et al. Effect of Aspirin on All-Cause Mortality in the Healthy Elderly; NEJM; 2018 Oct 18; 379(16): 1519–1528 DOI: 10.1056/NEJMoa1803955 https://www.nejm.org/doi/full/10.1056/NEJMoa1803955

1073. nejm.org / The ASCEND Study Collaborative Group. Effects of Aspirin for Primary Prevention in Persons with Diabetes Mellitus; NEJM; 2018 Oct 18; 379(16): 1529–1539 DOI: 10.1056/NEJMoa1804988 https://www.nejm.org/doi/full/10.1056/NEJMoa1804988

1074. nejm.org / The ASCEND Study Collaborative Group. Effects of n–3 Fatty Acid Supplements in Diabetes Mellitus; NEJM; 2018 Oct 18; 379(16): 1540–1550 DOI: 10.1056/NEJMoa1804989 https://www.nejm.org/doi/full/10.1056/NEJMoa1804989

1075. cnn.com / Vitamin D supplements don't improve bone health, major study finds. Tara John, October 5, 2018 https://www.cnn.com/2018/10/05/health/vitamin-d-no-benefits-bone-density-intl/index.html

1076. thelancet.com / Bolland MJ, et al. Effects of vitamin D supplementation on musculoskeletal health: a systematic review, meta-analysis, and trial sequential analysis; The Lancet Diabetes & Endocrinology; 2018 Oct 04 online DOI: https://doi.org/10.1016/S2213-8587(18)30265-1 https://www.thelancet.com/journals/landia/article/PIIS2213-8587(18)30265-1/fulltext

1077. thelancet.com / Vitamin D and bone density, fractures, and falls: the end of the story? J. Chris Gallagher, October 04, 2018 https://www.thelancet.com/journals/landia/article/PIIS2213-8587(18)30269-9/fulltext

1078. bbc.com / Fish oil supplements for a healthy heart 'nonsense'. July 18, 2018 https://www.bbc.com/news/health-44845879

1079. cochrane.org / New Cochrane health evidence challenges belief that omega 3 supplements reduce risk of heart disease, stroke or death. July 18, 2018 https://www.cochrane.org/news/new-cochrane-health-evidence-challenges-belief-omega-3-supplements-reduce-risk-heart-disease

1080. cochranelibrary.com / Abdelhamid AS, et al. Omega-3 fatty acids for the primary and secondary prevention of cardiovascular disease; Cochrane Library Cochrane Database of Systematic Reviews; 2018 Jul 18; DOI: 10.1002/14651858.CD003177.pub3 https://www.cochranelibrary.com/cdsr/doi/10.1002/14651858.CD003177.pub3/full

1081. eurekalert.org / Probiotic use is a link between brain fogginess, severe bloating. Medical College of Georgia at Augusta University, Public Release: August 6, 2018 https://www.eurekalert.org/pub_releases/2018-08/mcog-pui080318.php

1082. nature.com / Rao SS, et al. Brain fogginess, gas and bloating: a link between SIBO, probiotics and metabolic acidosis; Nature Clinical and Translational Gastroenterology; 2018 Jun 19; 9(162) https://www.nature.com/articles/s41424-018-0030-7

1083. whec.com / 32 children's medicines recalled due to possible life-threatening contamination. August 23, 2018 https://www.whec.com/news/3 2-childrens-medicines-recalled-due-to-contamination-/5042879/

1084. forbes.com / How One Class Of Diabetes Medications May Lead To Flesh-Eating Genital Infections. Bruce Y. Lee, September 1, 2018 https://www.forbes.com/sites/ brucelee/2018/09/01/how-one-class-of-diabetes-medications-may-lead-to-fles h-eating-genital-infections/#38e22c127619

1085. fda.gov / FDA: U.S. Food & Drug / FDA warns about rare occurrences of a serious infection of the genital area with SGLT2 inhibitors for diabetes https://www.fda.gov/ Drugs/DrugSafety/ucm617360.htm

1086. khn.org / Hidden Drugs And Danger Lurk In Over-The-Counter Supplements, Study Finds. Rachel Bluth, October 12, 2018 https://khn.org/news/hidden-drug s-and-danger-lurk-in-over-the-counter-supplements-study-finds/

1087. jamanetwork.com / Tucker J, et al. Unapproved Pharmaceutical Ingredients Included in Dietary Supplements Associated With US Food and Drug Administration Warnings; JAMA Network Open; 2018;1(6): e183337 DOI: 10.1001/jamanetworkopen.2018.3337 https://jamanetwork.com/journals/jamanetworkopen/fullarticle/2706496

1088. thelancet.com / Chekroud SR, et al. Association between physical exercise and mental health in 1·2 million individuals in the USA between 2011 and 2015: a cross-sectional study; The Lancet Psychiatry; 2018 Sep 01; 5(9): 739–746 DOI: https:// doi.org/10.1016/S2215-0366(18)30227-X https://www.thelancet.com/journals/ lanpsy/article/PIIS2215-0366(18)30227-X/fulltext

1089. theconversation.com / Why stretching is (still) important for weight loss and exercise. August 6, 2018 https://theconversation.com/why-stretching-is-still-important-f or-weight-loss-and-exercise-97814

1090. arstechnica.com / Doctors fear urgent care centers are wildly overus-ing antibiotics—for profit. Beth Mole, July 17, 2018 https://arstechnica. com/science/2018/07/doctors-fear-urgent-care-centers-are-wildly-ov erusing-antibiotics-for-profit/

1091. jamanetwork.com / Palms DL, et al. Comparison of Antibiotic Prescribing in Retail Clinics, Urgent Care Centers, Emergency Departments, and Traditional Ambula-tory Care Settings in the United States; JAMA Internal Medicine; 2018 Sep; 178(9): 1267–1269 DOI: 10.1001/jamainternmed.2018.1632 https://jamanetwork.com/jour-nals/jamainternalmedicine/article-abstract/2687524

1092. consumerreports.org / Safety of Probiotic Supplements Is Not Guaran-teed, Study Says. Sally Wadyka, July 16, 2018 https://www.consumerre-ports.org/dietary-supplements/safety-of-probiotic-supplements-is-no t-guaranteed-study-says/

1093. medicalxpress.com / Jury still out on probiotics. Dennis Thompson, July 17, 2018 https://medicalxpress.com/news/2018-07-safety-probiotics-prebiotics.html

1094. annals.org / Bafeta A, et al. Harms Reporting in Randomized Controlled Trials of Interventions Aimed at Modifying Microbiota: A Systematic Review; Annals of Internal Medicine; 2018 Aug 21; 169(4): 240–247 DOI: 10.7326/M18-0343 http:// annals.org/aim/article-abstract/2687953/harms-reporting-randomized-controlle d-trials-interventions-aimed-modifying-microbiota-systematic

1095. livescience.com / Will Baby Poop Bacteria Become the New Probiotic? Mindy Weis-berger, August 24, 2018 https://www.livescience.com/63421-baby-poop-probiotic. html

1096.   nature.com / Nagpal R, et al. Human-origin probiotic cocktail increases short-chain fatty acid production via modulation of mice and human gut microbiome; Scientific Reports; 2018 Aug 23; 8(12649) https://doi.org/10.1038/s41598-018-30114-4 https://www.nature.com/articles/s41598-018-30114-4 https://www.nature.com/articles/s41598-018-30114-4.pdf

1097.   gizmodo.com / For Some People, Taking Probiotics May Actually Harm Normal Gut Bacteria. Ed Cara, September 6, 2018 https://gizmodo.com/for-some-people-taking-probiotics-may-actually-harm-no-1828858007

1098.   inverse.com / Probiotics Unexpectedly Backfire in Gut Health Study. Yasmin Tayag, September 8, 2018 https://www.inverse.com/article/48746-word-is-still-out-on-probiotics-for-gut-health

1099.   cell.com / Zmora N, et al. Personalized Gut Mucosal Colonization Resistance to Empiric Probiotics Is Associated with Unique Host and Microbiome Features; Cell; 2018 Sep 06; 174(6): 1388–1405.E21 DOI: https://doi.org/10.1016/j.cell.2018.08.041 https://www.cell.com/cell/fulltext/S0092-8674(18)31102-4

1100.   cell.com / Suez J, et al. Post-Antibiotic Gut Mucosal Microbiome Reconstitution Is Impaired by Probiotics and Improved by Autologous FMT; Cell; 2018 Sep 06; 174(6): 1406–1423.E16 DOI: https://doi.org/10.1016/j.cell.2018.08.047 https://www.cell.com/cell/fulltext/S0092-8674(18)31108-5

1101.   theguardian.com / Probiotic goods a "waste of money" for healthy adults, research suggests. Damien Gayle, May 10, 2016 https://www.theguardian.com/science/2016/may/10/probiotic-goods-a-waste-of-money-for-healthy-adults-research-suggests

1102.   genomemedicine.biomedcentral.com / Kristensen NB, et al. Alterations in fecal microbiota composition by probiotic supplementation in healthy adults: a systematic review of randomized controlled trials; Genome Medicine; 2016; 8(52) https://doi.org/10.1186/s13073-016-0300-5 https://genomemedicine.biomedcentral.com/articles/10.1186/s13073-016-0300-5 https://genomemedicine.biomedcentral.com/track/pdf/10.1186/s13073-016-0300-5

1103.   npr.org / 'Predatory Bacteria' Might Be Enlisted In Defense Against Antibiotic Resistance. Richard Harris, September 6, 2018 https://www.npr.org/sections/health-shots/2018/09/06/643661823/predatory-bacteria-might-be-enlisted-in-defense-against-antibiotic-resistance

1104.   newsweek.com / Doctors Interrupt Patients, Stop Listening After 11 Seconds on Average, Study Says. Abbey Interrante, July 22, 2018 https://www.newsweek.com/doctor-patient-visits-1035514

1105.   link.springer.com / Ospina NS, et al. Eliciting the Patient's Agenda- Secondary Analysis of Recorded Clinical Encounters; Journal of General Internal Medicine; 2018 Jul 02 online https://doi.org/10.1007/s11606-018-4540-5 https://link.springer.com/article/10.1007/s11606-018-4540-5#citeas

1106.   techtimes.com / Pharmacist Admits To Filling Fake Opioid Prescriptions For Sexual Favors. Athena Chan, August 26, 2018 https://www.techtimes.com/articles/233760/20180826/pharmacist-admits-to-filling-fake-opioid-prescriptions-for-sexual-favors.htm

1107.   npr.org / Insulin's High Cost Leads To Lethal Rationing. Bram Sable-Smith, September 1, 2018 https://www.npr.org/sections/health-shots/2018/09/01/641615877/insulins-high-cost-leads-to-lethal-rationing

1108.   huffingtonpost.com / CVS, Aetna Win U.S. Approval For $69 Billion Merger. Diane Bartz and Caroline Humer, August 10, 2018 https://www.huffingtonpost.com/entry/cvs-aetna-win-us-approval-for-69-billion-merger_us_5bbe1fbee4b01470d057f4db

1109.   washingtonpost.com / CVS's $69 billion merger with Aetna is approved in deal that could transform health-care industry. Brian Fung, October 10, 2018 https://www.

washingtonpost.com/technology/2018/10/10/justice-department-approves-cvs s-billion-merger-with-insurance-giant-aetna/?noredirect=on&utm_term=. cec4279407aa

1110. gizmodo.com / Ancestry Sites Could Soon Expose Nearly Anyone's Identity, Researchers Say. Ed Cara, October 11, 2018 https://gizmodo.com/ancestry-site s-could-soon-expose-nearly-anyones-identit-1829685818

1111. science.sciencemag.org / Erlich Y, et al. Identity inference of genomic data using long-range familial searches; Science; 2018 Oct 11; 11: eaau4832 DOI: 10.1126/ science.aau4832 http://science.sciencemag.org/content/early/2018/10/10/science. aau4832

1112. bbc.com / C-section births surge to 'alarming' rates worldwide – study. Mal Siret, October 12, 2018 https://www.bbc.com/news/world-45834011

1113. thelancet.com / Boerma T, et al. Global epidemiology of use of and disparities in caesarean sections; The Lancet; 2018 Oct 13; 392(10155): 1341–1348 DOI: https://doi. org/10.1016/S0140-6736(18)31928-7 https://www.thelancet.com/journals/lancet/ article/PIIS0140-6736(18)31928-7/fulltext

1114. healthline.com / New Moms Who Smoke Pot Have THC in Breast Milk. Robert Curley, April 9, 2018 https://www.healthline.com/health-news/new-mom s-who-smoke-pot-have-thc-in-breast-milk#1

1115. nejm.org / May T. Sociogenetic Risks — Ancestry DNA Testing, Third-Party Iden- tity, and Protection of Privacy; NEJM; 2018 Aug 2; 379(5): 410–412 DOI: 10.1056/ NEJMp1805870 https://www.nejm.org/doi/full/10.1056/NEJMp1805870

1116. nejm.org / Bleich SN. A Road Map for Sustaining Healthy Eating Behavior; NEJM; 2018 Aug 9; 379(6): 507–509 DOI: 10.1056/NEJMp1805494 https://www.nejm.org/ doi/full/10.1056/NEJMp1805494

1117. nejm.org / Eisenstein L. To Fight Burnout, Organize; NEJM; 2018 Aug 9; 379(6): 509–511 DOI: 10.1056/NEJMp1803771 https://www.nejm.org/doi/full/10.1056/ NEJMp1803771

1118. nejm.org / Bhatt AS. Digesting New Developments in Biosensors; NEJM; 2018 Aug 16; 379(7): 686–688 DOI: 10.1056/NEJMcibr1806952 https://www.nejm.org/doi/ full/10.1056/NEJMcibr1806952

1119. nejm.org / Schramm C. Bile Acids, the Microbiome, Immunity, and Liver Tumors; NEJM; 2018 Aug 16; 379(7): 888–890 DOI: 10.1056/NEJMcibr1807106 https://www. nejm.org/doi/full/10.1056/NEJMcibr1807106

1120. nejm.org / Lamkin M. Physician as Double Agent — Conflicting Duties Aris- ing from Employer-Sponsored Wellness Programs; NEJM; 2018 Oct 4; 379(14): 1297–1299 DOI: 10.1056/NEJMp1804295 https://www.nejm.org/doi/full/10.1056/ NEJMp1804295

1121. nejm.org / Lewis M. Brain Change in Addiction as Learning, Not Disease; NEJM; 2018 Oct 18; 376(16); 1551–1560 DOI: 10.1056/NEJMra1602872 https://www.nejm. org/doi/full/10.1056/NEJMra1602872

1122. nejm.org / Chowkwanyun M, et al. "Precision" Public Health — Between Novelty and Hype; NEJM; 2018 Oct 11 379(15): 1398–1400 DOI: 10.1056/NEJMp1806634 https://www.nejm.org/doi/full/10.1056/NEJMp1806634

1123. nejm.org / Haendel MA, et al. Classification, Ontology, and Precision Medicine; NEJM; 2018 Oct 11 379(15): 1452–1462 DOI: 10.1056/NEJMra1615014 https://www. nejm.org/doi/full/10.1056/NEJMra1615014

1124. cbsnews.com / Not exercising may be even more deadly than smoking, diabetes, heart disease, study finds. Ashley Welch, October 22, 2018 https://www.cbsnews. com/news/not-exercising-more-deadly-than-smoking-diabetes-heart-dis- ease-study-finds/

1125.   jamanetwork.com / Mandsager K, et al. Association of Cardiorespiratory Fitness With Long-term Mortality Among Adults Undergoing Exercise Treadmill Testing; JAMA Netw Open. 2018 Oct 19;1(6): e183605. DOI:10.1001/jamanetworkopen.2018.3605 https://jamanetwork.com/journals/jamanetworkopen/fullarticle/2707428

1126.   hhs.gov / President's Council on Sports, Fitness & Nutrition / Physical Activity Guidelines for Americans 2018 https://www.hhs.gov/fitness/be-active/physical-activity-guidelines-for-americans/index.html

1127.   npr.org / Immigrating To The U.S.? Get Ready For A New Gut Microbiome (And Maybe More Pounds). Maanvi Singh, November 1, 2018 https://www.npr.org/sections/thesalt/2018/11/01/662652885/immigrating-to-the-u-s-get-ready-for-a-new-gut-microbiome-and-maybe-more-pounds

1128.   phys.org / Immigration to the US changes a person's microbiome. Cell Press, November 1, 2018 https://phys.org/news/2018-11-immigration-person-microbiome.html

1129.   cell.com / Vangay P, et al. US Immigration Westernizes the Human Gut Microbiome; Cell; 2018 Nov 01; 175(4): P962-972.E10 DOI: https://doi.org/10.1016/j.cell.2018.10.029 https://www.cell.com/cell/fulltext/S0092-8674(18)31382-5?_returnURL=https%3A%2F%2Flinkinghub.elsevier.com%2Fretrieve%2Fpii%2FS0092867418313825%3Fshowall%3Dtrue

1130.   nytimes.com / Microplastics Find Their Way Into Your Gut, a Pilot Study Finds. Douglas Quenqua, October 22, 2018 https://www.nytimes.com/2018/10/22/health/microplastics-human-stool.html

1131.   newatlas.com / First-of-a-kind study finds microplastics in human stool around the world. Nick Lavars, October 23rd, 2018 https://newatlas.com/microplastic-human-stool-samples/56908/

1132.   ajp.psychiatryonline.org / Morin JF G, et al. A Population-Based Analysis of the Relationship Between Substance Use and Adolescent Cognitive Development; The American Journal of Psychiatry; 2018 Oct 3; Published Online https://doi.org/10.1176/appi.ajp.2018.18020202 https://ajp.psychiatryonline.org/doi/10.1176/appi.ajp.2018.18020202

1133.   cnn.com / Applebee's is betting on stress eaters, and it's paying off. Danielle Wiener-Bronner, November 6, 2018 https://www.cnn.com/2018/11/03/business/applebees-turnaround/index.html

1134.   heart.org / New guidelines: Cholesterol should be on everyone's radar, beginning early in life. American Heart Association News, November 10, 2018 https://www.heart.org/en/news/2018/11/10/new-guidelines-cholesterol-should-be-on-everyones-radar-beginning-early-in-life

1135.   ahajournals.org / 2018 AHA/ACC/AACVPR/AAPA/ABC/ACPM/ADA/AGS/APhA/ASPC/NLA/PCNA Guideline on the Management of Blood Cholesterol; A Report of the American College of Cardiology/American Heart Association Task Force on Clinical Practice Guidelines; Circulation. 2018;000: e000–e000. DOI: 10.1161/CIR.0000000000000625 https://www.ahajournals.org/doi/pdf/10.1161/CIR.0000000000000625

1136.   usnews.com / High and Low BMI Linked to Increased Risk of Death. Alexa Lardieri, October 31, 2018 https://www.usnews.com/news/health-care-news/articles/2018-10-31/study-high-and-low-bmi-linked-to-increased-risk-of-death-from-all-major-causes

1137.   thelancet.com / Bhaskaran K, et al. Association of BMI with overall and cause-specific mortality: a population-based cohort study of 3·6 million adults in the UK; The Lancet Diabetes & Endocrinology; 2018 Oct 30; Published Online DOI: https://doi.

org/10.1016/S2213-8587(18)30288-2 https://www.thelancet.com/journals/landia/article/PIIS2213-8587(18)30288-2/fulltext

1138. gizmodo.com / American Lifespans Won't Get Much Longer by 2040, Report Finds. Ed Cara, August 17, 2018 https://gizmodo.com/american-lifespans-wont-get-much-longer-by-2040-report-1829817959

1139. thelancet.com / Foreman KJ, et al. Forecasting life expectancy, years of life lost, and all-cause and cause-specific mortality for 250 causes of death: reference and alternative scenarios for 2016–40 for 195 countries and territories; The Lancet; 2018 Aug 16 online DOI: https://doi.org/10.1016/S0140-6736(18)31694-5 https://www.thelancet.com/journals/lancet/article/PIIS0140-6736(18)31694-5/fulltext

1140. washingtonpost.com / Harvard investigation finds fraudulent data in papers by heart researcher. Carolyn Y. Johnson, October 15, 2018 https://www.washingtonpost.com/science/2018/10/15/harvard-investigation-finds-fraudulent-data-papers-by-heart-researcher/?noredirect=on&utm_term=.db04ea9c3344

1141. engadget.com / Brain implant lets paralyzed people turn thoughts into text. Rachel England, November 23, 2018 https://www.engadget.com/2018/11/23/brain-implant-lets-paralyzed-people-turn-thoughts-into-text/

1142. journals.plos.org / Nuyujukian P, et al. Cortical control of a tablet computer by people with paralysis; PLOS One; 2018 Nov 21; 13(11): e0204566 https://doi.org/10.1371/journal.pone.0204566 https://journals.plos.org/plosone/article?id=10.1371/journal.pone.0204566#sec009

About the Author

Dr. George Zahrebelski, MS, MD, is a board-certified Castle Connelly selected Top Doctor practicing gastroenterology, hepatology, and nutrition in the Northwest suburbs of Chicago, Illinois at the **Digestive Disorders & Liver Center** that he established in 1993.

His clinical interests include toxic drug and metabolic liver disorders including NASH, the Irritable Bowel Syndrome, inflammatory bowel diseases, the human gut microbiome, obesity, and using nutritional and lifestyle approaches to help the human body remain healthy and heal naturally.

Dr. Zahrebelski finished his fellowship in digestive and liver diseases and nutrition at the University of North Carolina Hospitals and Clinics at Chapel Hill, where he concentrated on how diet impacts human health and how drugs, environmental influences, social factors, and genetics affect the liver and the digestive and metabolic functioning of the human body. His fellowship training led to certification in gastroenterology and hepatology.

Prior to his fellowship, he completed a residency and internship in internal medicine at the University of Illinois at Chicago and Westside Veterans Administration Hospitals after earning his medical degree from the University of Illinois at Chicago.

Before pursuing his career in health care, Dr. Zahrebelski received a Bachelor of Arts degree with honors in chemistry from Loyola University in Chicago and attained a Master of Science degree in chemistry at the University of Illinois at Chicago, focusing his academic interests on studying organic chemistry and the metabolism and toxicity of drugs.

More recently, Dr. Zahrebelski founded the **Nutritional, Digestive and Liver Health Matters Institute** to direct his preventative health philosophy toward individualizing strategies to maintain health and manage weight naturally for those who are motivated and striving to attain the highest quality existence.

Made in the USA
Lexington, KY
26 March 2019